Diagnostic Imaging and Anatomy in Acute Care

Diagnostic Imaging and Anatomy in Acute Care

Edited by

Joshua Lauder
East Lancashire Hospitals NHS Trust
University of Central Lancashire
Clitheroe, UK and
University of Manchester
Skin & Bones Medical, Head of Imaging
Manchester, UK

Peter Driscoll
Faculty Lead for Clinical Anatomy
School of Medicine and Dentistry
University of Central Lancashire
Preston, UK

WILEY Blackwell

This edition first published 2025
© 2025 John Wiley & Sons Ltd

The right of Joshua Lauder and Peter Driscoll to be identified as the authors of the editorial material in this work has been asserted in accordance with law.

Registered Offices
John Wiley & Sons, Inc., 111 River Street, Hoboken, NJ 07030, USA
John Wiley & Sons Ltd, New Era House, 8 Oldlands Way, Bognor Regis, West Sussex, PO22 9NQ, UK

For details of our global editorial offices, customer services, and more information about Wiley products visit us at www.wiley.com.

Wiley also publishes its books in a variety of electronic formats and by print-on-demand. Some content that appears in standard print versions of this book may not be available in other formats.

Limit of Liability/Disclaimer of Warranty
While the publisher and authors have used their best efforts in preparing this work, they make no representations or warranties with respect to the accuracy or completeness of the contents of this work and specifically disclaim all warranties, including without limitation any implied warranties of merchantability or fitness for a particular purpose. No warranty may be created or extended by sales representatives, written sales materials or promotional statements for this work. This work is sold with the understanding that the publisher is not engaged in rendering professional services. The advice and strategies contained herein may not be suitable for your situation. You should consult with a specialist where appropriate. The fact that an organization, website, or product is referred to in this work as a citation and/or potential source of further information does not mean that the publisher and authors endorse the information or services the organization, website, or product may provide or recommendations it may make. Further, readers should be aware that websites listed in this work may have changed or disappeared between when this work was written and when it is read. Neither the publisher nor authors shall be liable for any loss of profit or any other commercial damages, including but not limited to special, incidental, consequential, or other damages.

Library of Congress Cataloging-in-Publication Data Applied for
Paperback ISBN: 9781119809449

Cover Design: Wiley
Cover Images: © Science Photo Library/Alamy Stock Photo, Courtesy of Josh Lauder, TK

Set in 10/12pt STIXTwoText by Straive, Pondicherry, India

Printed in Singapore
M117011_231224

CONTENTS

7 Heavy Painful Periods   50

Joshua Lauder, Onyibo Okafor, and Peter Driscoll

8 Severe Pelvic Pain   54

Joshua Lauder, Onyibo Okafor, and Peter Driscoll

9 Testicle Pain   59

Joshua Lauder, Patrick Green, and Peter Driscoll

Section 3 Respiratory Section 65

10 Thoracic Stabbing 67

Joshua Lauder, Aleksandr Valkov, Kris Philips, and Peter Driscoll

11 Blunt Chest Trauma 73

Joshua Lauder, Aleksandr Valkov, and Peter Driscoll

12 Acute Dyspnoea 77

Joshua Lauder, Aleksandr Valkov, and Peter Driscoll

13 Chronic Cough and Dyspnoea 83

Joshua Lauder, Aleksandr Valkov, and Peter Driscoll

17 Acute Shortness of Breath 111

Joshua Lauder, Aleksandr Valkov, and Peter Driscoll

Section 5 Abdominal Section 117

18 Blunt Trauma 119

Joshua Lauder, Benjamin Layton, and Peter Driscoll

19 Right Upper Quadrant Pain 124

Joshua Lauder, Benjamin Layton, and Peter Driscoll

20 General Abdominal Pain 130

Joshua Lauder, Benjamin Layton, and Peter Driscoll

21 Flank Pain 137

Joshua Lauder, Benjamin Layton, and Peter Driscoll

22 Back Pain 143

Joshua Lauder, Shofiq Al-Islam, Benjamin Layton, and Peter Driscoll

26 Back Pain and Fever   172

Joshua Lauder, Eoghan Donnelly, and Peter Driscoll

Section 7   Head Section   179

27 Sudden Severe Headache   181

Joshua Lauder, Aleksandr Valkov, and Peter Driscoll

28 Sudden Weakness   193

Joshua Lauder, Aleksandr Valkov, and Peter Driscoll

29 Head Injury   202

Joshua Lauder, Aleksandr Valkov, and Peter Driscoll

LIST OF CONTRIBUTORS

Dr Shofiq Al-Islam
MBChB, BSc, FRCR
East Lancashire Hospitals NHS Trust
Blackburn, UK

Dr Sanjay Banypersad
MBChB, BMedSci (Hons), FRCP
(London), MD (UCL)
East Lancashire Hospitals NHS Trust
Blackburn, UK

Mr Eoghan Donnelly
MBChB FRCSOrth
NHS Greater Glasgow and Clyde
Glasgow, UK

Professor Peter Driscoll
BSc (Hon), MSc, MD, FRCS(Ed), FRCEM
School of Medicine and Dentistry
University of Central Lancashire
Preston, UK

Mr Patrick Green
MBChB, Mres, MRCS
Alder Hey Children's NHS Foundation Trust
Liverpool, UK

Mr Lee Hoggett
MBChB (Hon), PGCert (Med Ed), FRCS, FHEA
Trauma and Orthopaedic Surgery Health Education
England North West
Preston, UK

Dr Joshua Lauder
MBChB, FRCR
East Lancashire Hospitals NHS Trust
University of Central Lancashire
Clitheroe, UK and
University of Manchester
Skin & Bones Medical Limited, Head of Imaging
Blackburn, UK

Dr Benjamin Layton
BSc, MSc, BMBS, FRCR
Morecambe Bay Hospitals Trust
Lancaster, UK

Dr Onyibo Okafor
MBChB, MPH, MRCGP, DRCOG, DGM
Skin & Bones Medical Limited
Blackburn, UK

Kris Phillips
BSc, PGCert
School of Medicine and Dentistry
University of Central Lancashire
Preston, UK

Dr Aleksandr Valkov
MSc, PGDip, MD, FRCEM, MRCS (Edin)
Salford Royal Hospital and University of Central
Lancashire
Salford, UK

There is a growing reliance upon imaging in medicine and surgery. Radiology is a rapidly expanding sector and with this expansion comes increasing complexity. This book will give the reader a contemporary overview of the differing radiology modalities: X-ray, CT, nuclear medicine, MRI, ultrasound and interventional. These will be explored using acute cases which commonly present to emergency and urgent care.

You will see there is a focus on pictures, allowing you to compare normal anatomy with pathology. Radiology relies heavily on pattern recognition, which humans are naturally good at. To help you with this natural talent, the images will be annotated with clinically relevant anatomy. As well as radiological images, there will be relevant anatomical images, allowing cross-reference with previous anatomical knowledge.

This book is designed to be accessible to many different readerships. Front-line clinicians involved in acute care should find the array of clinical cases relevant to their practice. Specialty doctors who would like to know more about imaging modalities will find this a useful starting point before more focused specialty-specific resources. Nurses and allied health professionals with an interest in anatomy and imaging will benefit from the variety of pathology and imaging displayed. Students of the above disciplines could use this as a starting point to learn about radiology.

After reading this book, you will have a greater understanding of different radiology modalities, their indications, advantages and limitations. You will also begin to able to recognise pathology on imaging, which you can apply to your clinical practice. Finally, the book will equip you with radiology terminology which will improve your understanding of radiology reports.

ACKNOWLEDGEMENT

We would like to acknowledge:

- Professor Ian Parkin
- the Anatomy department of UCLan
- the Radiology department at East Lancashire NHS Hospitals Trust, ELHT.

Thanks to them all.

ABBREVIATIONS

Abbreviation	In full
AAA	Abdominal Aortic Aneurysm
ADC	Apparent Diffusion Coefficient
AP	Anteroposterior
AXR	Abdominal X-ray – plain
CT	Computed Tomography
CT KUB	Computed Tomographic Kidney, Ureter and Bladder
CTPA	Computed Tomographic Pulmonary Angiogram
CXR	Chest X-ray – plain
DSA	Digital Subtraction Angiography
DVT	Deep Venous Thrombosis
DWI	Diffusion-weighted Imaging
eFAST	Extended Focused Assessment using Sonography in Trauma
ERCP	Endoscopic Retrograde Cholangiopancreatography
EVAR	Endovascular Aneurysm Repair
FIO$_2$	Fraction of Inspired Oxygen

Abbreviation	In full
FLAIR	Fluid-attenuated Inversion Recovery
HU	Hounsfield Unit
MEWS	Modified Early Warning Signs
MIP	Maximum Intensity Projection
MRA	Magnetic Resonance Angiography
MRCP	Magnetic Resonance Cholangiopancreatography
MRI	Magnetic Resonance Imaging
NICE	National Institute for Health and Care Excellence
PDFS	Proton Density with Fat Suppression
PERC	Pulmonary Embolism Rule out criteria
PET	Positron Emission Tomography
SpO$_2$	Oxygen Saturation
STIR	Short Tau Inversion Recovery
US	Ultrasound
V/Q	Ventilation Perfusion Scan

This book is accompanied by a companion website:

www.wiley.com/go/DiagnosticImaginginAcuteCare
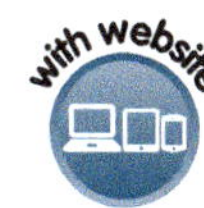

This website includes:

- Label the Diagram (Quiz images)
- Annotated Images in PPT format
- Un-annotated images in PPT format

CHAPTER 1

Radiology Introduction

Joshua Lauder[1] and Peter Driscoll[2]

[1] East Lancashire Hospitals NHS Trust, University of Central Lancashire and University of Manchester, UK
[2] School of Medicine and Dentistry, University of Central Lancashire, Preston, UK

1.1 Section/Chapter Order

The sections are arranged so they go through the various imaging modalities, starting with plain radiology, then ultrasound, CT and MR. The chapters in each section go from simple to more complex where information from the previous chapters is used.

This introductory chapter provides an overview of the different modalities covered in the book, the rationale for their use and an explanation of common terminology. Our advice is to scan this initially. Then, as you read other parts of the book, you will be encouraged to return to relevant parts in this chapter to refresh your memory.

Each of the remaining chapters starts with a clinical case and the images used in the acute situation. There are then questions asking for a differential diagnosis and preliminary interpretation of the images. The imaging modality is then explained along with a review of the relevant anatomy. The chapter concludes with the questions being reviewed and answers provided.

1.2 Imaging Modalities

Through this book you will develop an overview of each imaging modality and its advantages and limitations. Often, the best way to learn this is using examples of normal anatomy and pathology so you will be referred to relevant images in the other chapters.

Don't get bogged down in the technical aspects of physics and scan acquisition (unless you are particularly interested). Radiology interpretation is primarily pattern based and appreciating the image is the most important bit.

Radiological terminology will be introduced here and throughout the book. It helps to understand what these terms mean as they crop up throughout radiology reports. Being able to link the terminology with what you can see in the image is a vital step in using these investigations appropriately.

1.3 Ionising Radiation

It helps to divide the imaging modalities into those which expose the patient to ionising radiation and those which don't.

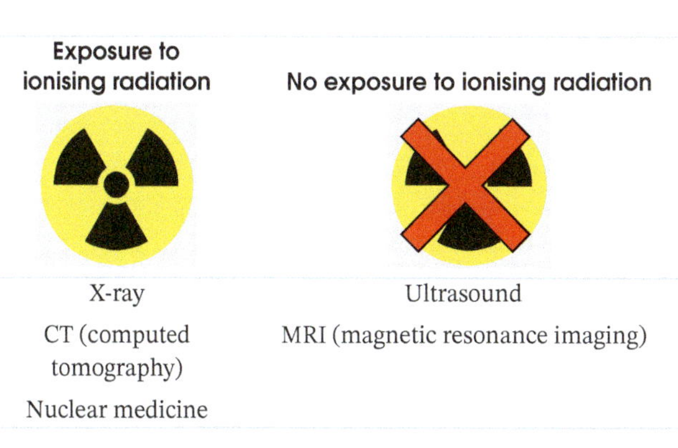

Ionising radiation is a type of energy released in the form of electromagnetic waves (e.g. gamma/X-rays) or particles (neutrons, beta or alpha). In diagnostic radiology, it is nearly all in the form of high-energy electromagnetic waves. Ionising particles are used more in clinical oncology.

As these waves are high energy, they can displace the electrons from atoms in the body, which causes them to ionise. This ionisation can cause mutations in DNA and has the potential to induce cancers at high doses or cumulative low doses. For this reason, any ionising radiation exposure must be justified.

Diagnostic Imaging and Anatomy in Acute Care, First Edition. Edited by Joshua Lauder and Peter Driscoll.
© 2025 John Wiley & Sons Ltd. Published 2025 by John Wiley & Sons Ltd.
Companion website: www.wiley.com/go/DiagnosticImaginginAcuteCare

> The benefit from the diagnostic test should outweigh the future cancer risk.

TABLE 1.1

Approximate radiation doses for various types of exposure.

Dental X-ray	0.005 mSv
100 g of Brazil nuts	0.01 mSv
Chest X-ray	0.014 mSv
Transatlantic flight	0.08 mSv
Nuclear power station worker average annual occupational exposure (2010)	0.18 mSv
V/Q perfusion component	1 mSv
Computed tomography (CT) scan of the head	1.4 mSv
UK average annual radiation dose	2.7 mSv
Low-dose CT chest	1.5 mSv
CT pulmonary angiography (CTPA)	6.1 mSv
Average annual radon dose to people in Cornwall (UK)	6.9 mSv
Whole-body CT	10 mSv
Positron emission tomography (PET)/CT	22 mSv

Source: Public Health England/Crown/Public domain.

Radiation dose in medicine is measured in millisievert units (mSv). As this is an abstract unit, it is useful to think about the dose in relation to the natural background radiation (Table 1.1). This varies from region to region, largely because of radon gas emission. Background radiation from the cosmos and ingested food also contributes. However, calculating the exact risk of developing cancer from a particular radiological test is an inexact process, extrapolated from the high doses of exposure at Hiroshima and Nagasaki. It is estimated that 1 mSv exposure has approximately a 1 in 20 000 risk of causing a fatal cancer.

1.4 X-ray (Plain Radiography)

This is the oldest of the radiology modalities and well recognised by most healthcare staff. A few key points are worth keeping in mind when looking at plain films.

- They are a 2D representation of the 3D structures of the body. Hence overlapping of structures is a common problem.
- High-density structures appear white. Other names for high density are opacity or opacification. A dense region in a bone is called sclerosis.
- Low-density structures appear black. Other names for low density are lucent or lucency. A low-density region in a bone is called lytic.

X-rays are still used a great deal and are very useful, particularly for assessing structures of very high density (**bones**, MSK Chapter 4 – Figure 4.10; **joints**, MSK Chapter 2 – Figure 2.1; **metal implants**, MSK Chapter 2 – Figure 2.4, etc.) or very low density (**lungs**, Resp Chapter 12 – Figure 12.2 or **bowel gas,** Abdo Chapter 20 – Figure 20.6). Another big advantage is their relatively low exposure to ionising radiation.

The limitations with plain radiographs become evident with intermediate-density structures, like **most organs, muscle, tendons** (MSK Chapter 5 – Figure 5.7) and **ligaments**. They tend to appear as homogenous grey shadows. **Joint effusions** are visible in certain joints (MSK Chapter 3 – Figure 3.12) but you will not be able to differentiate between simple fluid, pus or blood.

1.5 Computed Tomography

1.5.1 Scan Acquisition

> The annual number of CT scans performed in the NHS increased from 1 million to 6 million from 1997 to 2020.

CT relies on X-rays and so exposes the patient to ionising radiation. The method for acquiring an image is similar to plain radiography, with an X-ray source firing through the patient to a detector. In CT this X-ray source is rotated around the patient (tomography) as they are advanced through the scanner. This allows the whole body to be covered in a matter of seconds. The results are analysed electronically (computed) and the scan subsequently displayed in a picture archiving and communications system (PACS) system.

A CT scan contains hundreds (or sometimes thousands) of cross-sections through the patient. This is the key difference from plain radiography. A useful analogy is to think of a building. A traditional plain X-ray is like taking a photograph of a building, resulting in an image with 2D representation of a 3D structure. CT is like having the blueprints of the building, with detailed floor plans on every level.

1.5.2 Multiplanar Reformatting (MPR)

Each pixel of a CT image is actually a cube in 3D space, termed a voxel. Because of this, PACS software allows CT scans to be instantly reformatted into any desired anatomical plane. Axial, coronal and sagittal planes are the standard ones and are used at least 90% of the time. Occasionally it may be useful to create oblique planes along a certain part of anatomy (Figure 1.2).

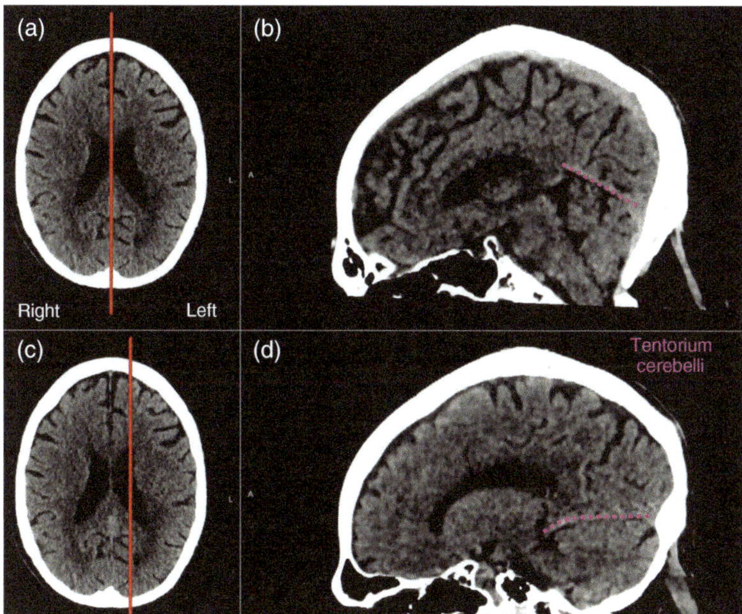

FIGURE 1.1 Axial (a) and sagittal views (b). The latter is taken in the midline as demonstrated by the red localiser line in image (a). When viewing a sagittal slice which is not in the midline (d), it is not always apparent which side of the body is being imaged. This is a common problem with neuro imaging as the brain and spine are anatomically symmetrical. By referring to the axial slice and localiser line (c), we can see that (d) is showing the left side.

1.5.3 Anatomical Planes and Orientation

The convention in radiology is that the image is viewed as if the patient is facing the practitioner. This initially applied to x-rays taken in a frontal projection but has been continued into CT imaging where the axial plane is predominantly used. Consequently, **the left-hand side of the screen will relate to the patient's right-hand side** (Figure 1.3). The convention also applies if you are viewing MRI or ultrasound. Note, however, that this rule is used when interpreting images taken in the axial and coronal planes. Orientating images in the sagittal plan is different and will be discussed below.

1.5.3.1 Sagittal Plane When viewing a CT or MRI in the sagittal plane, it is necessary to have the image linked to a different plane (axial or coronal) so you can tell whether the left or right of the midline is being examined. A localiser line can then be used to cross-reference the location on the sagittal image (Figures 1.1 and 1.4).

1.6 Reformatting 3D

Modern CT also allows 3D reformatting of scans, allowing the viewer to inspect the anatomy from any angle. This works best for dense structures, like bones (Head Chapter 29 – Figure 29.6) or angiograms (Abdo Chapter 22 – Figure 22.2). It is less effective at viewing organs or low-density structures (e.g. tendons).

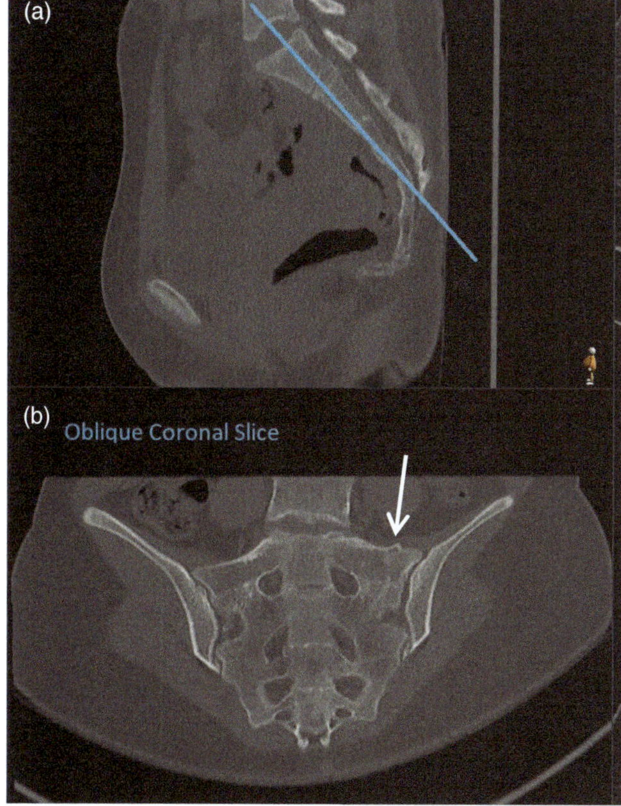

FIGURE 1.2 CT sacrum – bone window: (a) sagittal view (b) oblique coronal slice. CT scans can be manipulated so oblique images can be produced. This is demonstrated in (b) with the orientation of the oblique plane shown on the sagittal image (a). This type of manipulation is undertaken when searching for a suspected abnormality which is not visible on the classic axial, coronal and sagittal planes. In this case, using the oblique orientation enables a fracture of the left sacral ala (white arrow) to be seen more clearly.

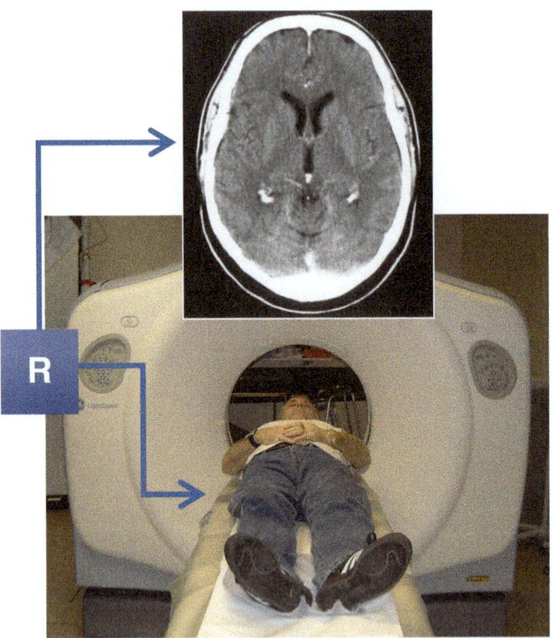

FIGURE 1.3 Orientation of a patient in the CT scanner and axial cranial scan. The scan is interpreted as if you are looking up to the patient's head, from their feet. Hence **the right side of the patient is on the left side of the screen**. Source: Driscoll et al. (2023)/John Wiley & Sons.

3D reformatting is useful in certain areas, for instance spotting skull fractures (Head Chapter 29 – Figure 29.10). However, it has poor resolution compared to the 2D CT slices, so should not be relied upon on its own.

1.6.1 Maximum Intensity Projection (MIP)

This is a software tool which provides a better overview of structures which extend over multiple adjacent slices, for example vessels (Head Chapter 27 – Figure 27.5). The slice thickness of the image is increased and only the brightest voxel across the thickened slice is shown. As a result, a winding vessel can be viewed along its course.

1.7 Density of Tissues and Hounsfield Units

1.7.1 Density of Tissues

Density on CT follows the same pattern as plain radiography, i.e. bones are **high density** so appear white and lungs are **low density** so appear black. The difference

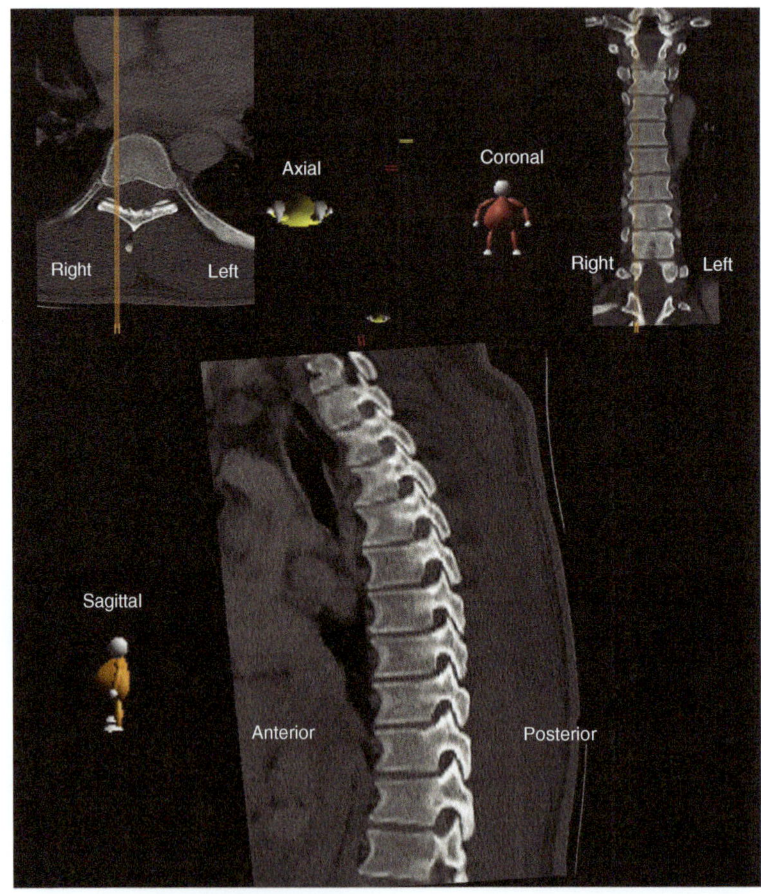

FIGURE 1.4 First observe the sagittal image. On its own, it is very difficult to appreciate whether we are viewing the left- or right-sided facet joints. We need to use the localiser line (orange) on the axial or coronal plane to confirm the position of the sagittal slice. In this case we are viewing the right-sided facet joints.

Hounsfield Units	Structure
−1000	Air
−100 to −50	Fat
0	Water
10 to 40	Soft tissue
25	White matter
40	Grey matter
30 to 80	Blood
100 to 300	Contrast
700 to 3000	Bone
3000	Metal

FIGURE 1.5 The Hounsfield Unit (HU) scale. Water is fixed at 0 and air is fixed at −1000, the density values of other substances lying accordingly along the scale. Hence structures appear darker on the image as HU decreases. Note that the density of blood changes depending on whether it is flowing, clotted or chronic (see 'blood density' section below).

with CT is that this density can be measured and given a value on the Hounsfield unit scale (Figure 1.5).

1.7.2 Hounsfield Units

1.7.2.1 Windowing Windowing changes the brightness and contrast to aid inspection of certain structures. It is useful to have common windowing presets for, for example, **brain** (Figure 1.6), **soft tissue**, **lung** (Resp Chapter 10 – Figure 10.2) and **bone**. For convenience, these will usually have hot keys on the keyboard (typically numbers).

While using the **brain windows**, the brain parenchyma is readily apparent and contrasts with cerebrospinal fluid (CSF) which appears black (Figure 1.6a). However, on this window, the bone appears as a featureless white mass. For greater detail, for example inspecting the skull vault's inner and outer tables, the **bone window** must be used (Figure 1.6b). Note, however, that when using this setting, the brain cannot be clearly seen. Therefore, the viewer needs to make an **active decision** which window setting to use when inspecting different parts of the body. This is one of the fundamental differences between inspecting a plain xray and a CT scan.

Using an inappropriate CT window to view a structure increases the chance of missing abnormalities.

1.7.3 Blood on CT

The density of blood on CT changes depending on its state (Figure 1.7). Flowing blood has the same density as soft tissues such as the brain (30–40 HU). After clotting, this increases to a maximum of around 90 HU. Over several weeks it declines as the haematoma is broken down and is either resorbed or becomes a seroma with the density of water (HU = 0).

It is possible to have a combination of densities. Figure 1.8a shows the density of an acute blood clot with areas of unclotted active bleeding.

In summary, an acute blood clot is bright on CT, making it easy to spot, especially in the cranium (Head Chapter 29 – Figure 29.8). Delayed presentations of bleeding are more challenging as the blood will start to break down and become darker (Figure 1.8b). The same concept applies whether the blood is intra-arterial (Head Chapter 28 – Figure 28.9a), venous or extravascular (Figure 1.8).

1.8 Contrast

Intravenous contrast is an extremely important addition to CT scans as it significantly improves the detection of pathology. Indeed, for certain studies contrast is mandatory, for example trauma CT (Abdo Chapter 18) and CTPA (Cardiac Chapter 17).

Depending on the clinical question, different contrast phases (i.e. timings) will be used to emphasise certain regions of anatomy (Table 1.2). The contrast is introduced via a vein, usually in the arm. The contrast flows into the superior vena cava (SVC) and right side of the heart before filling the pulmonary arteries. CTPAs are taken at this stage, which usually occurs around 30 seconds after injection. It is possible to trigger CT scans when the contrast is in the desired location. This is called **bolus tracking** (Cardiac Chapter 17 – Figure 17.2). Contrast then continues to the left side of the heart and into the systemic arterial tree. Subsequently, it is taken up by capillary beds in organs before filling the venous system (including the portal veins).

After 10 minutes, most of the contrast will have been excreted by the kidneys and lie in the ureters and bladder.

1.9 Artefacts

1.9.1 Movement

Although CT is performed relatively quickly, movement is still an issue. This may be an unco-operative patient moving during the scan (Figure 1.9) or unavoidable

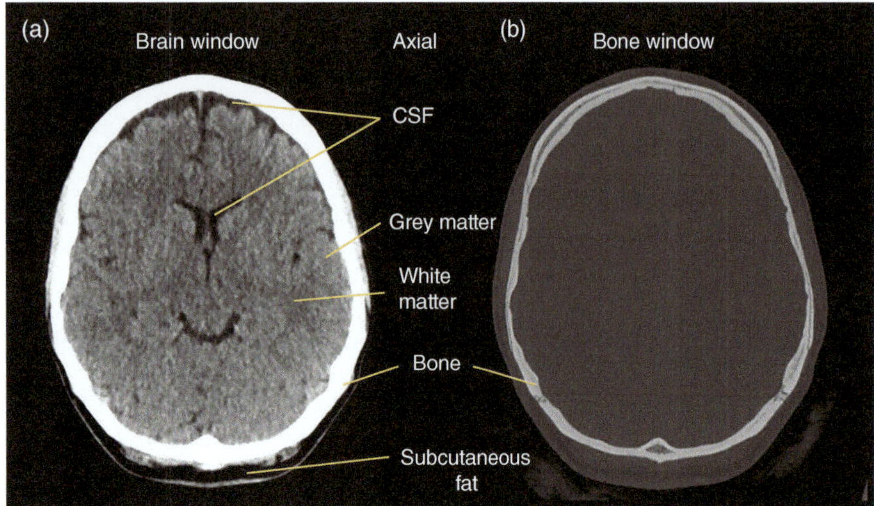

FIGURE 1.6 Axial CT head on brain (a) and bone (b) windows – unenhanced. Familiarise yourself with the appearance of the brain and CSF spaces on CT. Remember it is necessary to use **brain windows** to properly see the brain and CSF. **Bone windows** are required to assess for skull fractures (Head Chapter 29).

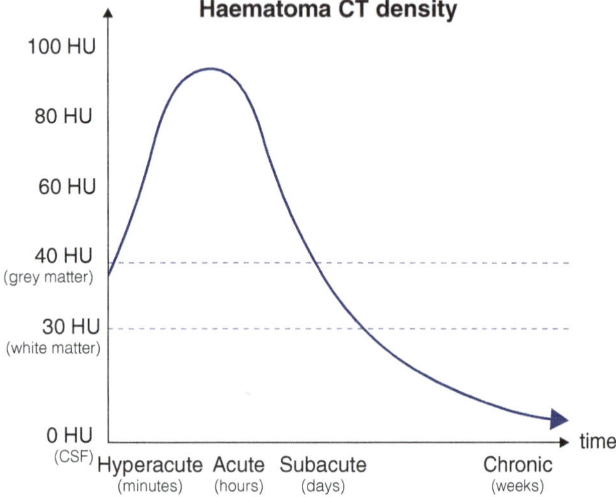

FIGURE 1.7 Changes in density of blood on CT over time.

respiratory or cardiac motion (Cardiac Chapter 16 – Figure 16.2). There are several techniques which help minimise these problems and these will be discussed in the relevant chapters.

1.9.2 Photon Starvation

If foreign objects are present and of sufficient density and thickness (e.g. hip replacement, Figure 1.10), they can block the X-ray beam and result in a '**photon starvation**' artefact. This manifests as black bands radiating out from the offending object which can mask nearby anatomy.

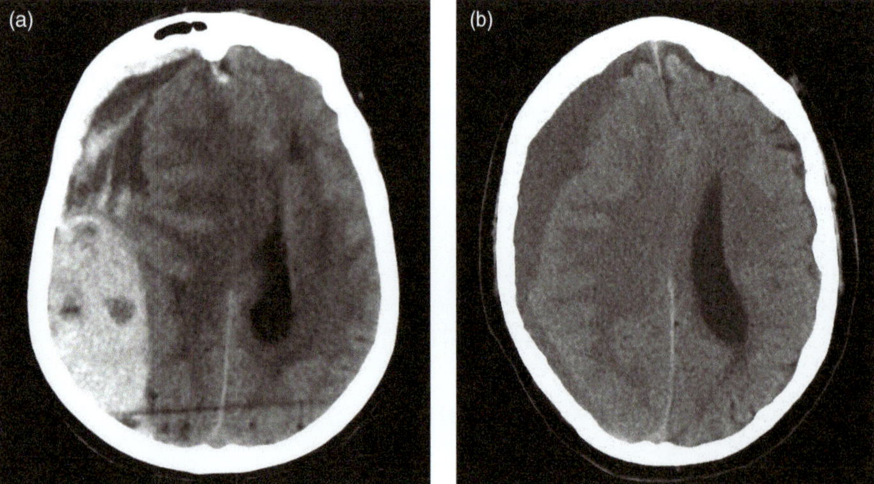

FIGURE 1.8 (a) CT head – brain window – axial view. This unenhanced CT head demonstrates a large right-sided subdural extending from the occipital to the frontal area. (b) CT head – brain window – axial view. This is a different patient with a right subacute, subdural haematoma (1–2 weeks old). Note the density is similar to that of brain tissue (isodense), making these more difficult to appreciate.

Contrast phase, timing and use.

Contrast phase	Timing of scan after IV contrast bolus	Use
Non-enhanced/ unenhanced	No contrast given	Head CTs are usually taken without contrast to improve detection of intracranial haemorrhage (Head Chapter 29 – Figure 29.8).
		Spine and MSK CT is also performed without contrast, as the primary interest is fractures and dislocations (Spine Chapter 25 – Figure 25.3; MSK Chapter 4 – Figure 4.11).
		In the torso, unenhanced scans are used to detect calcification, e.g. renal calculi (Abdo Chapter 21 – Figure 21.6).
Pulmonary arterial phase	30 seconds	CTPA scans are performed in this phase to look for pulmonary emboli (Cardiac Chapter 17 – Figure 17.5).
Arterial phase	40 seconds	Useful to identify arterial bleeding (Abdo Chapter 22 – Figure 22.5), arterial occlusions (Head Chapter 28 – Figure 28.11) and dissection.
Portal venous phase	70–80 seconds	Useful in the abdomen and pelvis in acute surgical patients (Abdo Chapter 20 – Figure 20.5).
Delayed phase	6–10 minutes	Used to identify damage to the urinary tract (not shown).

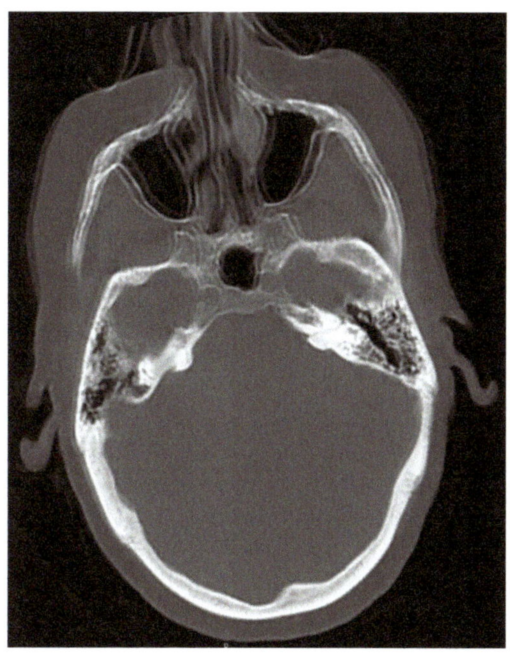

FIGURE 1.9 Axial CT head on bone windows showing movement artefact. The image appears blurry, significantly reducing the detection of facial bone fractures.

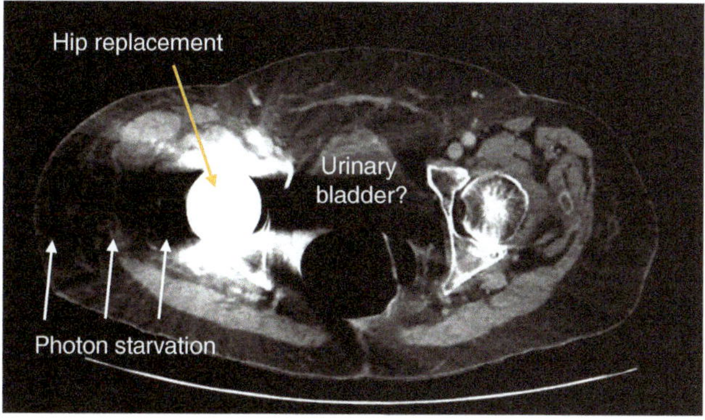

FIGURE 1.10 Axial CT pelvis on soft tissue windows showing photon starvation from a right hip replacement. The dense material blocks the whole X-ray beam, resulting in black bands across the image, masking organs like the urinary bladder.

from the patient with areas of increased radioactivity described as '**avid**' or '**hot**'.

Nuclear medicine studies show functional information about the body, but have much less anatomical definition compared to X-ray and CT.

1.10 Nuclear Medicine

This modality also exposes patients to ionising radiation, but it differs from X-ray and CT because the patient takes in the radioactive pharmaceuticals. This could be via intravenous injection, inhalation or by mouth.

The patient is then positioned inside a special detector called a gamma camera. This records the radiation emitted

1.11 V/Q Scan (Ventilation/ Perfusion)

This is used to investigate pulmonary embolism in patients under 40 years with a normal chest X-ray. It is preferable to CTPA because the radiation dose is lower (Table 1.1). It involves injecting radiopharmaceuticals into the veins and observing which segments of the lungs are perfused (Cardiac Chapter 17 – Figure 17.3). It is also possible to get the patient to inhale radioactive gas to see if there is a ventilation/perfusion mismatch. This component is not always performed as ventilation is likely to be normal if the chest X-ray is normal.

1.12 Positron Emission Tomography (PET)

This is used extensively in cancer care. The patient is injected with a radiopharmaceutical called fluorodeoxyglucose F18 (FDG) which mimics glucose in the body. Any region with increased metabolic activity will attract the FDG and become avid. Normal metabolically active tissues such as the brain and myocardium can be ignored, as can the urinary tract, where FDG is naturally secreted.

Any additional areas of metabolic activity could represent malignancy; for certain cancers (e.g. squamous cell carcinomas), this is highly sensitive for metastatic disease spread. However, the specificity of PET is limited, as pathologies such as infection and inflammation also increase metabolic activity.

PET images are invariably combined with CT scans (PET/CT). This overcomes the anatomical limitations of the PET images to give highly accurate anatomical and functional information (Resp Chapter 13 – Figure 13.2). The downside of PET/CT is a relatively high radiation dose (Table 1.1).

1.13 Magnetic Resonance Imaging (MRI)

1.13.1 Basic Physics

Magnetic resonance imaging does not expose patients to ionising radiation. Instead, the patient is exposed to a strong magnetic field and radio waves, neither of which poses a long-term health risk.

All the hydrogen atoms in the body align along the plane of the magnetic field. The radio waves then knock the atoms out of alignment. By recording the way that the atoms realign to the field, it is possible to build an image which shows information about the composition of different tissues.

MRI scans take longer than CT, usually in the order of 20–60 minutes, and are loud. Hearing defenders are therefore routinely offered to all patients. The scanner is also narrower and longer so claustrophobic patients can become distressed. Some may require sedation or even general anaesthetic to undergo an MRI.

1.13.2 Contraindications

Because of the strong magnetic field, ferrous metals cannot be taken near the scanner. In practice, most modern medical implants and prosthetics are MRI compatible, but there are certain cases which still pose issues.

- *Recent surgery*: it is standard practice to wait six weeks after surgery before performing MRI scans, regardless of whether any device has been implanted.
- *Active implantable metal devices (e.g. pacemakers, nerve stimulators, drug infusion pumps, shunts and cochlear implants)*: most modern versions of these devices are MRI conditional, meaning they can be scanned under certain circumstances. Due to the internal power and electrical circuits, MRI scanning can reset or reprogram the device. Provisions should therefore be made before scanning, such as having an appropriate technician available to reset the device.
- *Non-active implantable metal devices (e.g. joint replacements, heart valves, aneurysm clips and stents)*: these are generally OK to scan but will cause localised artefact, affecting image quality (Figure 1.11a).
- *Metallic fragments around the eyes* (e.g. from welding incidents) are an absolute contraindication. When there is a relevant history, an orbital X-ray of the orbits will be performed to assess for this prior to MRI.

Tattoos are nearly always safe, even if they contain traces of metal.

1.13.3 Basic Sequences

It is not necessary to understand the physics underlying each MRI sequence. However, knowing the brightness of the tissues of the body is fundamental to interpreting the images (Table 1.3). Structures such as cortical bone and tendons (MSK Chapter 2 – Figure 2.6) will be dark on all MRI sequences, simply because there is a lack of hydrogen atoms to return a signal (MSK Chapter 3 – Figures 3.6 and 3.8).

1.13.3.1 T1 Often termed the anatomical sequence, T1 is good for reviewing normal anatomy (MSK Chapter 3 – Figure 3.6). As **fat is bright**, the subcutaneous tissue and bone marrow will be bright. The white and grey matter of the brain therefore have appropriate relative shades (grey matter is darker than white matter) (Head Chapter 28 – Figure 28.3). **Fluid is dark on T1.**

A limited number of tissues are bright on T1. Knowing this list can be useful for problem solving.

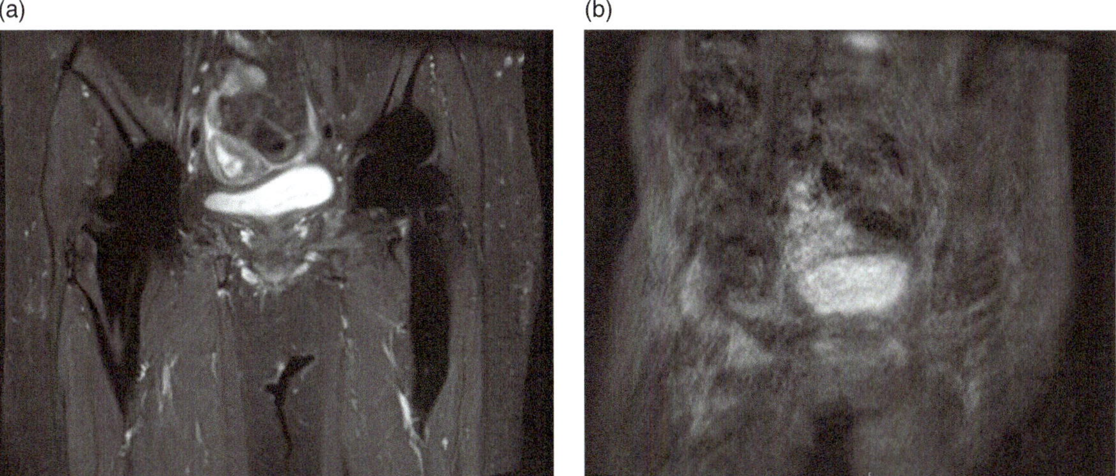

FIGURE 1.11 (a) Coronal MRI STIR sequence of the pelvis. There are bilateral hip replacements resulting in **metal artefact**. (b) Coronal MRI STIR sequence of the pelvis. There is significant **movement artefact** resulting in blurring.

TABLE 1.3

MRI sequences.

Standard sequences		Fluid	Fat	Tendons and cortical bone
T1		Dark	Bright	Dark
T2		Very bright	Bright	Dark
FLAIR (used in neuro imaging)		Dark	Bright	Dark
Fat-saturated sequences				
PD FS (used in MSK imaging)		Bright	Dark	Dark
STIR (used in MSK imaging)		Very bright	Dark	Dark
Special sequences				
DWI (used mainly in neuro imaging)	DWI trace (B1000)	Dark	Dark	Dark
	ADC trace	Bright	Dark	Dark

- Fat
- Blood breakdown products (Figure 1.12)
- Melanin
- Proteinaceous fluid
- Contrast agents

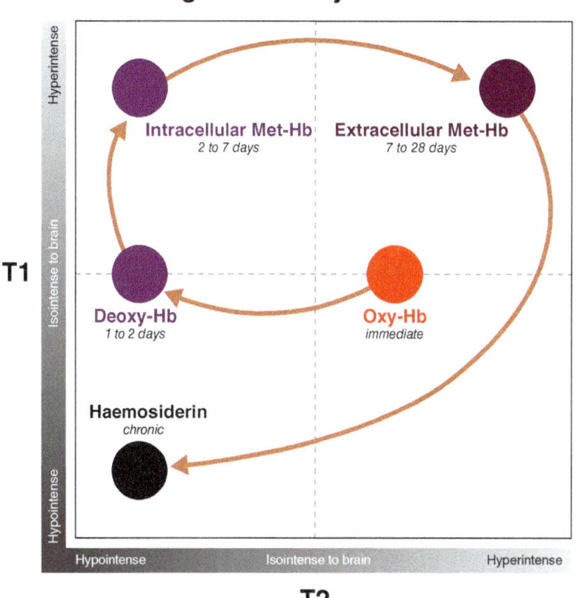

FIGURE 1.12 MRI signal intensity of haematomas. Hyperacute haemorrhage (hours old): T1 intermediate and T2 intermediate. Acute haemorrhage (1–2 days old): T1 intermediate and T2 dark. Subacute haemorrhage (2–7 days old): T1 bright and T2 dark. Late subacute haemorrhage (1–4 weeks old): T1 bright and T2 bright. Chronic haemorrhage (older than a month): T1 dark and T2 dark.

1.13.3.2 T2 The key difference with a T2 sequence is that **fluid is bright**. Hence it is also termed a fluid-sensitive sequence. This can be remembered with the aide mémoire '**WW2 (Water White 2)**'. For this reason, T2 is used to look for pathology (which usually manifests as oedema). On a standard T2 sequence fat remains bright. Consequently, this sequence is most often used for neuro imaging, where fat is separated from the anatomy of interest (Head Chapter 28 – Figure 28.3 and Spine Chapter 25 – Figure 25.5).

1.13.3.3 Fluid Attenuated Inversion Recovery (FLAIR) This type of T2 sequence is used mainly in neuro imaging. With FLAIR, the brightness of most tissues is exactly the same as T2 but the **CSF is suppressed** (becomes dark). This helps to pick up oedema in parts of the brain which are adjacent to CSF (Head Chapter 28 – Figures 28.3 and 28.8).

1.13.3.4 Short Tau Inversion Recovery (STIR) This is used extensively in MSK and spine imaging. It is also a type of T2 sequence but unlike FLAIR, the **fat is suppressed** (becomes dark) (Spine Chapter 25 – Figure 25.5). With fat in the soft tissues and bone marrow being suppressed, it is possible to pick up oedema in these tissues. This makes STIR highly sensitive for traumatic injuries (Spine Chapter 25 – Figure 25.7).

1.13.3.5 Proton Density Fat Suppression (PDFS) This is also a popular sequence in MSK imaging. The fat is suppressed (i.e. becomes dark). Fluid is bright (but not quite as bright as it is on T2 or STIR). This allows assessment of oedema from injuries. It also nicely shows the hyaline cartilage in joints so can be used to assess for early joint disease (MSK Chapter 3 – Figure 3.11).

1.13.3.6 Diffusion Weighted Imaging (DWI) This shows the relative movement of water molecules on a microscopic level. Certain pathologies result in restricted diffusion, so this is a useful sequence to characterise abnormalities previously identified on other sequences. DWI is extremely sensitive to strokes (Head Chapter 28 – Figures 28.4 and 28.12). However, it has poor spatial resolution compared to other sequences and is prone to artefacts at the skull base. Consequently it should not be used in isolation.

1.13.4 **Appearance of Blood on MRI**

Just as with CT, the appearance of blood on MRI varies depending on its age. However, this is a more complicated assessment, requiring the use of both T1 and T2 signal (Figure 1.12). This combined analysis can only be relied upon in the brain. If there are bleeds elsewhere in the body then other chemical processes disrupt the reliable evolution of a haematoma.

1.13.5 **Artefacts**

1.13.5.1 Metal Artefact Metal implants (even non-ferrous types) will stop the magnetic field being uniform and thus affect image quality. This effect is most pronounced next to the implant (Figure 1.11a).

1.13.5.2 Movement Because MRI scans take a long time to acquire, they are even more susceptible to movement artefact than CT. Furthermore, the process of producing the image means its quality is affected by any body movement in the scanner, not just in the part being moved.

It is not uncommon for the scan to be abandoned due to excessive patient movement. This should be a consideration when selecting patients for MRI, with adequate pain relief and sedation provided beforehand.

1.13.5.3 DWI – T2 Shine-through The DWI sequence must always be viewed in conjunction with the apparent diffusion coefficient (ADC). This is because bright areas on the DWI can be caused by an artefact called 'T2 shine-through' (Figure 1.13). The ADC is required to exclude this and confirm true diffusion restriction (compare this figure with Head Chapter 28 – Figure 28.13).

1.14 Ultrasound

1.14.1 **Basic Physics**

Ultrasound **does not** expose patients to ionising radiation. Instead, high-frequency vibrations are used which have no long-term health risk.

The ultrasound probe surface vibrates millions of times a second. Therefore, its frequency is measured in megahertz (MHz). When applied to the skin with a coupling gel, these vibrations travel through the body and reflect off tissues, returning to the probe. The returning vibrations are detected and processed to form an image which is a 2D fan shape.

This analysis takes into account how strong the return signal is and how far it has travelled (Pelvis Chapter 6 – Figure 6.3).

1.14.2 **Using the Machine**

Various types of ultrasound machine exist, from large cumbersome units to handheld pocket devices. Regardless of the type, they all have similar components and are used in a similar way.

1.14.2.1 Probe or Transducer This is where the ultrasound is emitted from. The side touching the patient may be straight (linear) or curved (curvilinear). Either way, there should be a marker at one end, which corresponds to the orientation on the screen (Figure 1.14).

Ultrasound is usually performed through the skin but probes exist to perform internal ultrasound (Pelvic Chapter 7 – Figure 7.2) and endoscopic ultrasound.

1.14.2.2 Screen This is where the image is viewed. Some handheld machines will link to mobile phone screens or tablets.

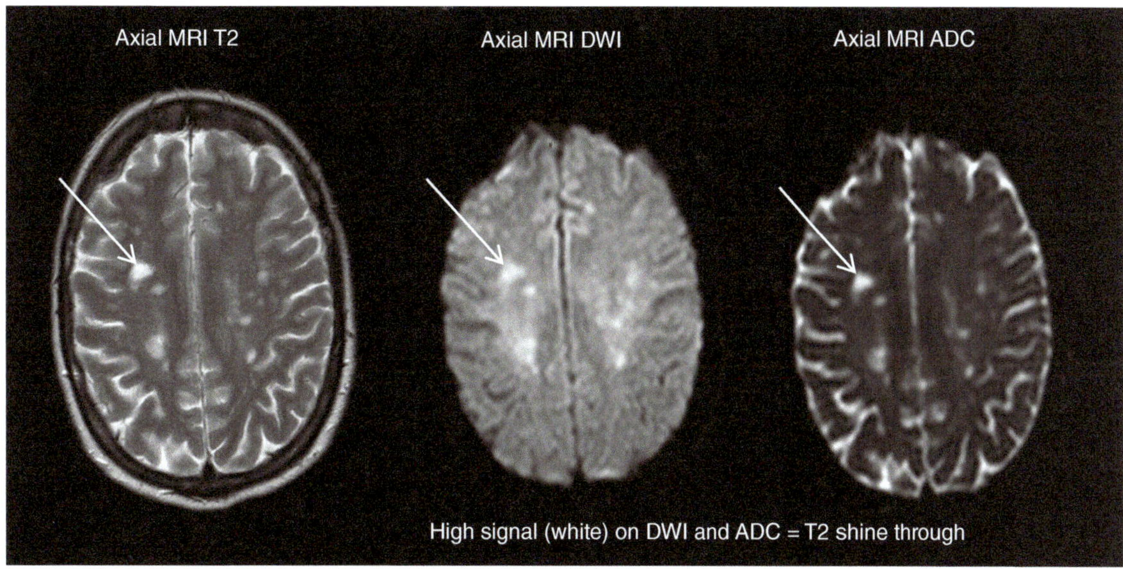

FIGURE 1.13 Axial MRI T2, DWI and ADC sequences, demonstrating 'T2 shine-through'. The T2 sequence shows multiple high-signal T2 lesions in the white matter, the largest in the right frontal lobe (white arrow). These lesions are high-intensity signals (white) on the DWI. However, before this can be called diffusion restriction, correlation with ADC is required. These lesions are also bright on ADC. This therefore represents represents a 'T2 shine-through' artefact, rather than true diffusion restriction. In this case the lesions represent chronic small vessel disease.

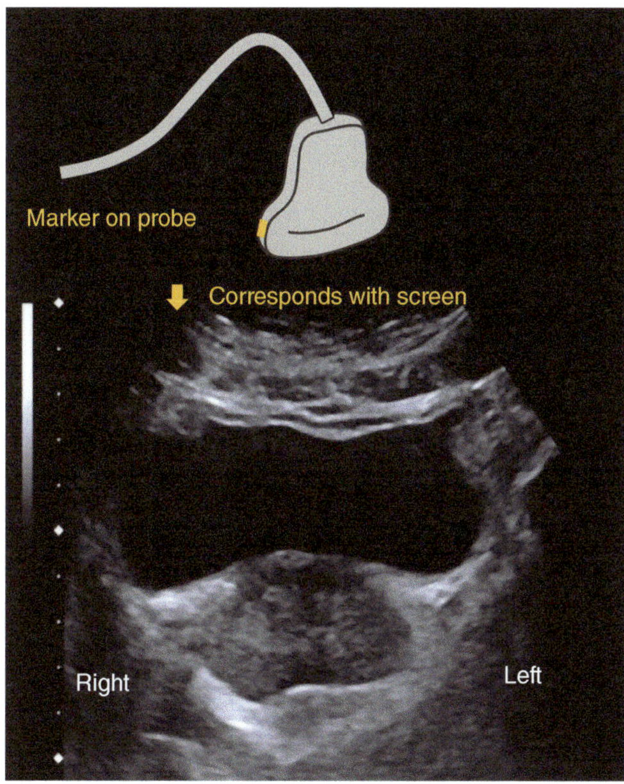

FIGURE 1.14 Axial ultrasound of the pelvis, showing orientation of the probe. In keeping with the imaging convention elsewhere, the patient's right side is on the left side of the screen. In the longitudinal plane, the cranial side goes on the left side of the screen by convention (Pelvis Chapter 7 – Figures 7.2 and 7.4).

1.14.2.3 Buttons There will be a way to manipulate the image; this could be via real buttons or a touch screen interface. Below are listed the commonly used buttons.

- *Depth*: controls the depth of tissues visible on the screen. Reducing depth to focus on anatomy of interest improves the image quality.
- *Frequency modulation*: higher frequency shows more detail. Lower frequency gives better penetration of deeper tissues. One of the operator skills is judging the optimal balance between these conflicting properties.
- *Zoom*: electronically zooms into a section of the screen. Beware, this does not improve image quality.
- *Gain*: changes the brightness of the image but does not alter overall image quality.
- *Doppler mode*: this enables the direction of blood flow to be seen (Pelvis Chapter 8 – Figure 8.2 and Cardiac Chapter 15 – Figure 15.6).

Dedicated ultrasound machines will also have a keyboard to label the images.

1.14.3 Terminology

- *Anechoic*: black appearance on an ultrasound image. This suggests either fluid content (Pelvic Chapter 6 – Figure 6.3) or a lack of ultrasound waves returning from this region (Abdo Chapter 19 – Figure 19.9).
- *Hypoechoic*: dark grey appearance on ultrasound image. This usually suggests a solid structure which allows some vibrations to pass through. Many organs appear like this, for example the prostate (Pelvis Chapter 6 – Figure 6.3).
- *Isoechoic*: middle grey appearance on ultrasound image. Slightly more reflective than hypoechoic

tissues but still allows passage of the ultrasound waves.

- *Hyperechoic*: bright grey or white on the ultrasound image. Structures which completely block the vibration transmission appear white because more of the sound waves are returning to the probe. Examples include gas and bone. As the vibrations are completely reflected, the deeper tissues will appear black (Pelvic Chapter 7.2 – Figure 7.2, bowel gas).

1.14.4 Artefacts

1.14.4.1 Posterior Acoustic Shadowing This is what happens when the ultrasound beam hits a completely reflective surface. All the waves are reflected back to the probe and the deeper tissues become black. It is often the result of calcification (Abdo Chapter 19 – Figure 19.9) or bone (Resp Chapter 10 – Figure 10.10).

1.14.4.2 Posterior Acoustic Enhancement This can be thought of as the opposite to posterior acoustic shadowing. The waves can travel through fluid with zero reflections, which results in a stronger signal returning from deeper tissues (Pelvis Chapter 9 – Figure 9.3). A fluid-filled cyst is one common example of a structure demonstrating posterior acoustic enhancement

1.14.4.3 Edge Artefact If the ultrasound beam hits a rounded object, the edges will reflect the ultrasound beam downwards and away from the probe, reducing the return signal and creating vertical dark bands (Pelvis Chapter 9 – Figure 9.3).

1.14.5 Ultrasound in Trauma

1.14.5.1 eFAST (Extended Focused Assessment Using Sonography in Trauma) Scanning This is a quick systematic scan of the torso, looking for life-threatening conditions. It can detect:

- pneumothorax
- haemothorax
- cardiac tamponade (Cardiac Chapter 14 – Figure 14.6)
- free fluid (peritoneal haemorrhage) (Abdo Chapter 18 – Figure 18.7).

Its limitations include the following.

- It is operator dependent (i.e. it is only as good as the practitioner holding the probe).
- It may miss small volumes of fluid (less than 200 ml).
- It is unlikely to show the source of the bleeding, especially in the abdomen.
- There may be limited views if there is excessive surgical emphysema or free gas in the abdomen.
- It has poor sensitivity in deeper regions like the thoracic aorta and retroperitoneum.

1.15 Take-home Tips on Radiology Modalities

- *Plain radiology*: ubiquitous but only provides static 2D images. It is good for looking at bone, lungs and bowel gas but has limited resolution of soft tissues.
- *CT*: this is much more versatile than plain radiology, especially if contrast is given. However, greater radiation doses are used and it requires the viewer to manipulate the image. Compared to MRI, it provides a poor view of the spinal cord.
- *Nuclear medicine*: provides functional information about the body but has much less anatomical definition compared to X-ray and CT. It is also unlikely to be available within the time frame in which the acute physician works.
- *MRI*: this is very good for viewing soft tissues in neuro and MSK systems. The disadvantage is that it takes longer than X-ray, CT and US and is not tolerated well by unstable or claustrophobic patients.
- *Ultrasound*: this is increasingly available inside and outside hospital. The limitations are that the US beam is blocked by gas and bone and the image quality is very dependent on the skill of the operator.

Further Resources

Driscoll, P.A., Goode, P.N. and Skinner, D.B. (2023) ABC of major trauma: Rescue, resuscitation with imaging, and rehabilitation. Hoboken, NJ, USA: Wiley Blackwell.

www.radiologyinfo.org/en/info/safety-xray

www.gov.uk/government/publications/medical-radiation-patient-doses

www.gov.uk/government/publications/ionising-radiation-dose-comparisons/ionising-radiation-dose-comparisons

Diagnostic Imaging Dataset Annual Statistical Release 2021/22 Version 1. www.england.nhs.uk/statistics/wp-content/uploads/sites/2/2022/12/Annual-Statistical-Release-2021-22-PDF-1.3-MB.pdf

Extremity Section

CHAPTER 2

Painful Hip

Joshua Lauder[1], Eoghan Donnelly[2], and Peter Driscoll[3]

[1] East Lancashire Hospitals NHS Trust, University of Central Lancashire and University of Manchester, UK
[2] NHS Greater Glasgow and Clyde, Glasgow, UK
[3] School of Medicine and Dentistry, University of Central Lancashire, Preston, UK

2.1 Primary Case

2.1.1 Presentation

Chronic progressive right hip pain.

2.1.1.1 History of Presenting Complaint A 65-year-old female presents to her GP with a six-month history of a gradual increase in pain in the right groin area. The pain initially occurred with walks over a mile but now it is present at shorter distances (around 1/4 mile). More recently, she has developed a limp but regular, simple analgesics provide temporary relief for a few hours.

Pain features (SOCRATES)

- S – Site: right groin.
- O – Onset: gradual increase in discomfort, initially noticed after a long walk. Now noticed after walking upstairs and at the end of the day.
- C – Character: dull ache.
- R – Radiation: into the anterior thigh.
- A – Associations.
  - Minimal morning stiffness, lasts under 10 minutes.
  - Disturbed sleep if she lies on the right side.
- T – Time course: gradually getting worse over the last year.
- E – Exacerbating/relieving factors: unable to sit cross-legged.
- S – Severity: 7/10 (0 = no pain; 10 = worse pain imaginable).

PMH: none.
SH: nil.

DH: paracetamol and naproxen. Dihydrocodeine has been recently started by her GP – no allergies.

2.1.2 Examination

OE:

- Overweight.
- Antalgic gait with an unwillingness to weight bear on the right side.
- Has started using a stick in the left hand which helps.
- Tenderness over the right groin on deep palpation.
- All movements of the right hip are reduced due to pain (active greater than passive). The range of movement (ROM) most restricted was internal rotation (10° v 40° active and 12° v 45° passive).
- Lumbar spine and knee – NAD.
- PNS – NAD.

Modified early warning signs (MEWS):

- Respiratory rate 18 bpm.
- SpO_2 95% on room air.
- Temp 37.2 °C.
- HR 90 bt/min.
- BP 130/80 mmHg.
- Alert.

2.1.3 Investigations

2.1.3.1 X-ray An X-ray was performed (Figure 2.1).

Diagnostic Imaging and Anatomy in Acute Care, First Edition. Edited by Joshua Lauder and Peter Driscoll.
© 2025 John Wiley & Sons Ltd. Published 2025 by John Wiley & Sons Ltd.
Companion website: www.wiley.com/go/DiagnosticImaginginAcuteCare

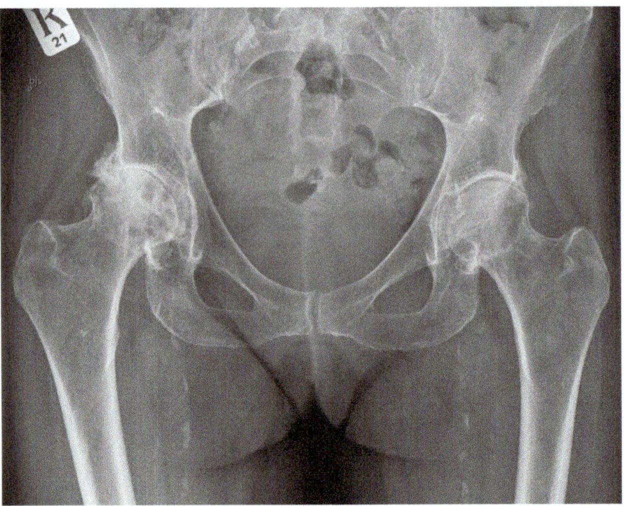

FIGURE 2.1 Patient A. AP pelvis X-ray.

Clinical Case Questions
- What is your differential diagnosis? Why?
- What abnormalities do you note on the plain X-ray?
- When might an MRI be of use?
- What is your final diagnosis?

2.2 Radiology Self-assessment

2.2.1 Technical

2.2.1.1 X-ray

- What does a synovial joint look like on X-ray?
- What are the X-ray signs of arthritis?

2.2.2 Correlation of Gross Anatomy to Imaging

2.2.2.1 Joint and Bones

- Which bones make up the pelvis?

2.3 Key Radiology Review

2.3.1 X-ray Pelvis

A correlation of the key gross anatomy with the plain X-ray is shown in Figure 2.2.

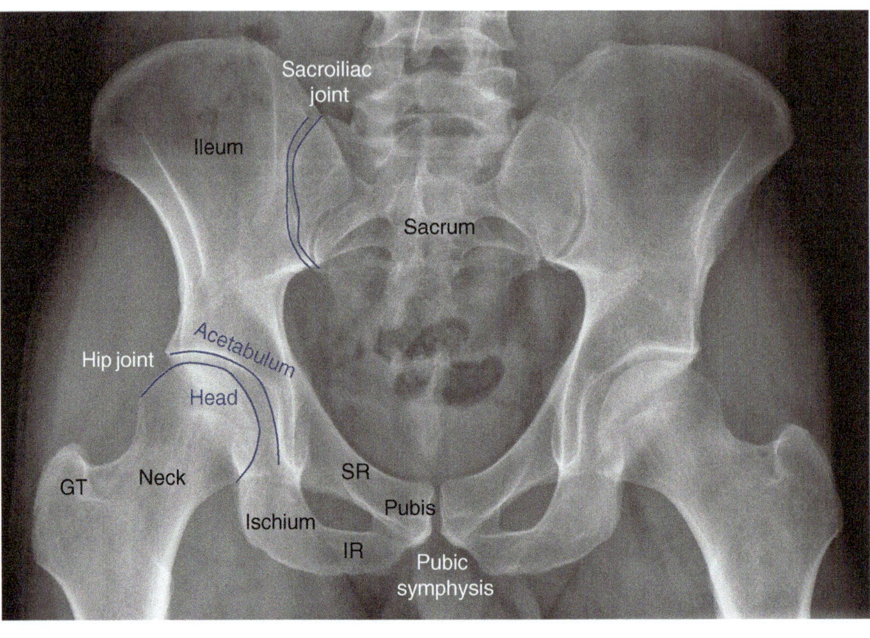

FIGURE 2.2 Normal pelvis X-ray. A normal synovial joint will have a gap visible on X-ray between the bone articular surfaces. This is where hyaline cartilage lies so the bone surfaces should be smooth. GT, greater trochanter; SR, superior pubic ramus; IR, inferior pubic ramus.

2.4 Review of the Clinical Case

2.4.1 What is Your Differential Diagnosis? Why?

- *Degenerative (osteoarthritis [OA])*: this is characterised by chronic progressive pain and has four classic radiological features (Figure 2.3).
- *Inflammatory (e.g. rheumatoid) arthritis*: usually this is in younger patients. It is often associated with morning stiffness and may have other autoimmune symptoms. Features on plain X-ray differ from those of osteoarthritis and are characterised by periarticular osteopaenia and erosions (Figure 2.4).
- *Crystal (gout and pseudogout).*
  - Gout is usually more acute than OA, coming to peak severity in several days. Acute gout causes minimal radiological changes so the plain X-ray may appear normal. In contrast, chronic gout is characterised by large erosions at the edge of the joint which may have a sclerotic rim (Figure 2.5).
  - Pseudogout appears very similar to OA but can affect different joints (such as the patellofemoral joint). Pseudogout is suspected radiographically if there is chondrocalcinosis, most often seen in the menisci of the knees and triangular fibrocartilage complex of the wrist (Figure 2.6).

2.4.2 When is Imaging Indicated?

If arthritis is suspected clinically then plain radiology can help to quantify the severity and sometimes characterise the cause. That said, OA is very common and the diagnosis can often be made in primary care without any imaging. If intervention is planned (for example, injections or joint replacement; Figure 2.7) then imaging is always required.

Ultrasound is used to assess the synovium, which can become inflamed in inflammatory arthropathies. Ultrasound or fluoroscopy can also be used to guide joint injections.

2.4.3 What Abnormalities are Identified on X-ray (Figure 2.3)?

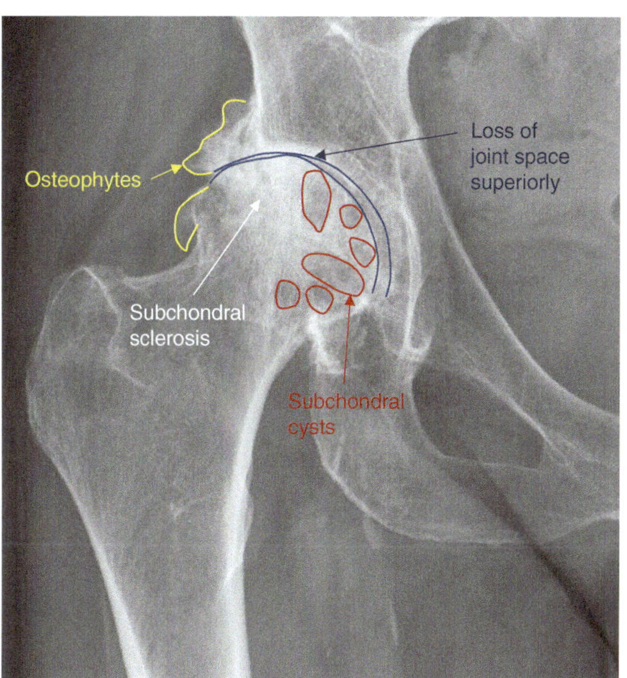

FIGURE 2.3 Patient A. AP right hip X-ray, annotated. The four radiological features of osteoarthritis are present. The earliest sign is usually **loss of joint space**, as the cartilage is eroded. Inflammatory mediators in the joint promote new bone growth resulting in **osteophytes**, which typically occur at the edge of the joint. When the full thickness of cartilage is lost it will begin to affect the underlying bone with **cysts** and **sclerosis** developing.

2.4.4 What is Your Final Diagnosis?

Osteoarthritis of the right hip. Note that there are early OA changes visible in the left hip as well.

Patient A went on to have a total hip replacement (Figure 2.7).

2.4.5 Other Arthropathies to Consider as Part of the Differential Diagnosis

See Figures 2.4–2.6.

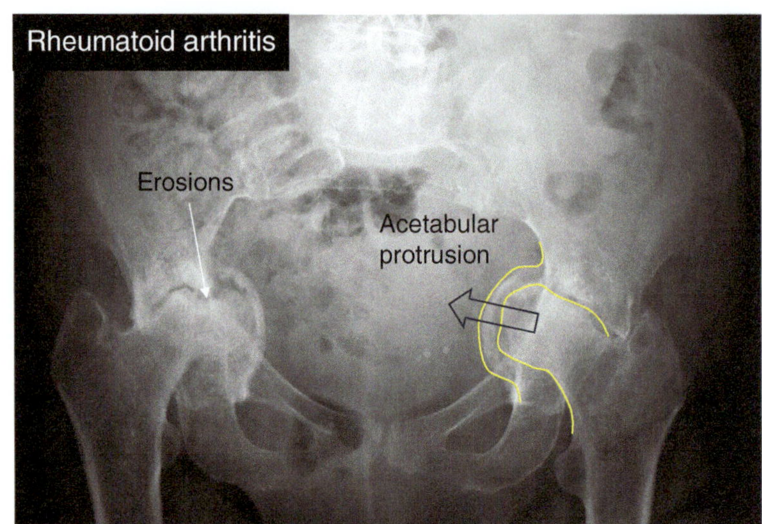

FIGURE 2.4 AP pelvis X-ray, rheumatoid arthritis. This patient has a long-standing history of rheumatoid arthritis affecting both hips. The femoral heads and acetabulae have migrated medially (protrusio acetabulae). There are also large erosions in the femoral heads. In bilateral disease this is called otto pelvis.

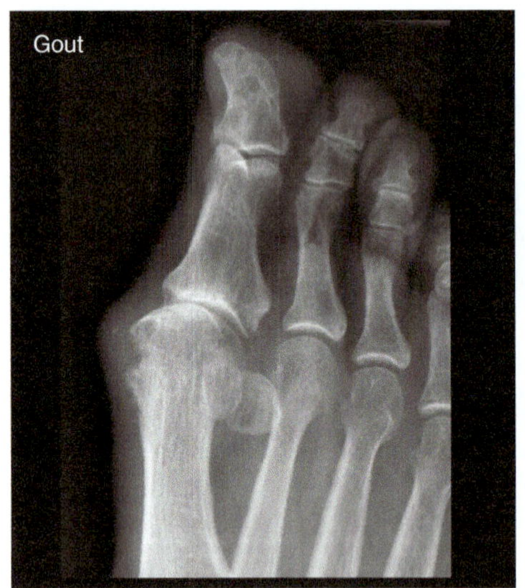

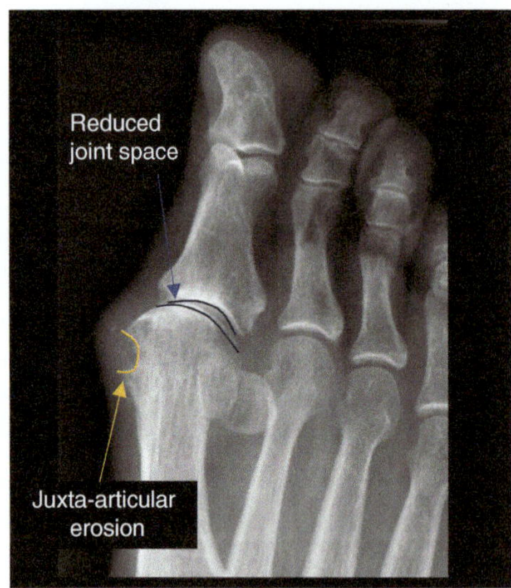

FIGURE 2.5 Oblique X-ray hallux showing gout in the first metatarsophalangeal joint. Compare the unmarked image to the annotated one. There is reduced joint space with a juxta-articular (i.e. next to joint) erosion. This contrasts with the subchondral cysts in OA, which occur centrally in the joint surface.

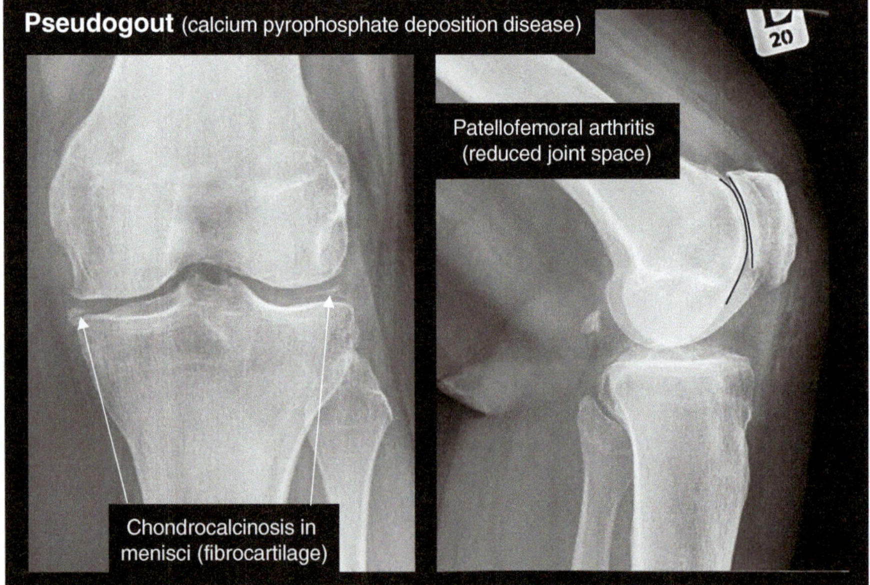

FIGURE 2.6 AP and lateral knee X-ray showing pseudogout or calcium pyrophosphate deposition disease (CPPD). This is characterised by calcification in the fibrocartilage, commonly seen in menisci of the knee, triangular fibrocartilage of the wrist and pubic symphysis. This causes secondary osteoarthritis which has the same features as osteoarthritis in Figure 2.3 but occurs in unusual joints, the patellofemoral joint being a classic location.

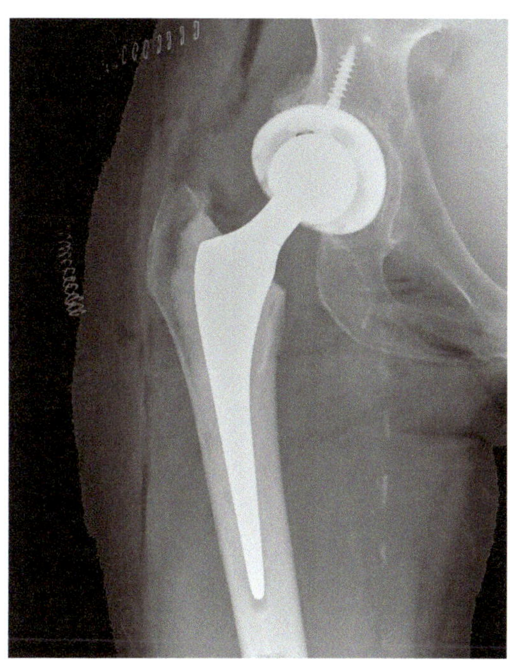

FIGURE 2.7 Patient A following total hip replacement. AP right hip X-ray. This is an example of a 'hybrid' total hip replacement. These have an uncemented acetabular cup with a screw and a cemented stem. Both components are metallic so appear bright (white) on X-ray. The cement around the stem can also be seen on X-ray as it contains either barium sulfate or zirconium dioxide which is used as a radio-opacifier. This is useful as it allows assessment of the bone/cement and cement/implant interfaces which can be used to determine whether the implant is loose.

2.5 Take-home Message – Arthritis

- If history is typical for osteoarthritis and conservative management is pursued then no imaging is required.

- Plain radiology is the first-line investigation in arthritis and usually the only investigation required.
- Ultrasound is used to look for active synovitis if inflammatory arthritis is suspected.

Further Resources

Helms, C.A. (2020). *Fundamentals of Skeletal Radiology*. Philadelphia: Elsevier.

CHAPTER 3

Hot, Swollen Knee

Joshua Lauder[1], Eoghan Donnelly[2], Lee Hoggett[3], and Peter Driscoll[4]

[1] *East Lancashire Hospitals NHS Trust, University of Central Lancashire and University of Manchester, UK*
[2] *NHS Greater Glasgow and Clyde, Glasgow, UK*
[3] *Trauma and Orthopaedic Surgery Health Education England North West, Preston, UK*
[4] *School of Medicine and Dentistry, University of Central Lancashire, Preston, UK*

3.1 Primary Case

3.1.1 Presentation

A 30-year-old unkempt male attends with a swollen and excruciatingly painful left knee. He is a poor historian and is unsure if he had an injury recently but states that he has been unable to weight bear for the past six hours due to pain.

3.1.1.1 History of Presenting Complaint Pain features (SOCRATES)

- S– Site: left knee.
- O – Onset: started 12 hours ago – atraumatic.
- C – Character: agony and tightness.
- R – Radiation: does not radiate.
- A – Associations: feels systemically hot and clammy.
- T – Time course: started as mild throbbing pain which gradually worsened.
- E – Exacerbating/relieving factors: any movement of the knee is painful, no relieving factors.
- S – Severity: 10/10.

PMH: intravenous drug abuser, recently been injecting cocaine into his left thigh.
SH; nil.
DH: nil – no allergies.

3.1.2 Examination

OE: the red, hot, tense swollen left knee is extremely painful to touch. There is no range of active or passive movement (ROM).
Modified early warning signs (MEWS):

- Respiratory rate 20 bpm.
- SpO_2 93% on room air.
- Temp 38.2 °C.
- HR 110 bt/min.
- BP 125/80 mmHg.
- Alert.

3.1.3 Investigations

3.1.3.1 Blood Tests WCC 14×10^9/l CRP 57 mg/dl

3.1.4 Imaging

An urgent knee X-ray was performed (Figure 3.1).
Due to the vague history of trauma, the patient had an MRI scan of his left knee (Figure 3.2).

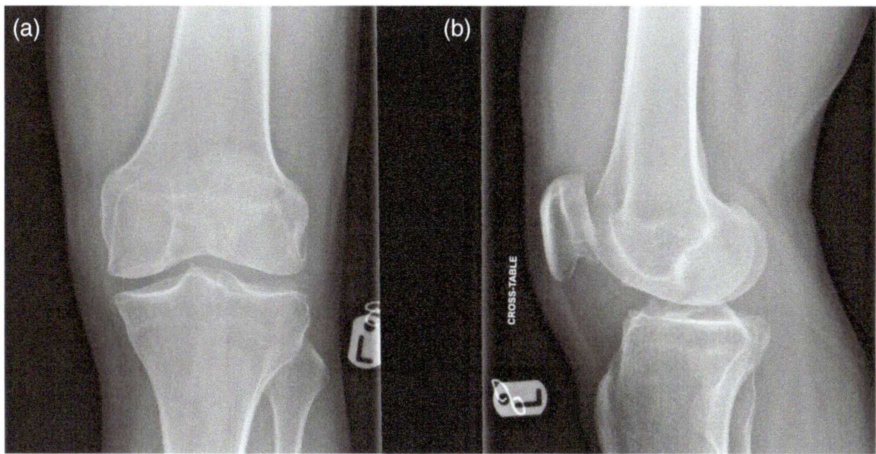

FIGURE 3.1 Patient A. Left knee X-ray anterior posterior (AP) (a) and lateral (b) projections.

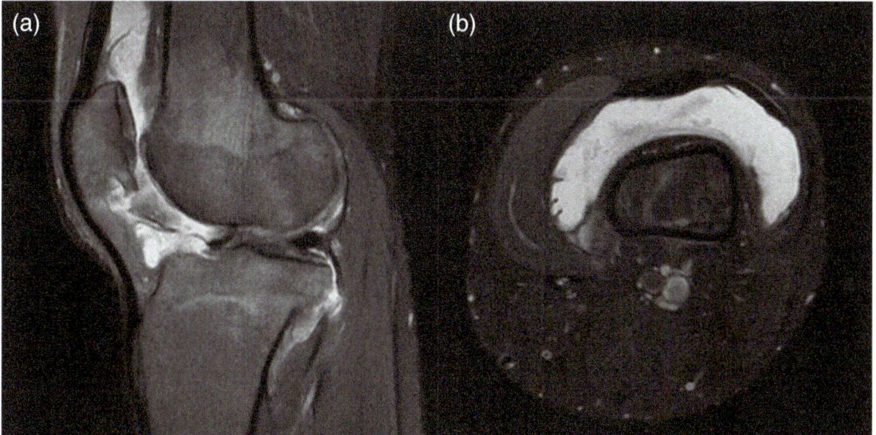

FIGURE 3.2 (a) Patient A. MRI left knee, sagittal PDFS; (b) axial PDFS. PDFS, proton density with fat suppression.

Clinical Case Questions

- What is your differential diagnosis? Why?
- What abnormalities do you note on the plain X-ray?
- What abnormalities do you note on the MRI scan?
- What is your final diagnosis?

3.2 Radiology Self-assessment

3.2.1 Technical

3.2.1.1 X-ray

- What density is fluid on an X-ray?

3.2.1.2 MRI

- What are the visual differences between T1 and T2 images?
- What is a proton density with fat suppression (PDFS) sequence?
- What is fat suppression imaging?
- What is STIR imaging?

3.2.2 Correlating Gross Anatomy to Imaging the Knee

3.2.2.1 Joint and Bones

- What is the extent of the joint capsule?
- What are the normal fat pads visible on plain X-ray?
- What are the T1 and STIR signal characteristics of normal bone marrow?

3.2.2.2 Ligaments

- What do the cruciate ligaments look like on MRI?
- What do the collateral ligaments look like on MRI?

3.2.2.3 Menisci

- What do the menisci look like on MRI?

3.3 Key Radiology Review

3.3.1 Correlating Gross Anatomy to Imaging

3.3.1.1 X-ray It is useful to have a system when interpreting an X-ray because it helps in cases where pattern recognition fails you. One such system is AABCS (Adequacy, Alignment, Bones, Cartilage, Soft tissues) which will be reviewed here using the knee as an example (Figure 3.3).

- *Adequacy*: this is primarily concerned with checking the **x-ray projection**. With the normal knee, the AP view allows assessment of the joint space with minimal overlapping of the femoral condyles on the tibial plateau. The lateral view should have superimposed femoral condyles. Penetration tends to be less of an issue with modern X-ray equipment as the radiation dose is electronically controlled and any poor quality in the image can often be improved with postprocessing.

- *Alignment* (i.e. are the joints and bones aligned normally?): significant forces are usually required to dislocate the knee (e.g. fall from a height/high-speed crashes) so it is often associated with other bone and soft tissue injuries. In contrast, less force is required to dislocate the patella and this is therefore seen more commonly. The patellar tendon should be approximately the length of the patella bone. **Valgus** or **varus** are other common malalignments, particularly in the context of arthritis (Figure 3.4).
- *Bones*: carefully inspect **every bone** on **every projection**. A fracture may only be visible on one projection.
- *Cartilage*: although the cartilage is not visible on an X-ray, the joint space should be. The knee has hyaline cartilage on the articular surfaces and fibrocartilage in the menisci.
- *Soft tissues*: this step also includes a review for soft tissue calcification and swelling. The joint capsule extends into the suprapatellar region and is the best place to check for a joint effusion (Figure 3.5).

3.3.1.2 MRI Sequences T1 and PDFS are the typical MRI sequencing techniques used for viewing musculoskeletal anatomy.

Fat has a high signal on T1 sequences, so both the subcutaneous tissue and bone marrow should be bright. Fluid is dark on this sequence. Compare this to a standard PDFS sequence where fat is dark, because it is suppressed, and fluid bright (Figure 3.6). Consequently, PDFS is effective at spotting MSK pathology because the commonly

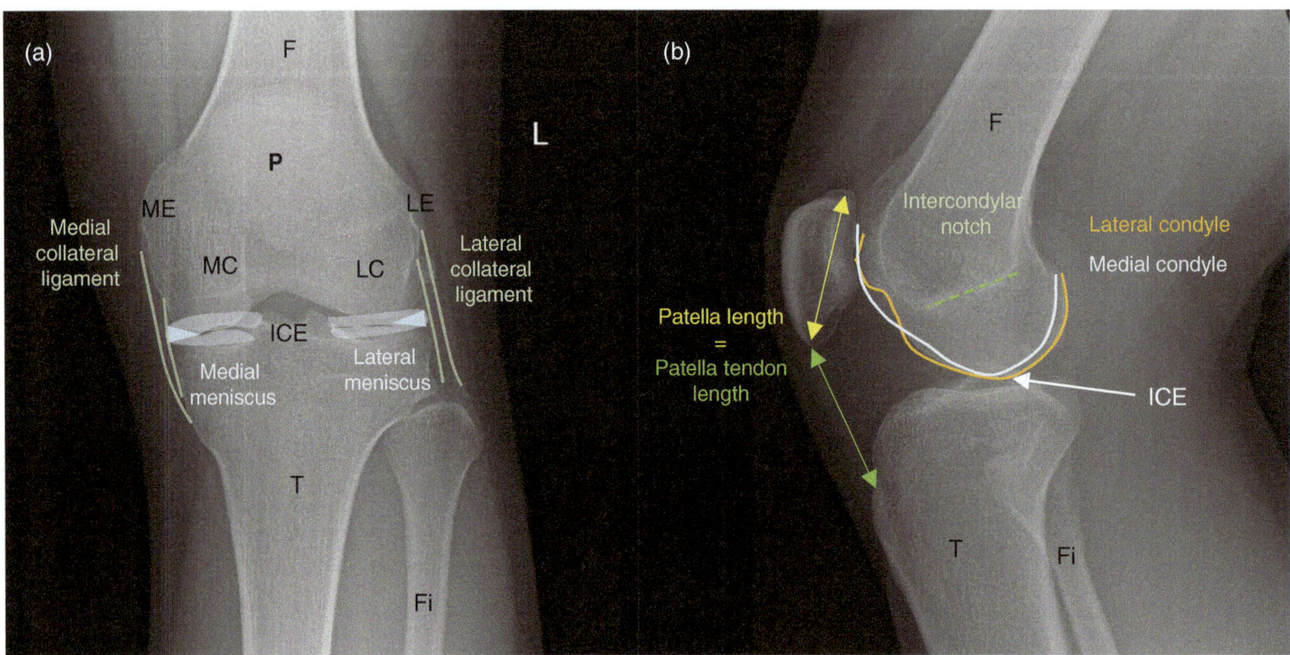

FIGURE 3.3 Normal knee X-ray, AP (a) and lateral (b) projections. F, femur; Fi, fibula; ICE, intercondylar eminence; LC, lateral condyle; LE, lateral epicondyle; MC, medial condyle; ME, medial epicondyle; P, patella; T, tibia.

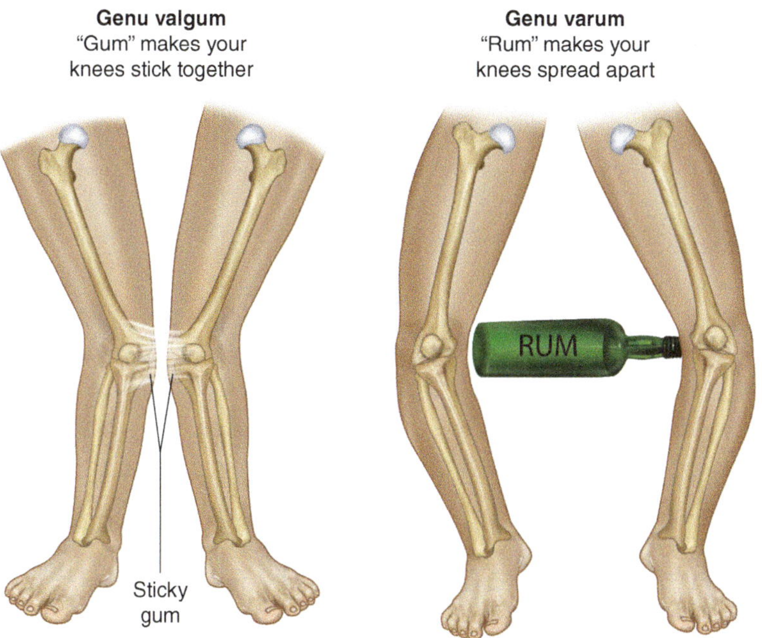

(a) (b)

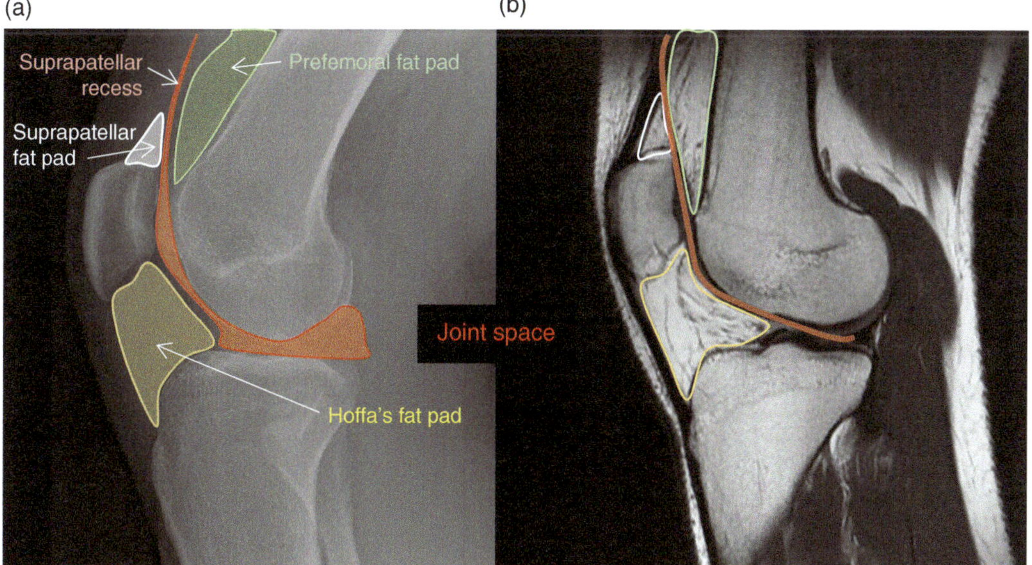

FIGURE 3.5 Normal knee. (a) Lateral plain X-ray. (b) Sagittal proton density (PD) MRI. The joint capsule extends superiorly beneath the patella to lie between the prefemoral and suprapatellar fat pad. This is called the suprapatellar recess and it extends a surprising distance superiorly above the patella (3–4 cm). If the gap between these two respective fat pads is over 1 cm on a lateral X-ray then there is likely an effusion. The prepatellar bursa cannot be seen in healthy knees, only when inflamed.

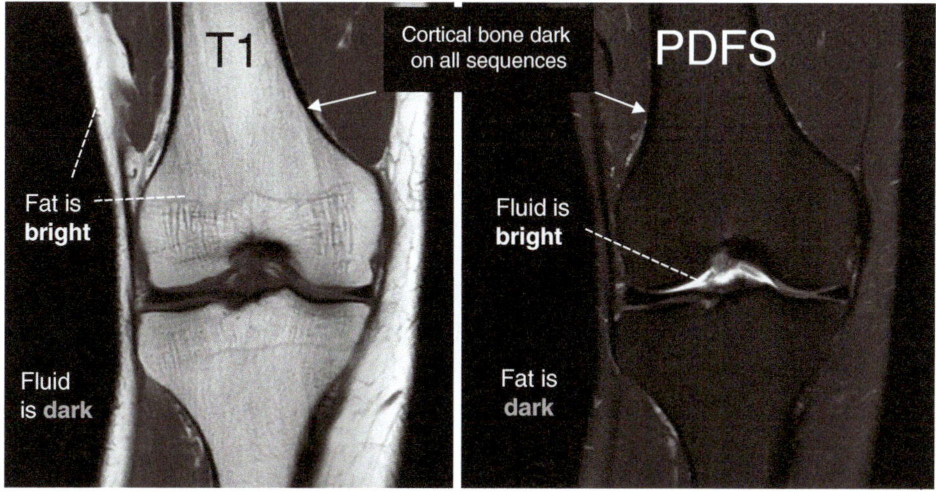

FIGURE 3.6 MRI view of a normal knee using T1 (left) and PDFS (right) sequencing.

(a)

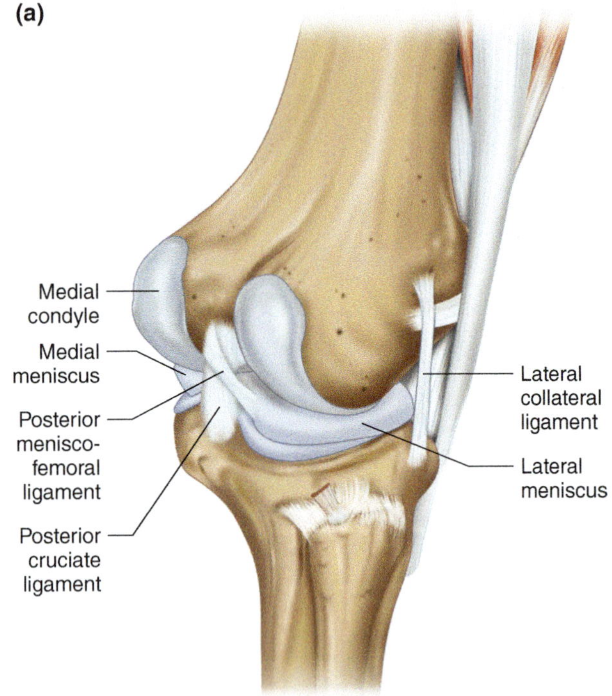

(b)

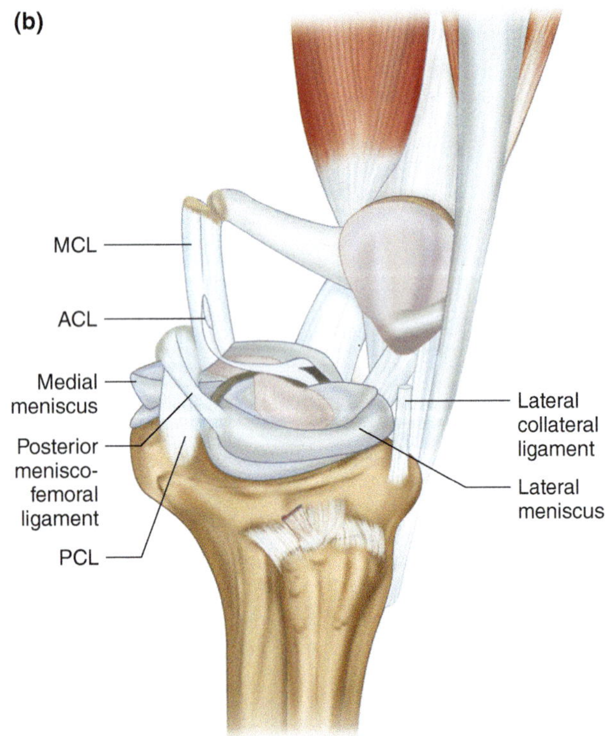

FIGURE 3.7 (a) Posterolateral view of the right knee with the femur in place. Note the posterior cruciate ligament (PCL) arises behind the intercondylar eminence. It runs upwards, forwards and medially to insert into the medial condyle of the femur. (b) Similar view to (a) but the femur has been removed. The anterior cruciate ligament (ACL) arises in front of the intercondylar eminence. Crossing the PCL, it runs posteriorly, upwards and laterally to insert into the lateral femoral condyle.

associated features of oedema and effusion appear bright and are not masked by fat.

Cortical bone, ligaments and tendons are dark on all sequences (Figures 3.6 and 3.8).

	T1	PDFS
Subcutaneous tissue and bone marrow (fat)	Bright (whiter)	Dark (blacker)
Fluid	Dark (blacker)	Bright (whiter)

3.3.1.3 Ligaments

3.3.1.3.1 Correlating Soft Tissue Anatomy with the MRI Image
Take a moment to revise the knee's main ligaments (Figure 3.7).

Now consider the same structures as they appear on an MRI (Figures 3.8 and 3.9).

3.3.1.4 Menisci Again, take a moment to revise the knee menisci (Figure 3.10).

Now consider the same structures as they appear on an MRI (Figure 3.11).

3.4 Review of the Clinical Case

3.4.1 What is Your Differential Diagnosis? Why?

- *Infection*: the most likely diagnosis and certainly the one to exclude early as it can cause irreversible damage to the joint.
- *Injury*: the patient is a poor historian and so it is not possible to exclude traumatic injury without investigating. In this case there would have to be a secondary cause for his systemic symptoms.
- *Gout/pseudogout*: these can be excruciatingly painful in the acute phase and develop quickly. It is also unlikely to be associated with this level of pyrexia.
- *Inflammatory arthritis*: this will often be polyarticular, more chronic and associated with other systemic symptoms.
- *Soft tissue or bony malignancy*: this can present as a knee effusion if intra-articular or in close proximity to the joint. It would not explain the pyrexia.
- *Osteoarthritis (OA)*: this can produce a hot, swollen joint. However, some movement is usually possible. The age of the patient and the lack of a previous history of OA also make it unlikely.

The diagnosis of septic arthritis is made from a joint aspiration, gram stain and culture, not imaging.

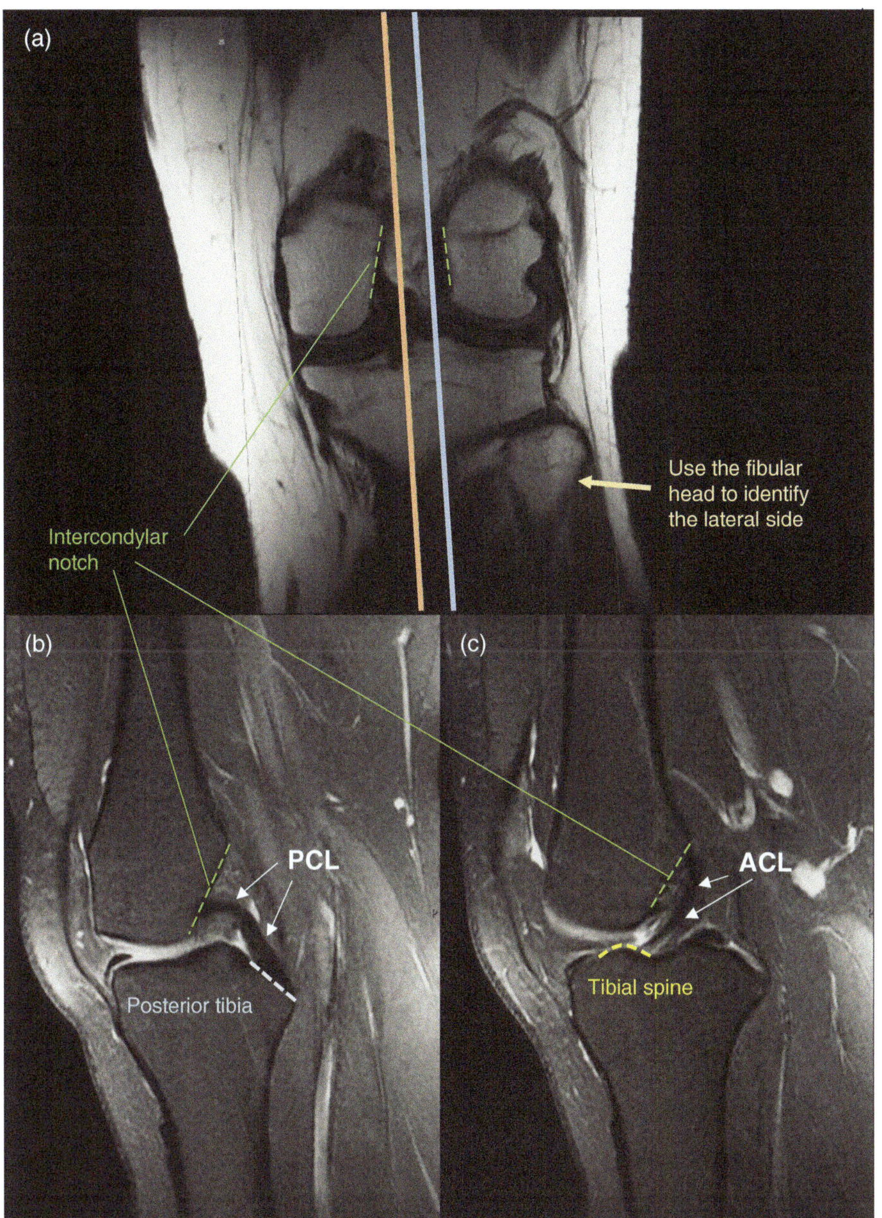

FIGURE 3.8 Normal knee. (a) Coronal T1 showing the relative slice positions. (b) Sagittal PDFS through the posterior cruciate ligament (PCL). (c) Sagittal PDFS through the anterior cruciate ligament (ACL) which lies lateral to the PCL. Normal ligaments are dark on all sequences. If they contain oedema from sprains or tears then they will become bright on PDFS.

3.4.2 When is Imaging Indicated?

A joint aspiration should be carried out urgently, before administration of antibiotics, when septic arthritis is the likely diagnosis, the reason being if pus is found, treatment can begin at once. If no aspirate can be obtained but septic arthritis is still suspected, it may be appropriate to use imaging to confirm effusion and guide aspiration (in the case of suspected hip septic arthritis, this is the only way to obtain an aspirate). This will often be done using ultrasound.

- Plain radiology is indicated in cases of trauma (when an underlying fracture is possible) and OA, if surgery is considered.
- CT is used mainly in trauma cases to plan surgery.

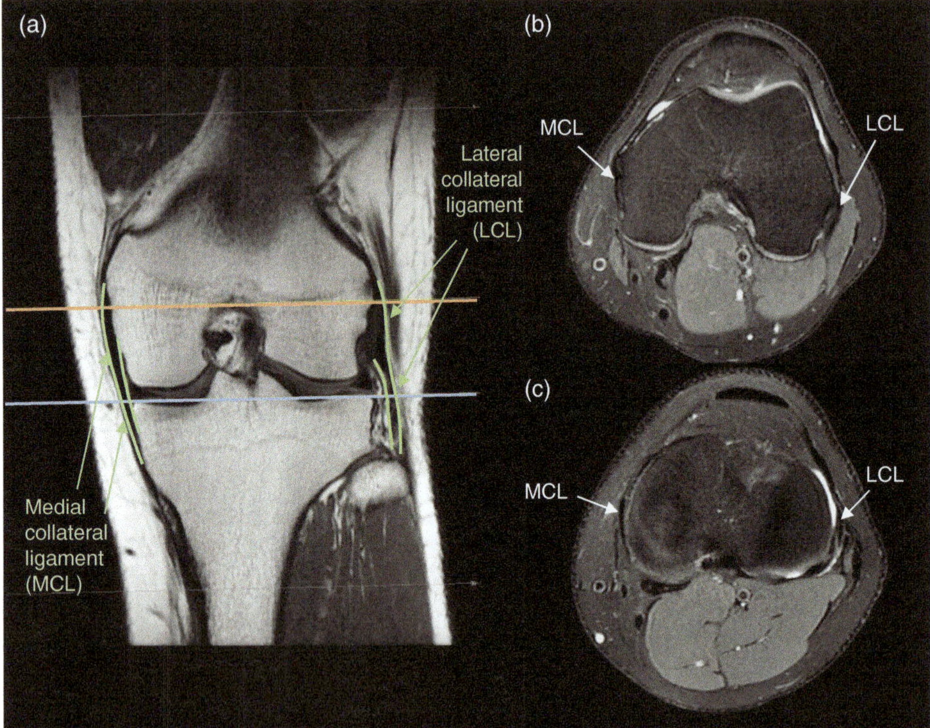

FIGURE 3.9 (a) Normal knee. Coronal T1 showing the course of the collateral ligaments and the relative slice positions.
(b) Axial PDFS through the femoral condyles showing the origin of the MCL and LCL as black bands of tissue.
(c) Axial PDFS through the tibial plateau showing the collateral ligaments continuing as black bands next to the bone.

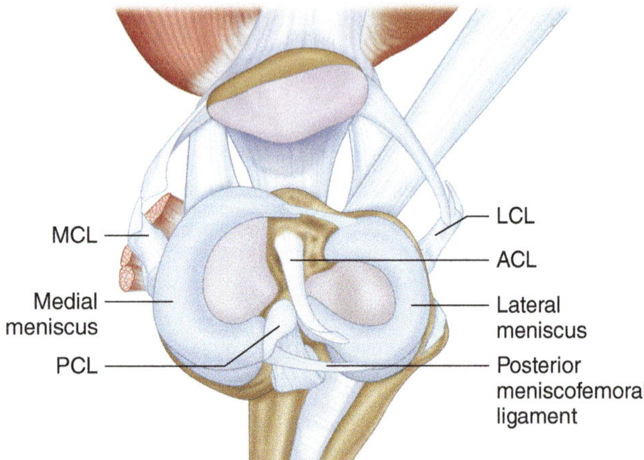

FIGURE 3.10 Superior view of the right tibial plateau. In comparison to the medial meniscus, the lateral meniscus is smaller, more C-shaped, not anchored to the LCL and has a connection by the posterior meniscofemoral ligament to the femur. All these are considered important in protecting it during twisting movements of the knee.

- MRI can be used to look for early signs of osteomyelitis and to investigate traumatic injury to the intrinsic knee ligaments and menisci.

3.4.3 What Abnormalities are Identified on the Plain X-ray?

Septic arthritis will appear as a joint effusion. Patient A does have a large suprapatellar effusion but this finding is non-specific (Figure 3.12). It can be seen in any condition that causes inflammation in the knee.

Osteomyelitis can be visible on X-ray as bony destruction (osteolysis) but the X-ray appearances typically lag behind clinical symptoms by several weeks (Figure 3.13).

3.4.4 What Abnormalities are Identified on the MRI Scan?

In view of the lack of a precise history in this case, an MRI scan was arranged (Figure 3.14).

The presence of an effusion with severe pain should be treated as septic arthritis until proven otherwise. A joint aspiration with urgent gram stain, microscopy and culture will be required for definitive diagnosis.

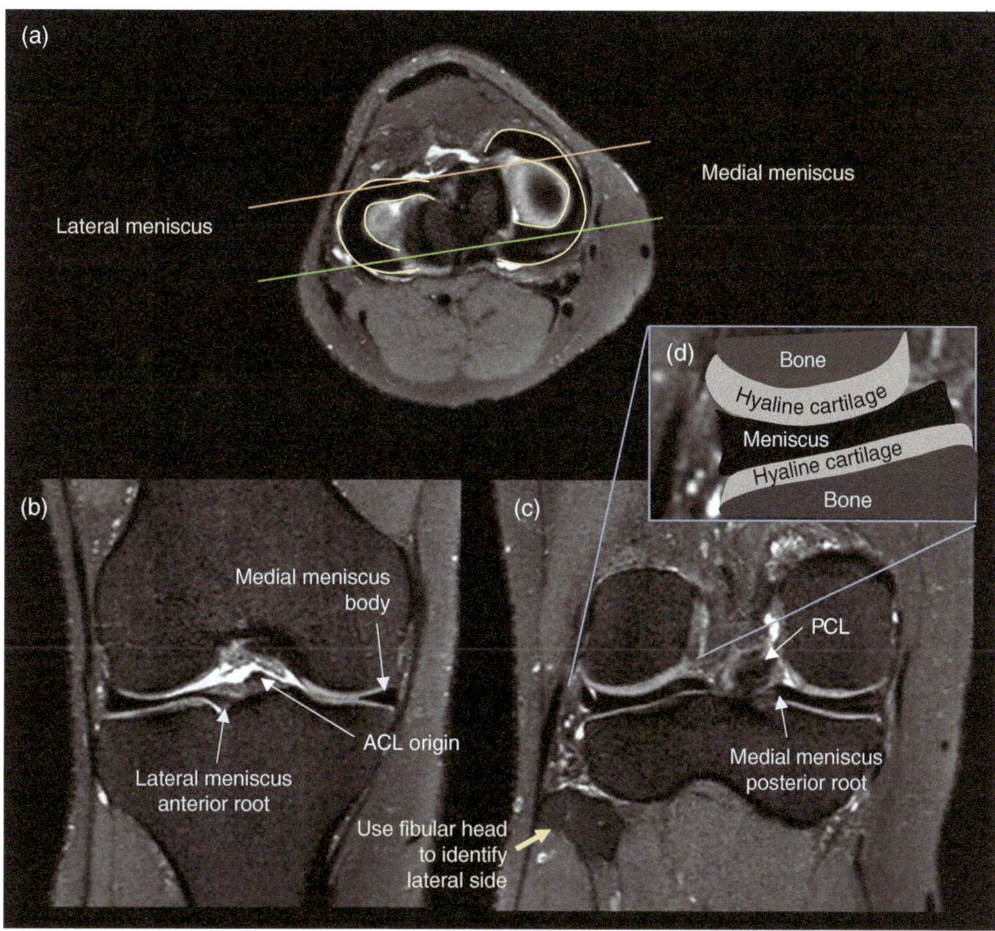

FIGURE 3.11 Normal right knee. (a) Axial PDFS through the menisci showing the 'C' shape of each meniscus. (b) Coronal PDFS through the anterior root of lateral meniscus, showing relationship to the ACL. (c) Coronal PDFS showing the posterior root of medial meniscus. (d) PDFS is a good sequence for assessing hyaline cartilage (also called the chondral surface of the joint). Hyaline cartilage is higher signal (brighter) than the fibrocartilage of the meniscus.

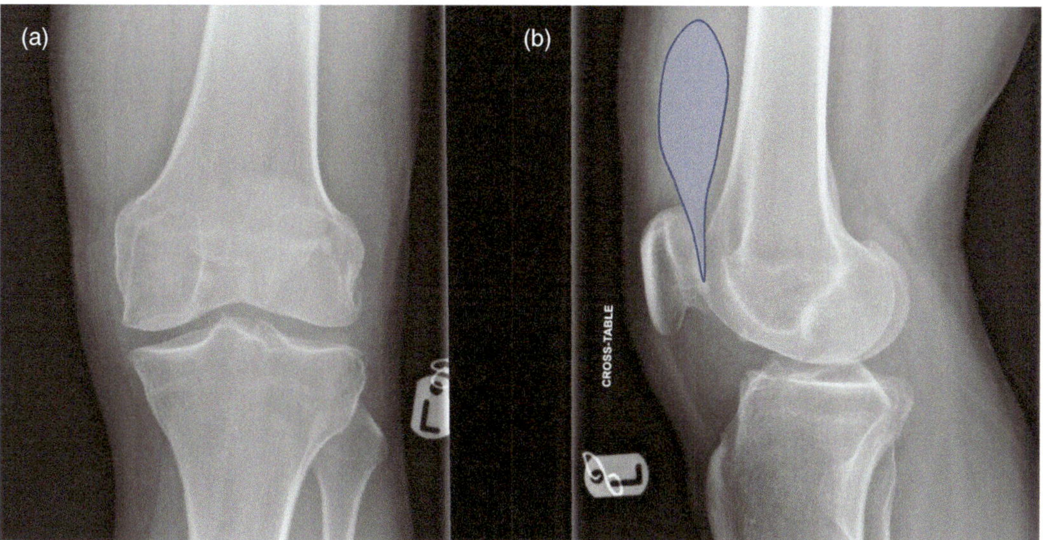

FIGURE 3.12 Patient A annotated. Left knee X-ray AP (a) and lateral (b) projections. There is a large suprapatellar joint effusion (blue). There is no osteolysis to suggest osteomyelitis at this stage (see Figure 3.12), although X-ray features lag behind clinical condition by several weeks.

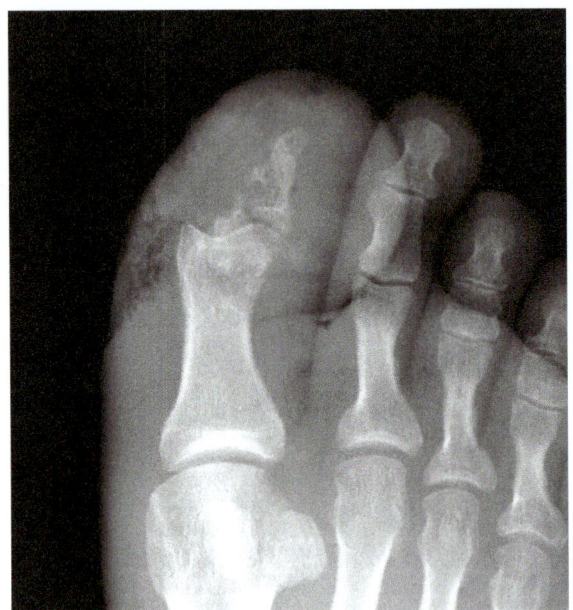

FIGURE 3.13 An AP X-ray of a different patient with osteomyelitis of the hallux. There is loss of the bone in the distal phalanx (osteolysis).

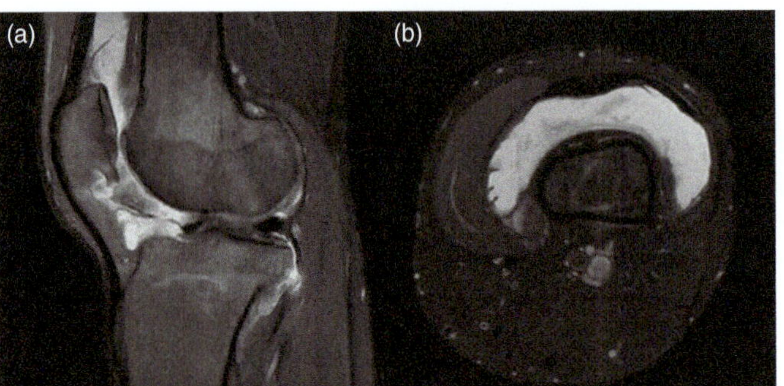

FIGURE 3.14 Patient A. MRI left knee, (a) sagittal PDFS; (b) axial PDFS. The effusion can be better appreciated on MRI, with the bright signal on PDFS suggesting pathological fluid. There is also thickening of the synovium surrounding the joint (compare it to normal synovium seen in Figure 3.15). The cruciate ligaments, collateral ligaments and menisci are intact.

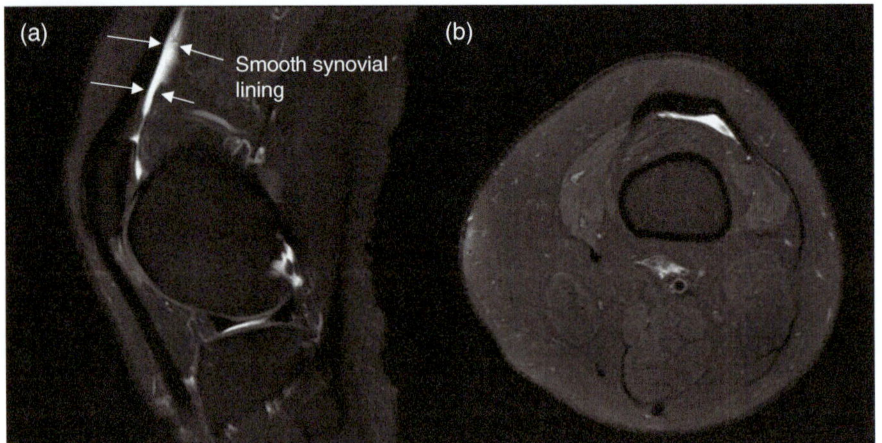

FIGURE 3.15 Normal comparison MRI knee, sagittal PDFS (a) and axial PDFS (b). It is normal to have a trace of fluid in the knee joint. In the healthy state, synovial lining of the joint should be smooth.

3.4.5 What is Your Final Diagnosis?

Septic arthritis of the knee joint.

3.5 Take-home Message – Septic Arthritis

- Advanced imaging (CT/MRI) is not indicated in septic arthritis. Urgent joint aspiration is required.

Further Resources

Ravn, C., Neyt, J., Benito, N. et al., for the Sanjo Guideline Group (2023). Guideline for management of septic arthritis in native joints (SANJO). *J Bone Joint Infect* 8 (1): 29–37.

CHAPTER 4

Shoulder Injury

Joshua Lauder[1], Eoghan Donnelly[2], and Peter Driscoll[3]

[1] *East Lancashire Hospitals NHS Trust, University of Central Lancashire and University of Manchester, UK*
[2] *NHS Greater Glasgow and Clyde, Glasgow, UK*
[3] *School of Medicine and Dentistry, University of Central Lancashire, Preston, UK*

4.1 Primary Case

4.1.1 Presentation

A 54-year-old male presents to the emergency department having developed severe pain in his right shoulder while lifting free weights at the gym. He has recently been trying to get fit again and previously played competitive rugby in his youth.

4.1.1.1 History of Presenting Complaint Pain features (SOCRATES)

- S – Site: right shoulder.
- O – Onset: sudden onset after feeling a clunk.
- C – Character: sharp pain initially, now constant throbbing.
- R – Radiation: no radiation.
- A – Associations: pins and needles around the shoulder.
- T – Time course: sudden onset.
- E – Exacerbating/relieving factors: pain increases with shoulder movement in any direction.
- S – Severity: 7/10 at rest, 10/10 on attempted movement.

PMH: hypertension; previous right shoulder injury many years ago.
SH: nil.
DH: ramipril – no allergies.

4.1.2 Examination

OE: the right shoulder looks obviously different in shape from the left and the patient's upper limb is held down by his side (Figure 4.1). The whole shoulder girdle is tender to touch generally and any attempt at movement is met with extreme pain.

On further examination, numbness is also noted on the lateral aspect of his shoulder but distally he has normal pulses and hand function.

Modified early warning signs (MEWS):

- Respiratory rate 16 bpm.
- SpO_2 98% on room air.
- Temp 36.5 °C.
- HR 112 bpm.
- BP 145/76 mmHg.
- Alert.

4.1.3 Investigations

4.1.3.1 X-ray An urgent right shoulder X-ray was performed (Figure 4.2).

> #### Clinical Case Questions
>
> - What is your differential diagnosis? Why?
> - What is the initial investigation of choice?
> - What abnormalities do you note on the plain X-ray?
> - When might a CT be of use?
> - What is your final diagnosis?

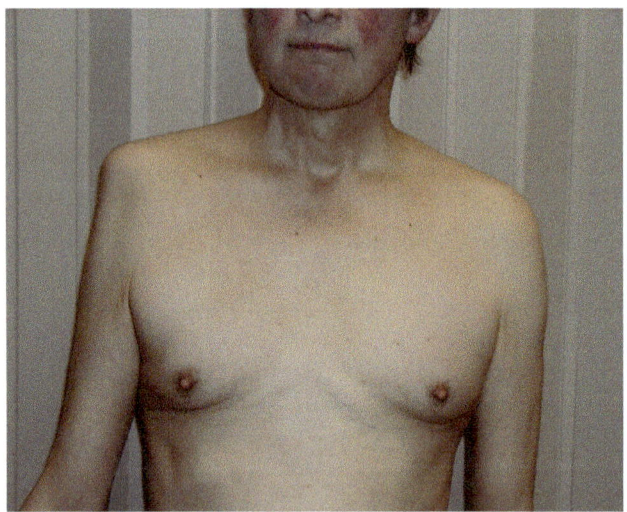

FIGURE 4.1 Clinical picture of Patient B on presentation to the Emergency Department. *Source:* Driscoll et al. (2023)/John Wiley & Sons.

4.2 Radiology Self-assessment

4.2.1 Technical

4.2.1.1 X-ray

- Why is it important to have two X-ray projections?
- Which X-ray projections are used in the shoulder?

4.2.1.2 CT

- Which window should be used to provide optimal bone images?
- What do bones look like on CT?

4.2.2 Correlating Gross Anatomy to Imaging

4.2.2.1 Joint and Bones

- Which joints make up the shoulder girdle?

4.2.2.2 Cartilage

- What cartilaginous structure helps maintain gleno-humeral alignment?

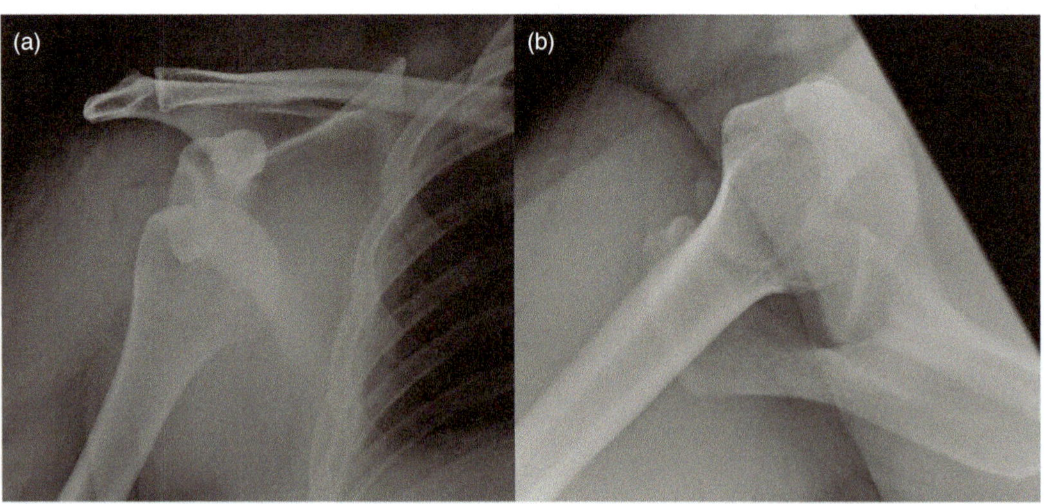

FIGURE 4.2 Patient B. Plain radiographs of the right shoulder. (a) AP projection. (b) Axial projection.

4.3 Key Radiology Review

4.3.1 X-ray Projections

It is vital to have two x-ray projections for the region of interest. This is to better localise pathology, including the direction of dislocations. With the glenohumeral joint, the AP view is typically utilised. A true lateral view of the shoulder cannot be performed as the thorax gets in the way (Figure 4.3). Instead, the axial and Y views are used to check glenohumeral alignment (Figure 4.4).

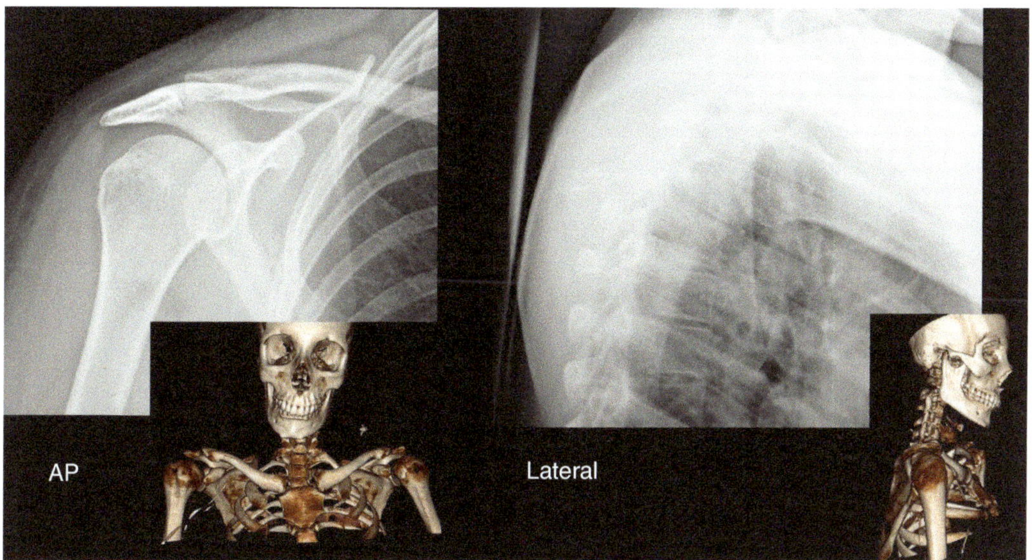

FIGURE 4.3 AP and lateral X-ray projections of the right shoulder. Recall that the shoulder girdle comprises three joints: the glenohumeral; the acromioclavicular and the sternoclavicular. Though most movement occurs at the glenohumeral joint, impairment in any of the articulations leads to reduced mobility. Be aware the plain radiograph cannot view all these joints on the same image. The radiographer therefore needs to know which one is under investigation so that the optimal images can be produced. The lateral view is useless for looking at the shoulder due to overlapping thorax and contralateral shoulder. Instead, the axial and Y views are used (see Figure 4.4).

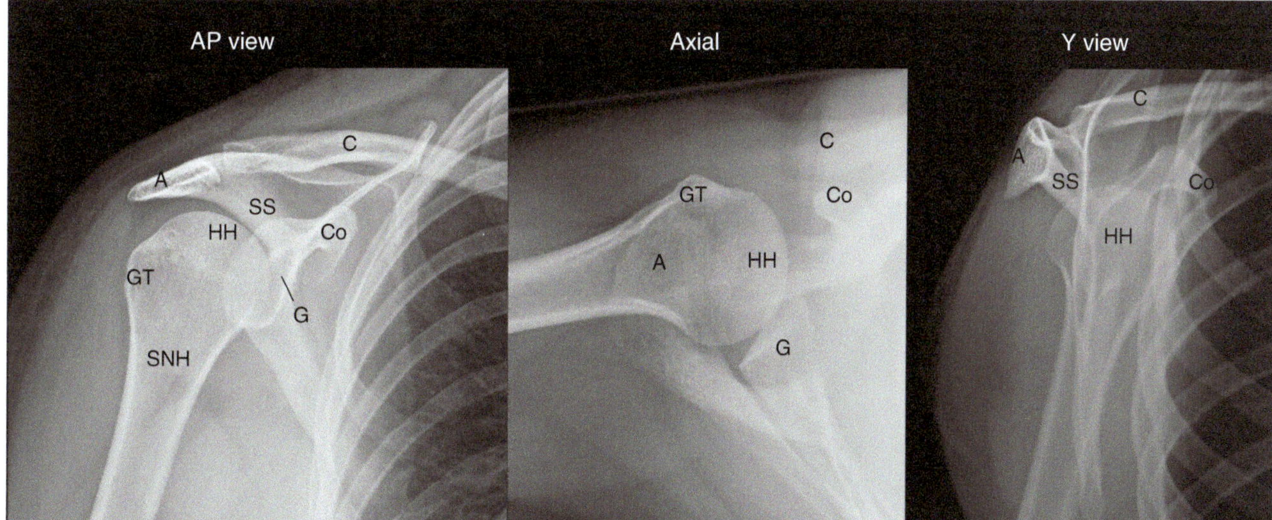

FIGURE 4.4 AP, axial and Y view are the three commonly used views in the shoulder. The main purpose of the axial and Y view is to assess glenohumeral joint alignment. Standard views of the shoulder girdle showing key anatomical landmarks. A, acromion; C, clavicle; Co, coracoid process; G, glenoid; GT, greater tuberosity; HH, humeral head; SNH, surgical neck of humerus; SS, scapular spine.

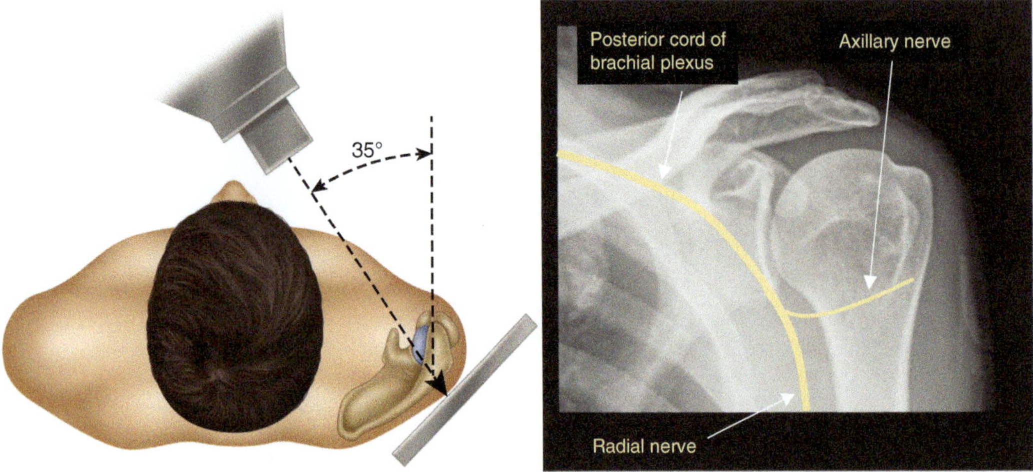

FIGURE 4.5 There is a further projection termed a 'true AP glenohumeral projection' or 'Grashey view'. This brings the glenohumeral joint into a perpendicular plane so the joint space can be assessed. The right image also shows the close relationship between the surgical neck of the humerus and the axillary nerve. As a result, this nerve is at risk following dislocation of the glenohumeral joint. This will compromise the innervation of deltoid muscle and the skin overlying the upper, lateral shoulder.

4.4 Correlation of Gross Anatomy to Imaging

4.4.1 Joint and Bones

4.4.1.1 X-ray The AABCS system introduced in the previous chapter can also be applied to the shoulder (Figure 4.6).

- *Adequacy*: this is primarily concerned with checking the **x-ray projection**. The upper third of the humerus, outer half of the clavicle and lateral aspects of the ribs should be visible.

- *Alignment*: check the humeral head is lying in (i.e. overlaps) the glenoid fossa. Then check for acromio-clavicular disruption by tracing the inferior border of the clavicle to the inferior border of the acromion on the AP view.
- *Bones*: carefully inspect **every bone** on **every projection.** A fracture may only be visible on one projection.
- *Cartilage*: although the cartilage is not visible on an X-ray, the joint space should be. Normally the distance from the humeral head to the anterior margin of the glenoid fossa is the same from top to bottom. Asymmetry could be a marker of a dislocation or fracture so recheck each view.

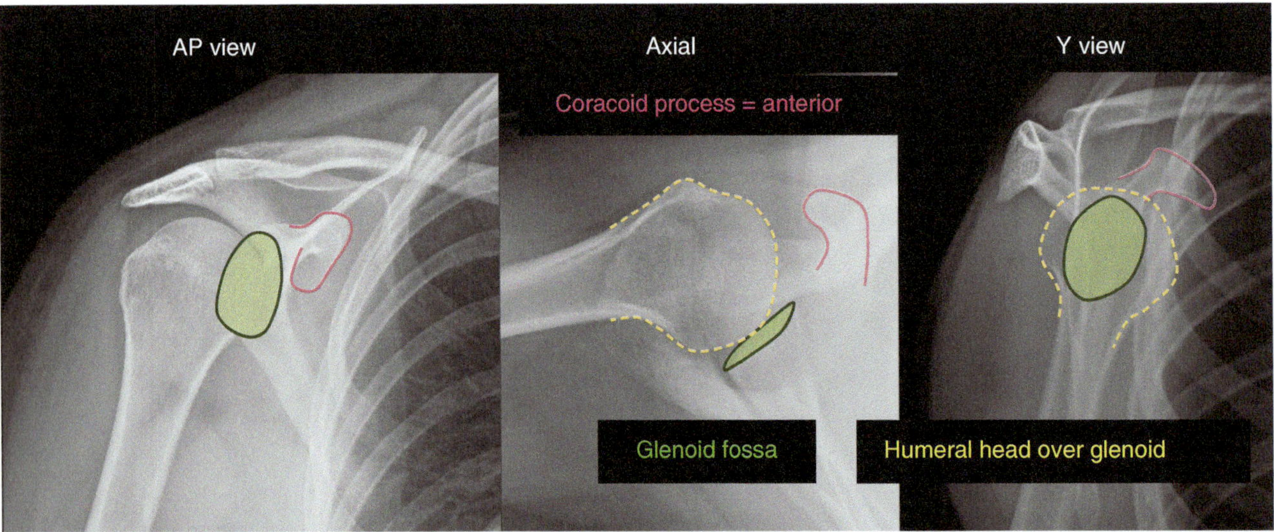

FIGURE 4.6 Annotated. AP, axial and Y view are the three commonly used views of the shoulder. The main purpose of the latter two is to assess glenohumeral joint alignment. Start by locating the coracoid process to identify the anterior aspect of the image. Then check the position of the humeral head. It normally lies over the glenoid fossa (as shown here). If it does not, determine if it has been displaced anteriorly or posteriorly.

- *Soft tissue*: this step includes a review for soft tissue calcification and swelling. The latter could be due to a lipohaemarthrosis (e.g. from a fracture) or effusion (e.g. from infection/inflammation).

4.4.2 **Soft Tissue**

4.4.2.1 Correlating the Soft Tissue Anatomy with the CT Image Take a moment to revise the ligaments and nerves associated with the glenohumeral joint (Figures 4.7 and 4.8) before inspecting the CT image (Figure 4.9).

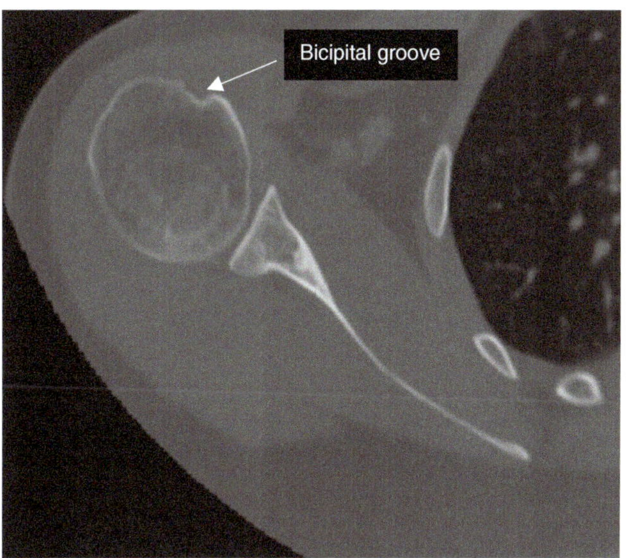

FIGURE 4.9 Axial CT on bone windows. The humeral head should sit on the glenoid, like a golf ball on a tee. Normally the humerus is rounded with no depression except for the bicipital groove anteriorly.

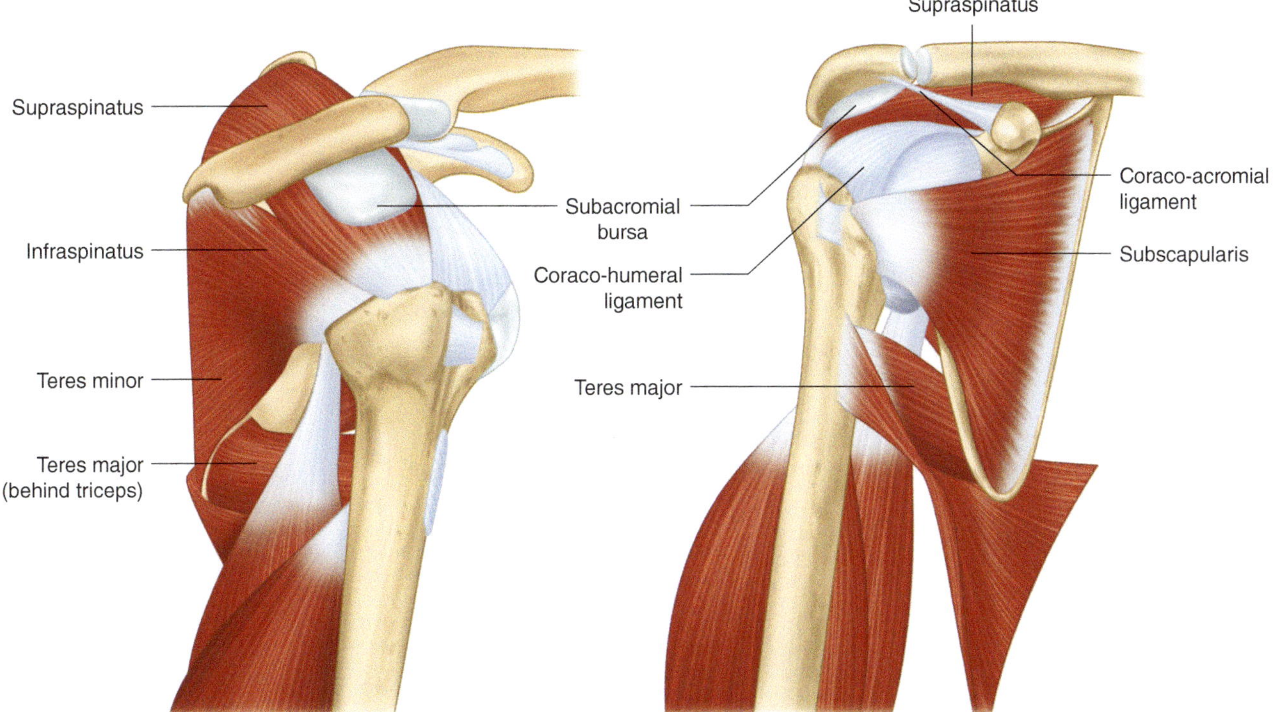

FIGURE 4.7 Anterior view of the right glenohumeral joint showing its relationship to the two heads of biceps, the axillary nerve and the circumflex humeral arteries. The attachment of the joint capsule to the adjacent bone margins is also demonstrated.

FIGURE 4.8 The right glenohumeral joint, subacromial bursa; supraspinatus and infraspinatus; fibrous capsule and ligaments (coracohumeral and coracoacromial). Left image – posterior view (supraspinatus, infraspinatus and teres minor). Right image – anterior view (supraspinatus, subscapularis and teres major).

4.5 Anatomical and Radiological Changes Following a Dislocation

4.5.1 Review of the Clinical Case

4.5.1.1 What is Your Differential Diagnosis? Why?

- Glenohumeral joint dislocation is the most likely diagnosis. Anterior dislocation is most common.
- Acromioclavicular joint dislocation – this is another consideration, but the elevated clavicle would usually be clinically apparent. A plain X-ray of the joint can easily distinguish between the two.
- Fracture of the proximal humerus. This may also result in deformity and can co-exist with a dislocation.
- Fracture of the clavicle. This can result in a deformity if significantly displaced.
- Rotator cuff tear. It is unusual to see a clinical deformity with this condition, unless the patient is thin, it is chronic and there is wasting of supraspinatus.

4.5.1.2 When is Imaging Indicated?

Plain radiographs when a dislocation or fracture is suspected. These should be performed both before and after an attempted reduction.

CT is used to demonstrate fracture patterns and assess glenohumeral anatomy in cases of recurrent dislocations. They are therefore required to aid in surgical planning.

Ultrasound and MRI can be used to assess suspected pathology in the rotator cuff and subacromial bursa. In addition, MRI will show bone marrow oedema (e.g. following arthritis or fracture).

All these modalities are ineffective at visualising the labrum and joint capsule which are important for stabilisation of the glenohumeral joint. If injury to these structures is suspected then a specialist will arrange an MRI arthrogram, where contrast is injected into the glenohumeral joint prior to MRI. This allows visualisation of labral tears and capsular ruptures.

4.5.1.3 What Abnormalities are Identified on X-ray?

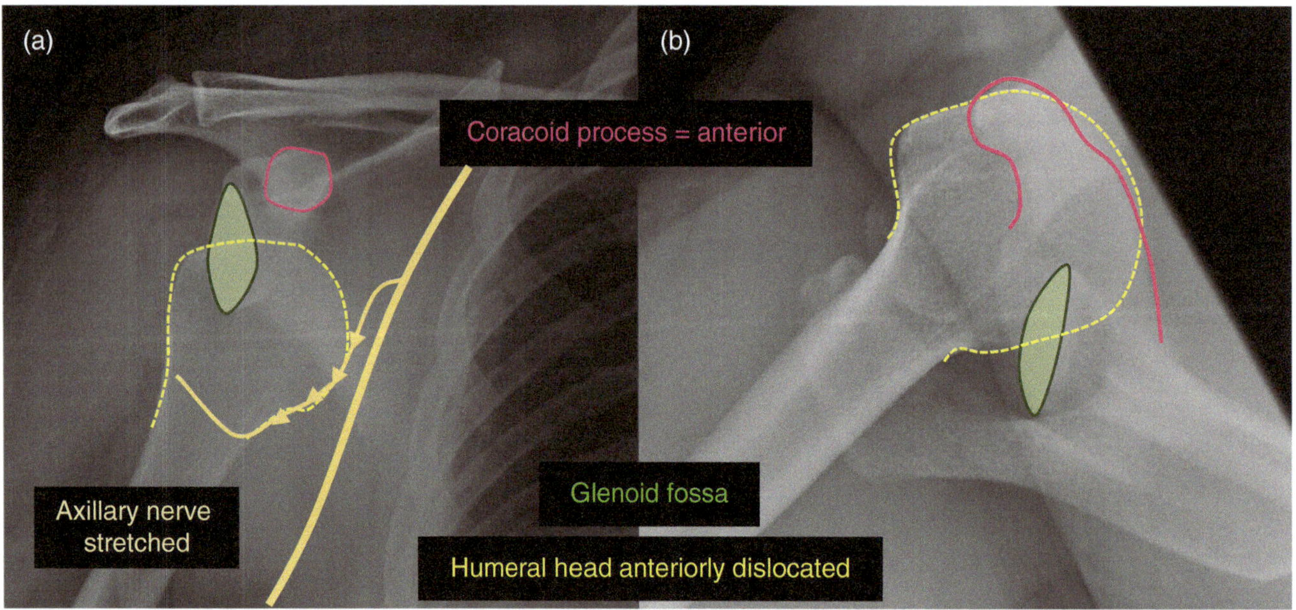

FIGURE 4.10 Patient B. Right shoulder X-ray AP (a) and axial (b) projections. Use the coracoid to orient the X-ray (pink). The humeral head (yellow) is dislocated anterior to the glenoid fossa (green) and is now lying in a subcoracoid position. The path of the axillary nerve is shown. Compare this to Figure 4.5 and note how this dislocation stretches the nerve.

4.5.1.4 What Abnormalities are Identified on CT?

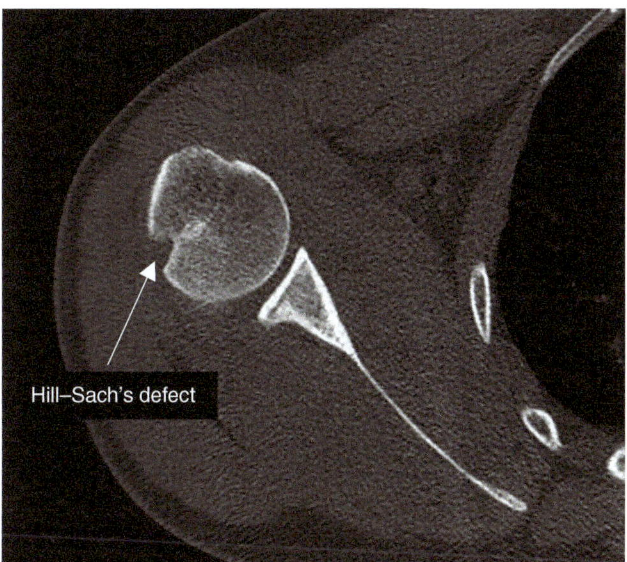

FIGURE 4.11 An axial CT on bone windows taken after the dislocation was reduced. There is a bony depression on the posterolateral humerus caused by the impact with the glenoid rim (Hill–Sachs defect). This can predispose to instability and repeated dislocations as the defect locks with the glenoid rim.

4.5.2 **What is Your Final Diagnosis?**

Anterior glenohumeral dislocation with associated Hill–Sachs defect and axillary nerve injury.

Tip: when reviewing dislocation, look for clues of soft tissue damage. This includes:

- markers of significant energy transfer (wide displacement); multiple fractures
- fractures of bony attachment of the joint ligaments
- bone deformity (e.g. Hill–Sachs, Figure 4.11).

In addition to the soft tissues involved in joint stability, there are also soft tissue structures, such as nerves and vessels, which run close to the joint which can be stretched and damaged following a dislocation. An example is the axillary nerve which runs around the surgical neck of the humerus (Figures 4.5 and 4.10). Evidence for its damage comes from checking the power of deltoid and the sensation of the overlying skin (badge area). This *must* be carried out during the initial assessment, and certainly before any attempted reduction.

A significant proportion of adults with shoulder dislocation have associated rotator cuff tears. The risk of this occurring increases with age and has implications for management. MRI or ultrasound can be used to assess for this complication (Figure 4.12). When there is rotator cuff

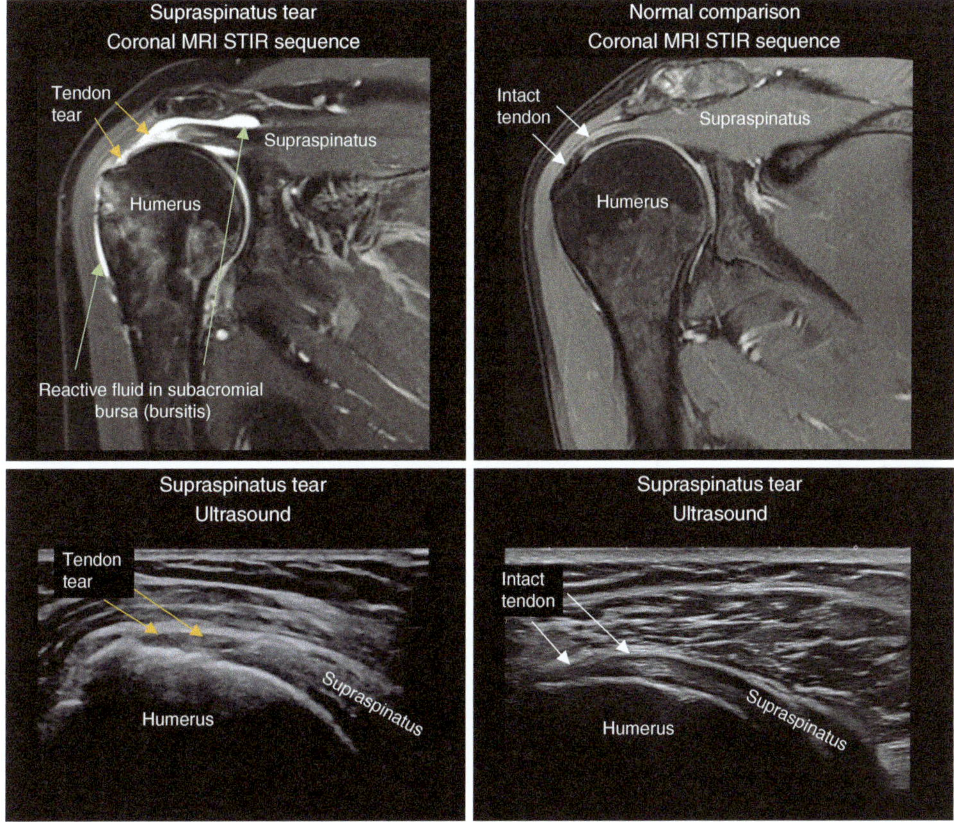

FIGURE 4.12 Coronal MRI STIR (upper) and ultrasound images (lower) showing an acute supraspinatus tendon tear (left) and normal comparison (right). Both MRI and ultrasound can be used to assess the rotator cuff. In a tear there is loss of continuity between the tendon and the greater tuberosity of humerus. This is commonly associated with reactive fluid in the subacromial bursa (bursitis). When these tears become chronic, the muscle belly will lose volume and be replaced by fat (atrophy).

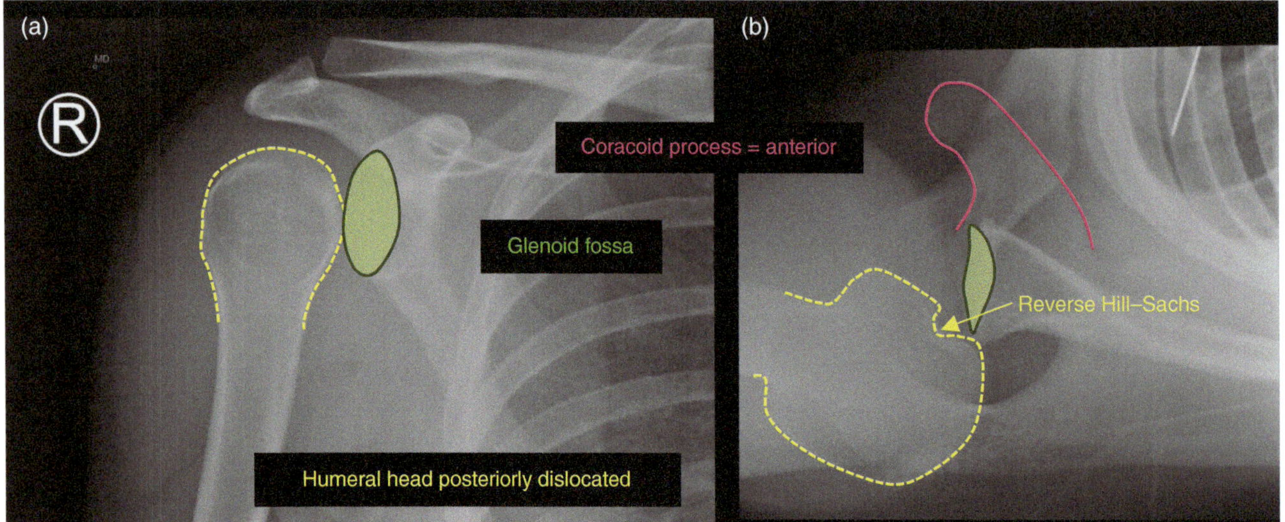

FIGURE 4.13 Right shoulder X-ray AP (a) and axial (b) projections. This shows a posterior shoulder dislocation. The humeral head internally rotates, resulting in a 'lightbulb'-shaped appearance on the AP projection. The axial projection shows the humeral head displaced posterior to the glenoid rim. There is a reverse Hill–Sachs defect on the anterior humeral head. This can be seen locking with the posterior rim of the glenoid.

pathology, it is common to have co-existing reactive subacromial bursitis (Figure 4.12).

Posterior dislocations of the glenohumeral joint are much less common than their anterior counterpart. Their relative rarity and subtle radiological signs (Figure 4.13) therefore mean they are more commonly missed. An important clue is the mechanism of injury – always suspect a posterior dislocation if the patient is complaining of a painful shoulder, with a reduced range of movement, following a general epileptic seizure, electrocution or the proximal humerus being subjected to a significant anterior force.

4.6 Take-home Message – Trauma

- Plain radiology is the first-line imaging in suspected bony trauma or dislocation.
- CT is often required for surgical planning. This is performed without contrast.
- MRI can be used to assess for soft tissue injury (tendons and ligaments). It is also more sensitive for microtrabecular fractures which may not be visible on X-ray.

CHAPTER 5

Painful Ankle

Joshua Lauder[1], Eoghan Donnelly[2], and Peter Driscoll[3]

[1]East Lancashire Hospitals NHS Trust, University of Central Lancashire and University of Manchester, UK
[2]NHS Greater Glasgow and Clyde, Glasgow, UK
[3]School of Medicine and Dentistry, University of Central Lancashire, Preston, UK

5.1 Primary Case

5.1.1 Presentation

A 36-year-old male presents to the Emergency Department with left ankle pain. He was playing five-a-side football the previous evening. This was for the first time in many years and he describes hearing a sudden snapping noise followed by instant pain in the heel area. 'It felt like being kicked on the back of the ankle'. He was unable to continue and rested his leg overnight, considering it a simple sprain. However, after two days he is still unable to weight bear so has come to the Emergency Department.

On further questioning, the patient states that he has been bothered by posterior heel pain on and off for the past year and has received several steroid injections from a physiotherapist.

5.1.1.1 History of Presenting Complaint Pain features (SOCRATES)

- S – Site: generalised ankle pain. Worse posteriorly.
- O – Onset: shortly after hearing the snapping noise.
- C – Character: constant, dull ache.
- R – Radiation: does not radiate.
- A – Associations: unable to weight bear and ankle feels weak.
- T – Time course: since the incident.
- E – Exacerbating/relieving factors: relieved by not moving the foot, elevation and NSAIDs. Worse if he dorsiflexes or plantarflexes the foot.
- S – Severity: 7/10.

PMH: asthma.
SH: nil.
DH: inhalers – no allergies.

5.1.2 Examination

OE: pain, bruising and swelling around left ankle and heel areas. The resting position of the foot with the knees bent is in more dorsiflexion when compared with the contralateral side.

Plantarflexion of the foot is weak. There is no bony tenderness on palpation, but you can feel a gap over the Achilles tendon and Simmonds/Thompson test is abnormal (Figure 5.1).

Modified early warning signs (MEWS):

- Respiratory rate 14 bpm.
- SpO_2 98% on room air.
- Temp 36.5 °C.
- HR 86 bpm.
- BP 122/65 mmHg.
- Alert.

Diagnostic Imaging and Anatomy in Acute Care, First Edition. Edited by Joshua Lauder and Peter Driscoll.
© 2025 John Wiley & Sons Ltd. Published 2025 by John Wiley & Sons Ltd.
Companion website: www.wiley.com/go/DiagnosticImaginginAcuteCare

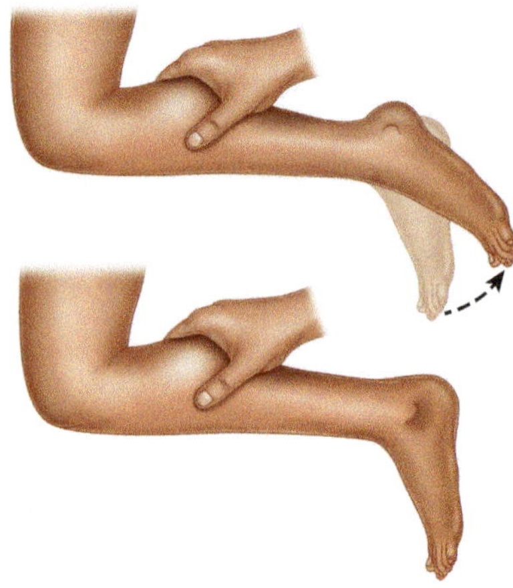

FIGURE 5.1 Simmonds test. The calf is squeezed while the foot is dangling off the bed or chair. In a normal patient, this action will induce plantarflexion. An abnormal result occurs if the foot remains motionless.

5.1.3 Investigations

5.1.3.1 X-ray An urgent X-ray was performed to exclude bony injury (Figure 5.2).

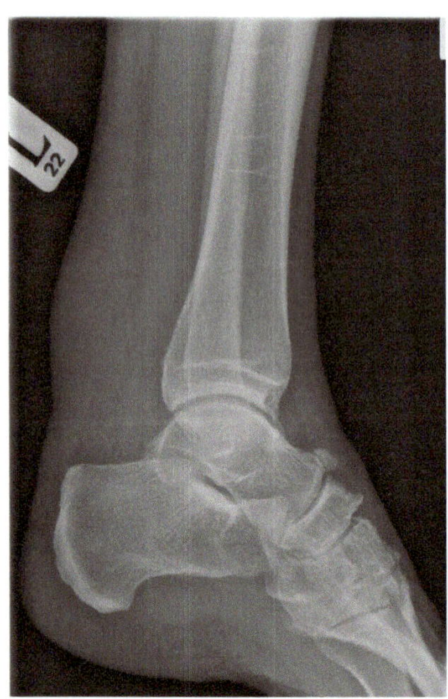

FIGURE 5.2 Patient A. Lateral ankle X-ray.

5.1.3.2 Ultrasound Subsequently, an ultrasound was performed (Figure 5.3).

> **Clinical Case Questions**
> - What is your differential diagnosis? Why?
> - What abnormalities do you note on the plain X-ray?
> - When might an MRI be of use?
> - What is your final diagnosis?

5.2 Radiology Self-assessment

5.2.1 Technical

5.2.1.1 X-ray
- What secondary signs of tendon injury can be seen on the plain X-ray?

5.2.1.2 Ultrasound
- What do tendons look like on ultrasound?

5.2.2 Correlating Gross Anatomy to Imaging

5.2.2.1 Joint and Bones
- Which bones make up the hind foot?

5.2.2.2 Tendons
- What is the anatomy of the Achilles tendon?

5.3 Key Radiology Review

5.3.1 X-ray Ankle

5.3.1.1 Correlating Gross Anatomy to Imaging (Figure 5.4)

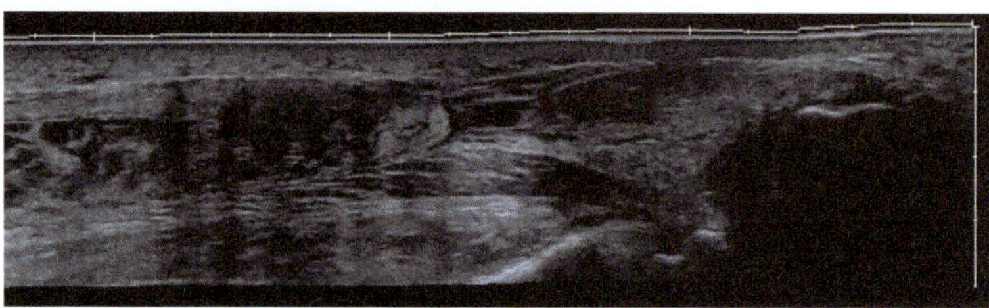

FIGURE 5.3 Patient A. Ultrasound of left Achilles tendon.

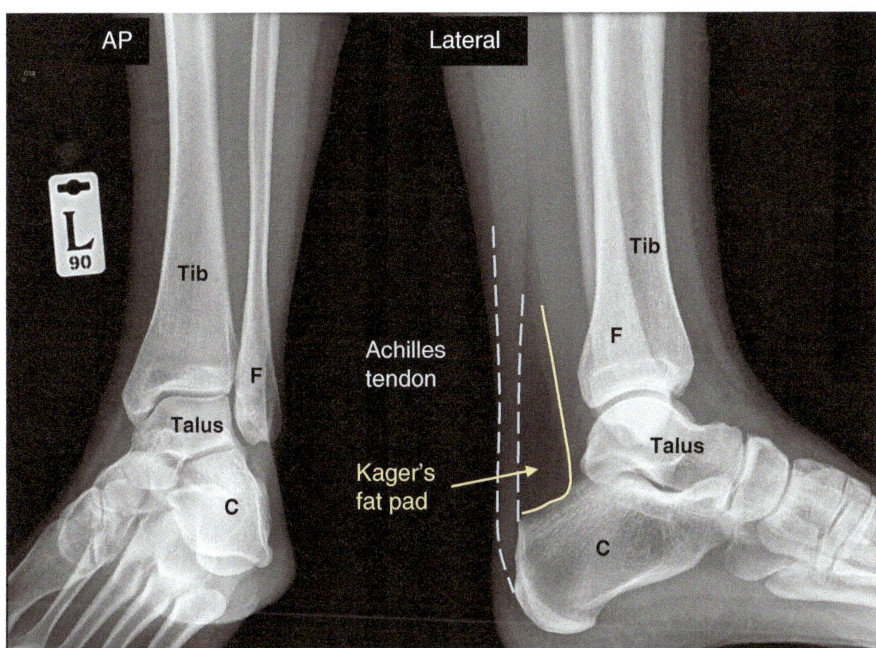

FIGURE 5.4 Normal ankle X-ray, AP and lateral. Tib, tibia; F, fibula; C, calcaneus. Even on a plain X-ray, the Achilles tendon can be seen as a relatively dense structure inserting into the calcaneus. Anterior to the tendon is Kager's fat pad and there should be a well-defined line between the two.

5.3.2 **Ultrasound** (Figures 5.5 and 5.6)

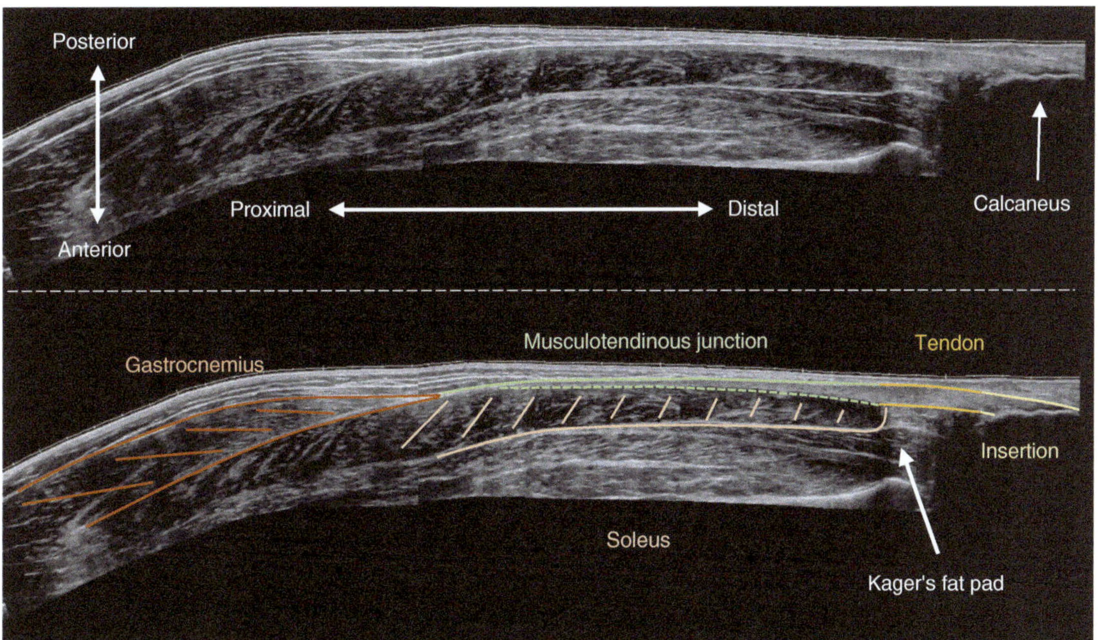

FIGURE 5.5 Normal long axis ultrasound of the Achilles tendon. Conventionally, on a long axis image, the left side is proximal and the right is distal. The tendon's insertion into the calcaneus can be seen on the right side of the image. Proximal to the insertion is the midsubstance part of the tendon. It is about 5 cm in length and has a relatively poor blood supply. Consequently, this area is the most susceptible to tears. More proximal still are the musculotendinous junctions of soleus and gastrocnemius.

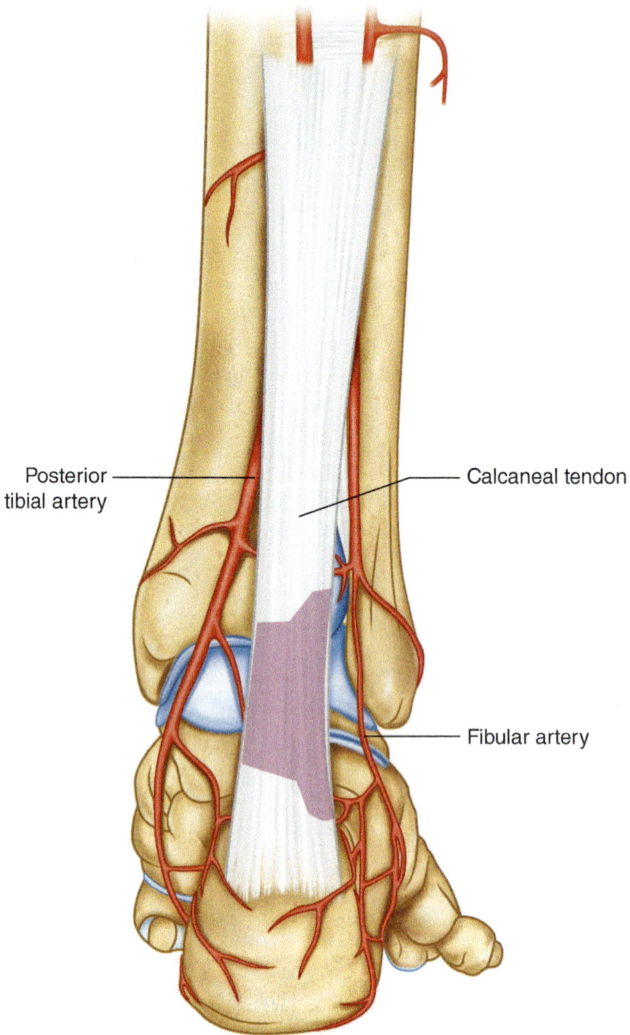

FIGURE 5.6 Posterior view of the right ankle showing the Achilles tendon and its area of relatively poor vascularity. The Achilles tendon is supplied by two arteries resulting in three vascular territories. The midsection (purple area) has the poorest blood supply. Consequently, this is where there is the highest risk of rupture and surgical complications because microtrauma here is very slow to repair.

5.4 Review of the Clinical Case

5.4.1 What is Your Differential Diagnosis? Why?

- Achilles tendon rupture – either at its insertional or midsubstance parts (see below).
- Tear or rupture of head or belly of gastrocnemius. This will usually present with more proximal pain in the calf and will not have palpable tendon gap.
- Tibialis posterior or fibularis tendon rupture. This will often present with pain behind the corresponding malleolus. Furthermore, plantarflexion at the ankle will be relatively well preserved.
- Fracture of medial/lateral/posterior malleolus. This is usually associated with localised tenderness on bony palpation.

Note – bruising around the ankle is non-specific and can be seen in all of the above conditions.

5.4.2 When is Imaging Indicated?

The classic history for Achilles tendon rupture is a sudden onset of pain accompanied by an audible snap behind the ankle during exercise. Typically, there is an immediate inability to weight bear. Certain risk factors significantly increase the risk of this condition, including taking fluoroquinolones and intratendinous steroid injection.

Clinically. three signs are used to establish the diagnosis of Achilles tendon rupture.

1. The resting foot position is no longer in slight plantarflexion. This is best seen with the foot dangling while kneeling on the edge of a chair.
2. A palpable gap in the tendon.

3. An abnormal Simmonds test (i.e. no plantarflexion on squeezing the calf).

If all three are present, with a convincing history, then imaging is not required. If there is any doubt over the diagnosis, then imaging can be used to confirm the diagnosis or look for an alternative diagnosis.

5.4.3 What Abnormalities are Identified on X-ray (Figure 5.7)?

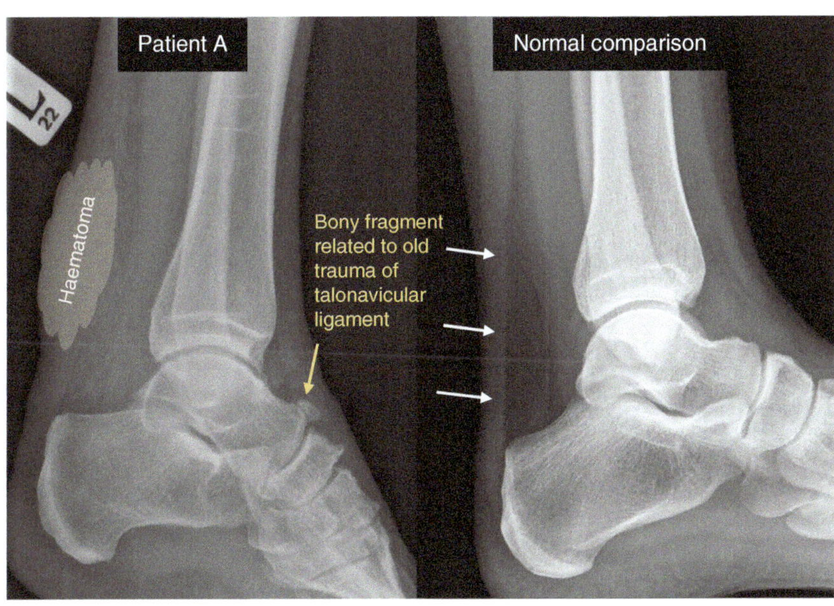

FIGURE 5.7 Lateral ankle X-ray for patient A and a normal comparison. There is loss of the clear demarcation between the Kager's fat pad and the tendon (demonstrated by the white arrows on the normal image). There is also soft tissue swelling in the region of the Achilles tendon (brown area). In combination with the above history, this is suspicious of an Achilles rupture because the tear fills with haematoma which extends into the surrounding fat.

5.4.3.1 What Abnormalities are Identified on Ultrasound (Figures 5.8 and 5.9)?

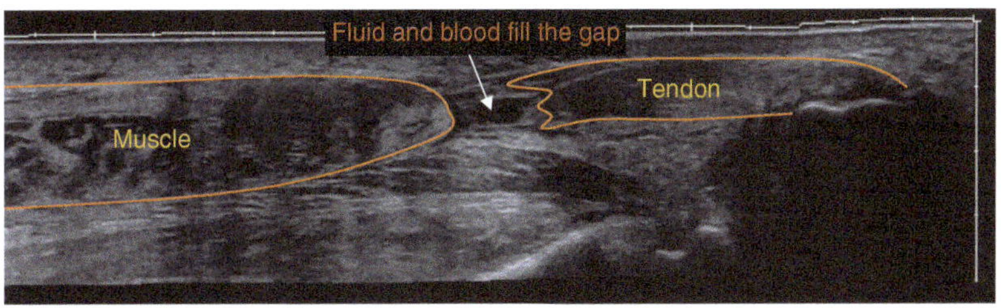

FIGURE 5.8 There is a tear in the Achilles tendon 4.5 cm from the insertion. The proximal muscle is retracted, with fluid and blood filling the gap.

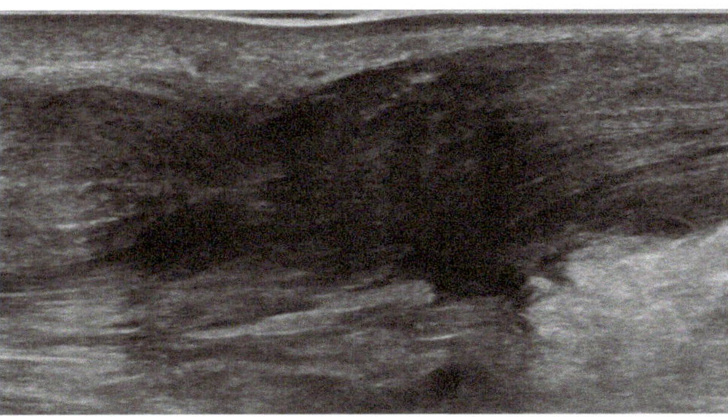

FIGURE 5.9 Close-up view of rupture area in Figure 5.8. One ultrasound feature of a torn tendon is that the edges become hypoechoic. This is due to anisotropy, as the fibres leave the horizontal orientation in relation to the ultrasound probe.

5.4.3.2 What is Your Final Diagnosis? Achilles tendon rupture with a tendon gap. Treatment options include conservative management in an equinus boot or surgical tendon repair, with the ultimate decision based on lifestyle requirements and co-existing medical problems.

In some cases it has been suggested that ultrasound may be useful in aiding decisions around operative management. This is achieved by measuring the size of the gap between the tendon ends with the foot in full plantarflexion, with larger gaps possibly being less amenable to conservative management.

5.5 Take-home Message – Tendon Rupture

- X-ray will usually be performed initially to exclude a bony injury or dislocation.
- Ultrasound or MRI can be used to assess for tendon injury. This should be performed on an urgent outpatient basis, so the choice of modality often depends on availability.

Further Resources

Pass, B., Robinson, P., Ha, A. et al. (2022). The Achilles tendon: imaging diagnoses and image-guided interventions – *AJR* expert panel narrative review. *Am J Roentgenol* 219 (3): 355–368.

Pelvis Section

CHAPTER 6

Urinary Retention

Joshua Lauder[1], Onyibo Okafor[2], and Peter Driscoll[3]

[1] *East Lancashire Hospitals NHS Trust, University of Central Lancashire and University of Manchester, UK*
[2] *Skin & Bones Medical Limited, Blackburn, UK*
[3] *School of Medicine and Dentistry, University of Central Lancashire, Preston, UK*

6.1 Primary Case

6.1.1 Presentation

A 74-year-old male presents to the Emergency Department with an acute onset of severe lower abdominal pain and associated confusion.

6.1.1.1 History of Presenting Complaint His wife reports that he has a history of nocturia and is known to spend a long time at the toilet due to a sluggish stream and dribbling after passing urine.

He is eating and drinking as normal but his wife says he has been constipated over the past week.

Today he has had increased confusion and progressively worsening lower abdominal pain. His wife reports that he has been going to the toilet more frequently due to a sensation of needing to urinate but not passing any urine. He was sweaty but when she checked his temperature, it was normal. She felt that due to his severe discomfort they had no alternative but to attend the ED.

PMH: Parkinson disease, overactive bladder. He also has mild memory loss and is being investigated for dementia.

SH: Lives with wife who is his carer. Ex-smoker; drinks approx. 10 units/week.

DH: co-careldopa; solifenacin; amlodipine.

6.1.2 Examination

Patient is lying on a trolley and appears distressed.
OE:

- Chest – clear
- Normal heart sounds.
- Tender palpable mass in the lower abdomen.
  - This is dull on percussion and extends to just below the umbilicus.
- Digital rectal examination identified a smooth enlargement of the prostate with a palpable normal sulcus.
- Glasgow Coma Scale: Eye opening 4; Verbal response 4; Motor response 6.

Modified early warning signs (MEWS):

- Respiratory rate 16 rpm.
- SaO_2 95% on room air.
- Tympanic temp 37.0 °C.
- HR 110 bpm.
- BP 162/92 mmHg.
- Alert.

6.1.3 Bloods

PSA three months ago was 5 ng/ml (normal range 1–1.5 ng/ml).

6.1.4 Bladder Scan

An urgent bladder scan was performed in the ED (Figure 6.1).

> ### Clinical Case Questions
> - What is your differential diagnosis?
> - Why is ultrasound indicated?
> - What is your final diagnosis and immediate management?

6.2 Radiology Self-assessment

6.2.1 Technical

- What basic US physics knowledge do I need for this case?
- How does a bladder scanner work?
- How can a bladder volume be measured on ultrasound?

6.2.2 Correlating Gross Anatomy with the US Image

- What is the anatomical relationship between the bladder, prostate and urethra?
- How do I orientate myself when carrying out a bladder volume assessment?

6.3 Key Radiology Review

6.3.1 Technical Aspects

6.3.1.1 Ultrasound Physics Ultrasound scanners rely on very high-frequency vibrations (waves) to obtain an image. The 'ultra' refers to this frequency being beyond the normal hearing range of 20–20 000 Hz (where a hertz is the number of vibrations per second). As medical devices generate vibrations in the order of millions of times per second, they are inaudible to humans.

It is the surface of the ultrasound probe which vibrates at this frequency. When it is applied to the skin with a lubricating gel, these waves travel through the body and reflect off tissues, returning to the probe (Figure 6.2). These returning vibrations are detected and processed to form an image which is a two-dimensional fan shape. This analysis takes into account how strong the return signal is and how far it has travelled (Figure 6.3).

6.3.2 Bladder Scanner

This type of scanner uses ultrasound technology for the sole purpose of finding the volume of urine in the bladder. Instead of a conventional ultrasound image, the screen shows arrows to direct the user in the direction of the bladder. When the bladder is central to the probe, the volume is automatically calculated and displayed on the screen. This is an excellent tool to have when assessing for urinary retention, but it is

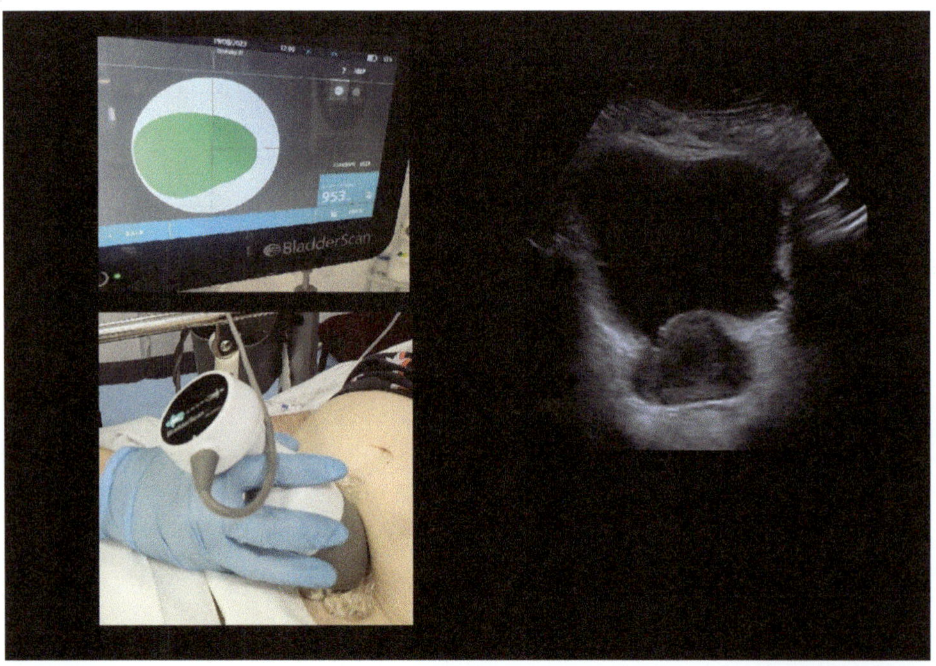

FIGURE 6.1 Bladder scan image (left) and a conventional ultrasound (US) which was also subsequently performed (right).

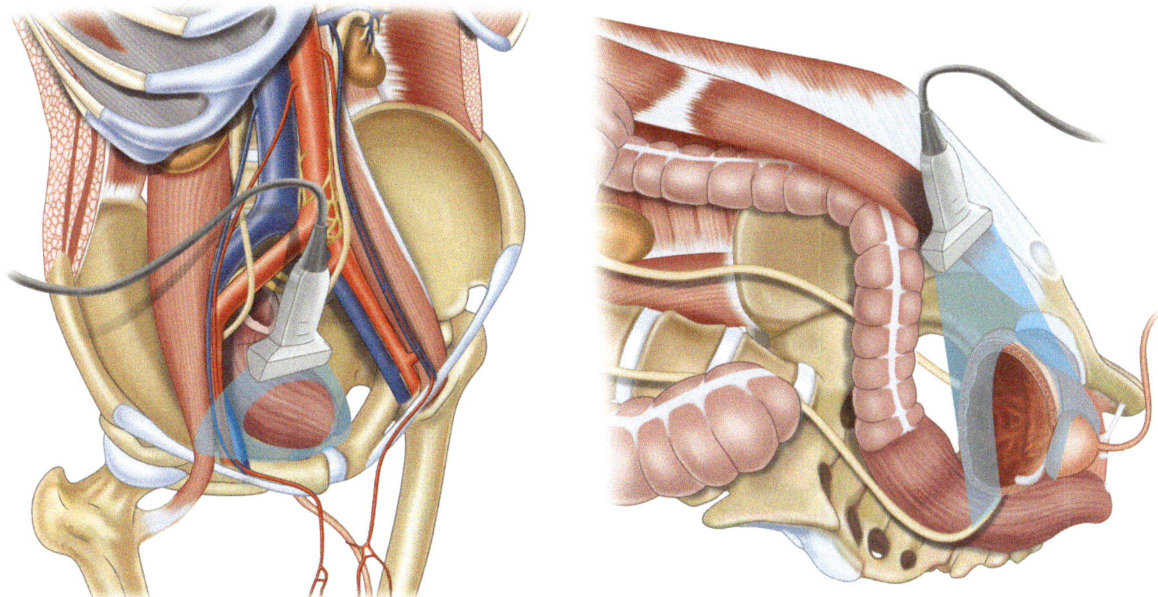

FIGURE 6.2 Diagram showing the transverse transabdominal view of the bladder, looking down into the pelvis from the patient's right side (abdominal anterior wall removed). Transverse view of the pelvis in a prone patient, showing the relationships of the bladder, prostate and rectum. The probe needs to be angled inferiorly to look into the pelvis and image the bladder.

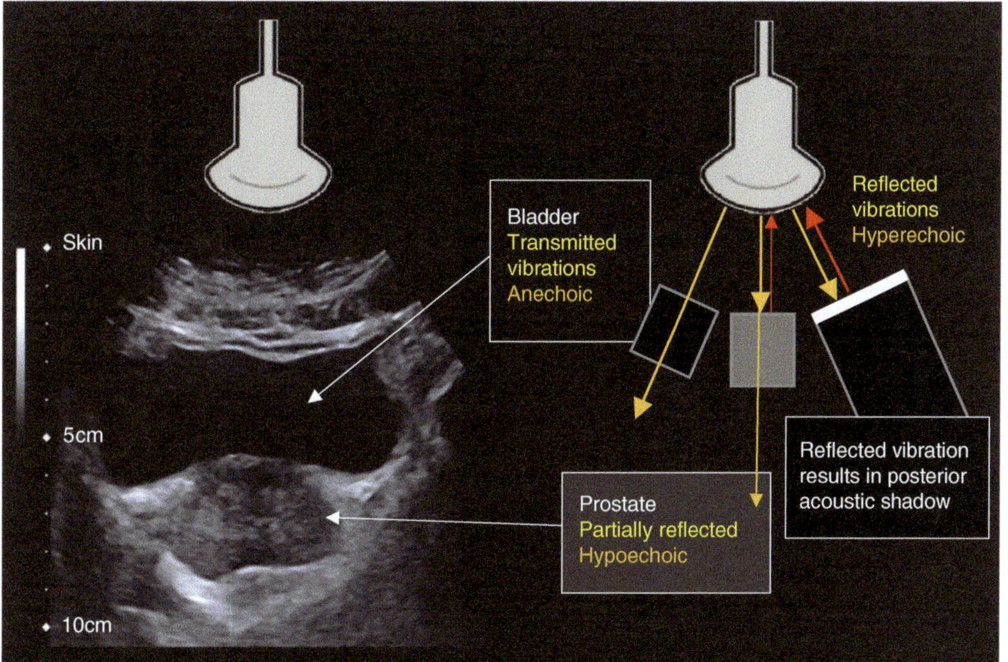

FIGURE 6.3 Transverse ultrasound of a normal bladder and prostate. By convention, the ultrasound image is displayed as if the probe was at the top of the screen. Hence this is where the skin is, with deeper structures being lower down on the image. There is a depth scale on the side of the image for reference. The echotexture of a tissue describes its brightness and is related to how well the sound waves bounce off its surface. This is given specific terminology as follows. *Anechoic*: no sound is reflected back because structures allow easy passage of the vibrations. As no sound wave is returning, the structure appears black on the image. This suggests the structure has a fluid composition, for example the urine in the bladder. *Hypoechoic*: solid structures which allow some vibrations to pass through will appear dark but not completely black. Many organs appear like this, for example the prostate. *Hyperechoic*: structures which completely block the vibration transmission appear white because more of the sound waves are returning to the probe. Examples include gas and bone (not shown on this image). As the vibrations are completely reflected, the deeper tissues will appear black. This is termed a posterior acoustic shadow and an example is shown in other chapters (see Figure 7.3 and Figure 19.9a).

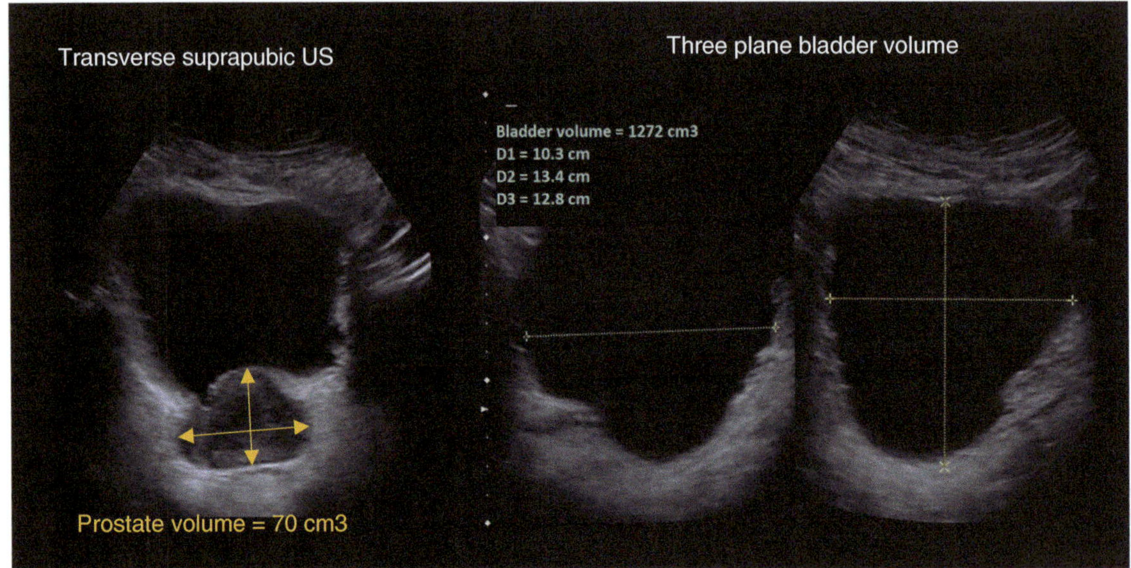

FIGURE 6.4 Patient A. Transabdominal bladder ultrasound. Three dimensions are measured. Two are in the transverse plane (anterior–posterior and side to side). The final one is measured in the sagittal plane (bladder height). In this case the bladder volume is 1272 cm³. This equates to 1.272 l of urine. Most people will feel a strong urge to urine at 0.6 l.

susceptible to false positives. For example, if there is a large adnexal cyst, this can be mistaken for the urinary bladder.

With a bit more skill, the volume of the bladder can also be calculated using a standard ultrasound machine (Figure 6.4).

6.4 Correlating the Anatomy with the US Image

6.4.1 Review of the Clinical Case

- What is your differential diagnosis?
- Why is US indicated?
- What is your final diagnosis and immediate management?

6.4.2 Differential Diagnosis

Lower abdominal pain can have a variety of causes. Urinary retention should always be excluded, especially in patients who are poor historians, as the history of reduced urine output may not be forthcoming. This becomes even more likely when there is a supra-added urinary infection leading to confusion.

It is also important to rule out a ruptured abdominal aortic aneurysm as this can commonly present with abdominal pain instead of back pain (Chapter 22).

Other important differentials to consider include:

- prostate pathology (benign prostatic hyperplasia [BPH] vs cancer)
- urinary tract infection
- diverticulitis
- cauda equina syndrome (Spine Chapter 26).

Once a bladder scan has confirmed urinary retention, a catheter should be inserted for symptomatic relief. BPH is by far the most common cause of bladder outflow obstruction in this age group. Other causes include urethral calculus, bladder cancers and some pelvic malignancies including cervical cancer and cauda equina syndrome.

6.4.3 Ultrasound

A bladder scan may be performed to confirm urinary retention. If this is not available, then catheterisation should not be delayed while waiting for a definitive US investigation (Figure 6.4).

When ultrasound is used, it can also assess the cause of urinary retention (Figure 6.4). In men, most of these will be the result of BPH. This gland's size can be calculated on ultrasound in the same way as the bladder volume. BPH can be diagnosed when it is bigger than 40 cm³ and there are associated urinary symptoms.

In patients presenting with the more chronic markers of bladder outflow obstruction (i.e. frequency, nocturia, incontinence), the postvoid bladder volume can help to predict overflow. Normal patients should have less than 50 ml residual urine in the bladder after voiding.

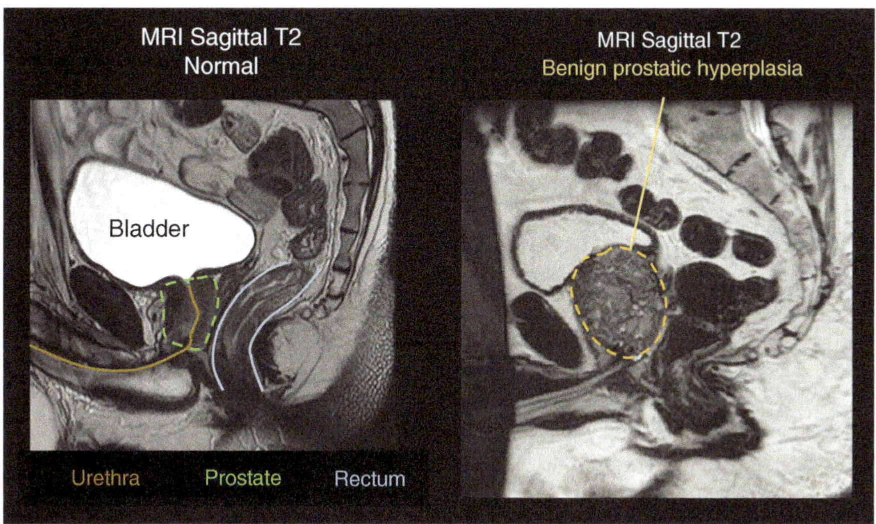

FIGURE 6.5 MRI sagittal T2 sequences showing normal anatomy (left) compared to BPH (right). In the latter, the prostate is compressing the urethra, limiting bladder emptying. Also note the close relationship between the prostate and rectum. Hence size and position of the gland can be detected by digital rectal examination. The posterior surface can also be palpated through the rectal wall, but not the anterior aspects.

6.5 Final Diagnosis

Acute urinary retention caused by BPH with supra-added infection.

6.6 Other Imaging

Suspected prostate cancer is investigated with MRI. BPH is very often encountered on these scans (Figure 6.5). Urinary tract calculi and other pelvic malignancies are usually investigated with CT.

6.7 Take-home Message – Imaging in Urinary Retention

- Ultrasound can be used to assess the size of the bladder but if acute urinary retention is suspected, catheterisation should not be delayed while waiting for a scan.
- Bladder scanners are useful as they can be immediately available at the point of care and require very little training to use.
- In more chronic urinary retention, a postvoid bladder volume can help diagnose overflow.

Further Resources

Alagiakrishnan, K. and Valpreda, M. (2009). Ultrasound bladder scanner presents falsely elevated postvoid residual volumes. *Can Fam Physician* 55 (2): 163–164.

Barrisford, G.W. and Steele., G. (2010). Urinary retention. In: *Decision Making in Medicine*, 3e (ed. S. Mushlin and H. Greene), 570–575. Philadelphia: Mosby Elsevier.

Lepor, H. (2004). Evaluating men with benign prostatic hyperplasia. *Rev Urol* 6 (Suppl. 1): S8–S15.

CHAPTER 7

Heavy Painful Periods

Joshua Lauder[1], Onyibo Okafor[2], and Peter Driscoll[3]

[1] East Lancashire Hospitals NHS Trust, University of Central Lancashire and University of Manchester, UK
[2] Skin & Bones Medical Limited, Blackburn, UK
[3] School of Medicine and Dentistry, University of Central Lancashire, Preston, UK

7.1 Primary Case

7.1.1 Presentation

A 45-year-old woman presents to a primary healthcare clinic with heavy painful periods.

7.1.1.1 History of Presenting Complaint This has been going for several months and is associated with deep dyspareunia and mild constipation. She has also found that she is having to pass urine more frequently. There has been no incontinence, but her partner has mentioned that she is always going to the toilet to pee.

Previously her periods were regular with bleeding for 4–5 days every four weeks. Now they are lasting for 7–9 days every three weeks and she has some occasional spotting in between her periods.

There has been no change in diet or medication and no nausea, vomiting or acid reflux. She describes now opening her bowels every other day rather than daily and is having to strain a bit more.

PMH: history of anaemia; nulliparous; smear up to date and normal.

SH: alcohol 20 units/week; non-smoker.

DH: Microgynon®.

7.1.2 Examination

Obs: stable.

Abdomen soft but some tenderness in the suprapubic region. No peritonitic symptoms.

Urine dip negative. Urine pregnancy test negative.

Internal examination was satisfactory with the cervix appearing normal. There are no vaginal masses or cervical excitation.

7.1.3 Bloods

Full blood count – microcytic anaemia.

Urea & electrolytes; liver function tests and C-reactive protein are all normal.

7.1.4 Ultrasound

An ultrasound (US) scan of the pelvis was arranged (Figure 7.1).

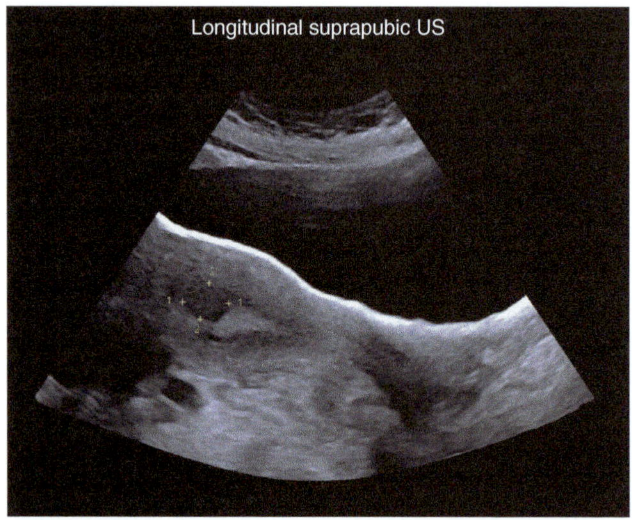

FIGURE 7.1 Patient A. Transabdominal ultrasound pelvis in the sagittal plane.

7.2 Radiology Self-assessment

7.2.1 Technical

- How is pelvic ultrasound performed?

7.2.2 Correlating Gross Anatomy to US

- What is the anatomical relationship between the bladder, vagina, cervix and uterus?

- How do I orientate myself when carrying out pelvic US assessment?

7.3 Key Radiology Review

7.3.1 Technical Aspects

7.3.1.1 Transabdominal vs Transvaginal Ultrasound

Examining the pelvic organs with ultrasound through the abdominal wall is difficult, owing to the anatomically narrow space, surrounding bones and overlying bowel gas. Scanning the patient with a full bladder can help to overcome this, as the bladder acts as a 'sonographic window'. This term is used to describe viewing an organ of interest through another structure. As the sound waves are readily transmitted through the bladder, it makes an ideal medium for a sonographic window. In some patients this could be enough to enable an adequate assessment of the uterus and ovaries to be made using a transabdominal approach (Figure 7.2).

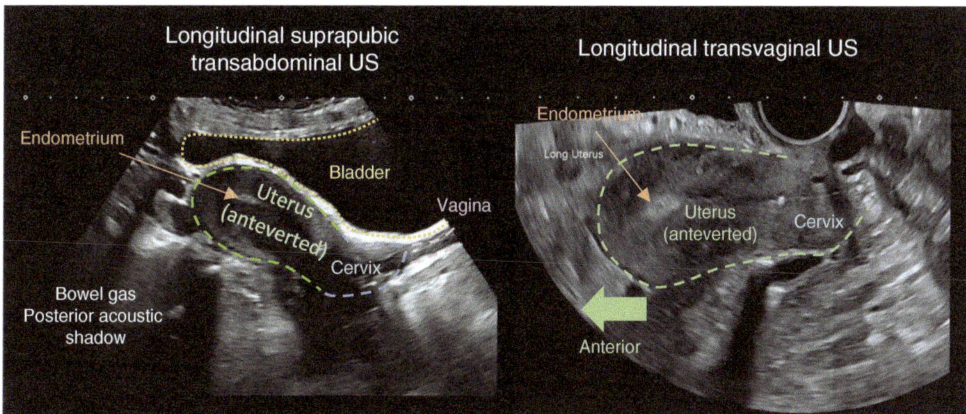

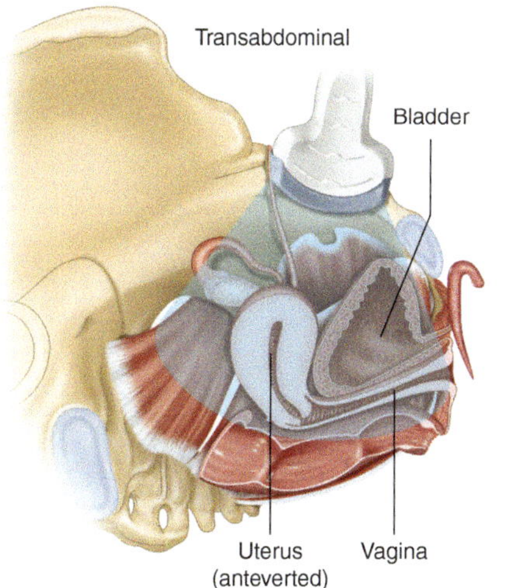

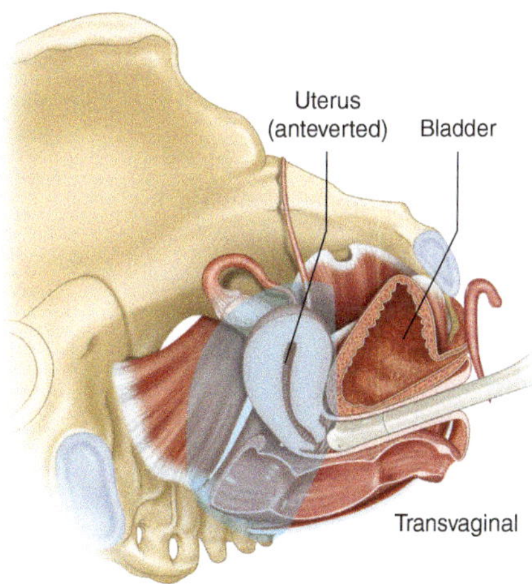

FIGURE 7.2 Anteverted uterine anatomy on transabdominal (left) and transvaginal ultrasound (right). The uterus may be anteverted or retroverted (see Figure 7.3). The myometrium should be homogenous with no focal lesions. The endometrial thickness varies depending on stage of menstrual cycle and menopause status.

Another option is transvaginal scanning. This is a more invasive procedure but overcomes the issues of depth and bowel gas. It is now considered a standard way to assess for uterine and adnexal pathology, if the transabdominal approach fails (Figure 7.2).

As well as assessing for uterine and cervical lesions, the endometrium can be checked. Abnormally thickened endometrium can be a sign of endometrial cancer.

7.3.1.2 Retroverted Uterus (Figure 7.3)

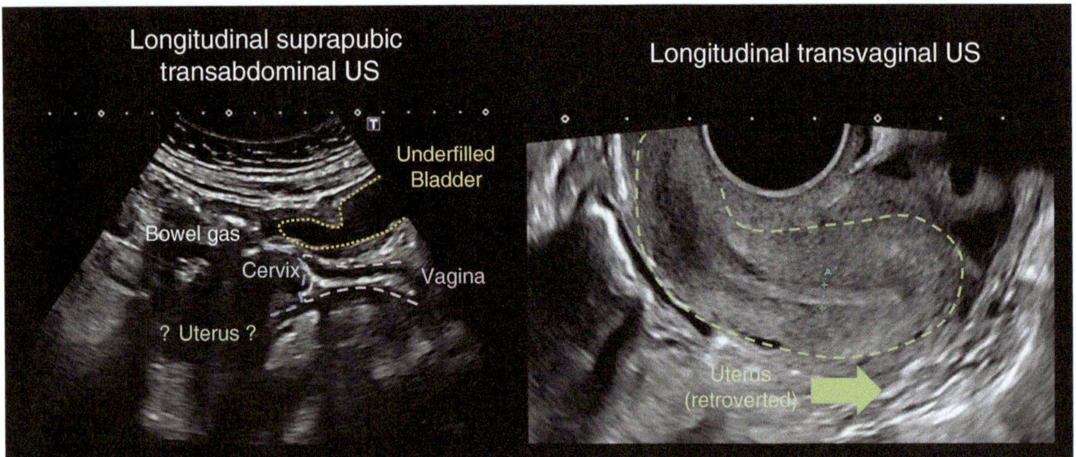

FIGURE 7.3 Retroverted uterine anatomy on transabdominal (left) and transvaginal ultrasound (right). The uterus is very difficult to assess on transabdominal ultrasound scans when it is retroverted or if the bladder is underfilled. In contrast, the transvaginal approach nicely visualises the uterus, regardless of position. The endometrial thickness is 4 mm, which is within normal range.

7.4 Review of the Clinical Case

- What is your differential diagnosis?
- Why is US indicated?
- What is your final diagnosis and immediate management?

7.4.1 Differential Diagnosis

In a woman of child-bearing age, it is important to rule out ectopic pregnancy as a matter of urgency. A positive pregnancy test associated with abdominal pain and vaginal bleeding will necessitate gynaecologist input. In these cases a transvaginal ultrasound is usually carried out in the first instance to improve the localisation of the ectopic.

Pelvic inflammatory disease is another important differential and should be considered if there are any infectious signs. Internal examination is important here to rule out cervical excitation.

Ovarian pathology including torsion, cyst haemorrhage and cyst rupture are important differentials, but would tend to have a more acute history.

In this woman, the most likely cause of her symptoms would be fibroids. However, as mentioned above there are important differentials that need to be considered and ruled out with careful assessment and use of appropriate imaging.

7.4.2 Ultrasound

Ultrasound is the first-line test for suspected uterine abnormality. It readily visualises the uterus and endometrial cavity. It is also possible to spot large cervical masses on ultrasound, although direct inspection is preferable.

7.4.3 MRI

Pelvic MRI is used for characterising unusual lesions and staging known malignancy. There is a limited role for pelvic MRI in the urgent care setting, but images are shown here to help demonstrate the pathology (Figure 7.4).

7.5 Final Diagnosis

Bleeding submucosal uterine fibroid.

7.5.1 Uterine Fibroids

These are classified according to their location (Figure 7.5). Submucosal fibroids tend to present with vaginal bleeding (see Figure 7.4), whereas intramural and subserosal fibroids present with pain and bloating. Both subserosal and submucosal fibroids can become pedunculated.

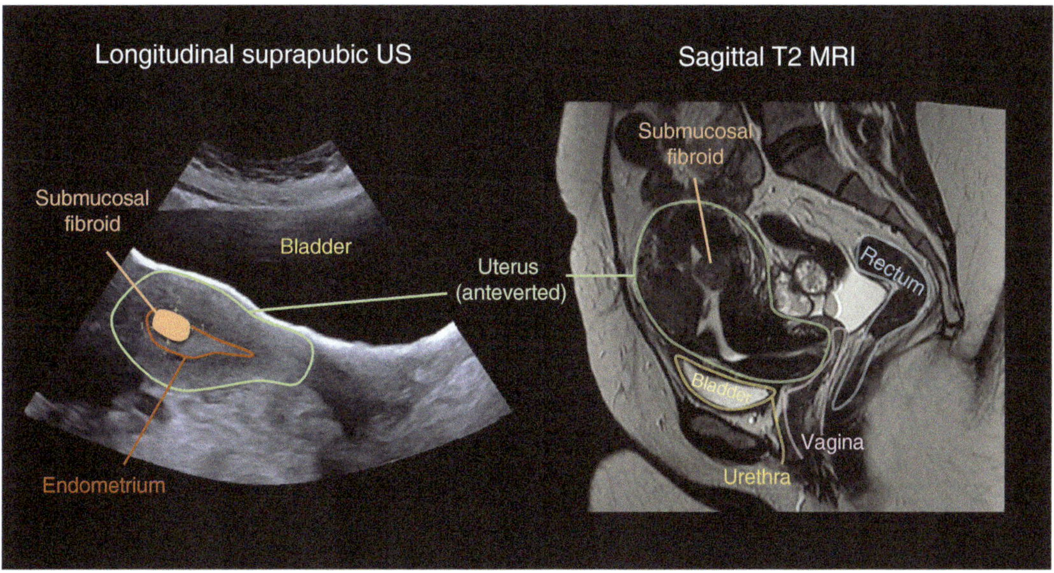

FIGURE 7.4 Patient A imaging review. Sagittal ultrasound pelvis (left), MRI sagittal T2 (right). There is a 2 cm submucosal fibroid bulging into the endometrial cavity, which is the source of the patient's bleeding (see Figure 7.5). The relative anatomy of the uterus, cervix and vagina is best appreciated on a sagittal MRI.

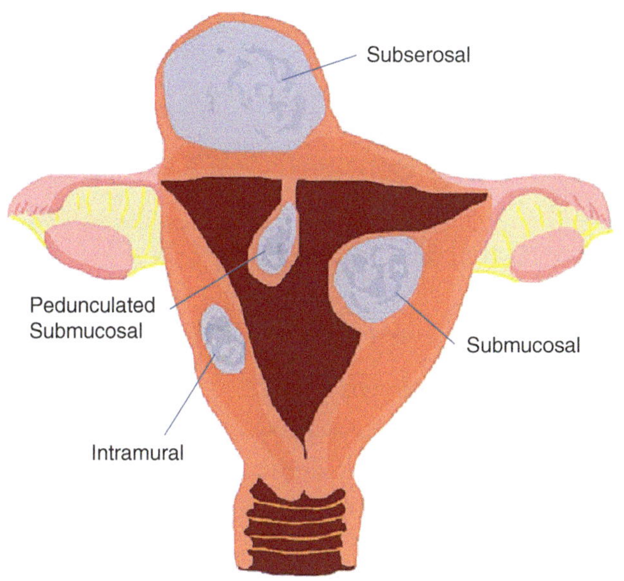

FIGURE 7.5 Diagram of types of uterine fibroid by anatomical location.

7.6 Take-home Message – Imaging of Uterus

- Transabdominal ultrasound can often locate the uterus and may identify pathology of the myometrium and endometrium. However, the view can be limited by bowel gas or if the uterus is retroverted.
- Transvaginal ultrasound is more sensitive for uterine pathology and is the standard investigation.
- Pelvic MRI is a specialist investigation, used to characterise and delineate suspicious lesions in the uterus and cervix.

CHAPTER 8

Severe Pelvic Pain

Joshua Lauder[1], Onyibo Okafor[2], and Peter Driscoll[3]

[1] *East Lancashire Hospitals NHS Trust, University of Central Lancashire and University of Manchester, UK*
[2] *Skin & Bones Medical Limited, Blackburn, UK*
[3] *School of Medicine and Dentistry, University of Central Lancashire, Preston, UK*

8.1 Primary Case

8.1.1 Presentation

A 38-year-old woman presents to the Emergency Department (ED) with acute severe pelvic pain that started during her morning high-intensity training class.

8.1.1.1 History of Presenting Complaint There have been two episodes of vomiting since the pain started two hours ago. Using the 111 emergency call service, she was advised go to the ED due to concerns about appendicitis. She describes the pain as being in her right iliac fossa (RIF). There have also been intermittent episodes of mild pain to the same area, especially during sexual intercourse and vigorous activity. For the past three months her periods have been heavier and irregular.

She denies any bowel or urinary symptoms. There has been no PV bleeding or fever and she has been eating and drinking as normal until the pain started today.

PMH: undergoing ovulation induction for infertility.
SH: non-smoker; social drinker, approx. 10 units/week.
DH: nil.

8.1.2 Examination

The patient is on a trolley, lying on her side and appears in discomfort.

RIF tenderness with a palpable mass and guarding.
Modified early warning signs (MEWS):

- Respiratory rate 16 rpm.
- SaO_2 98% (room air).
- Tympanic temp 37.0 °C.
- HR 105 bpm.
- BP 100/56 mmHg.
- Alert.

8.1.3 Bloods

Urine dip – clear.
Urine beta-HCG – negative.

8.1.4 Ultrasound

In view of the signs and symptoms, an urgent pelvic ultrasound (US) was arranged (Figure 8.1).

Clinical Case Questions

- What is your differential diagnosis?
- When is US indicated in pelvic pain?
- What is your final diagnosis and immediate management?

8.2 Radiology Self-assessment

8.2.1 Technical

- What is Doppler ultrasound?

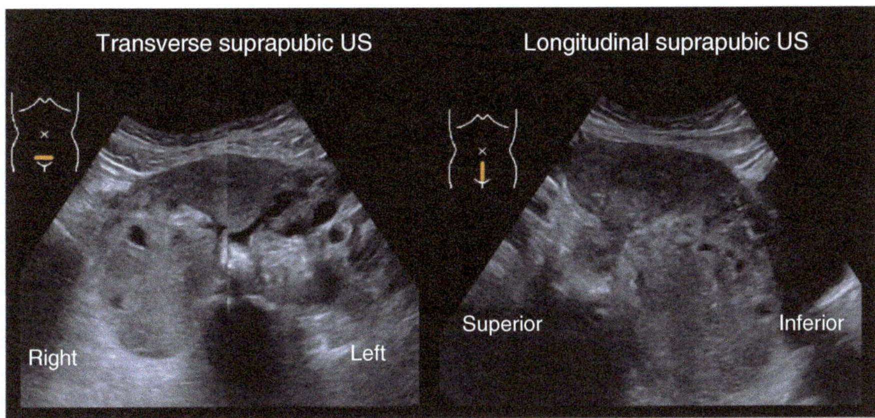

FIGURE 8.1 Patient A. Transverse (right) and sagittal (left) views from a transabdominal pelvic ultrasound scan.

8.2.2 Correlating Gross Anatomy with the US Image

- What is the anatomy of the ovary and fallopian tube?

8.3 Key Radiology Review

8.3.1 Technical Aspects

8.3.1.1 Doppler Ultrasound The Doppler effect allows detection of movement. In the case of ultrasound, Doppler detects the movement of blood and hence blood flow. It is sensitive enough to detect both arterial and venous flow (Figure 8.2a), as well as generalised hyperaemia in a tissue, which can be a sign of inflammation (Figure 8.2b) or vascularity in tumours. It is important to be aware that the probe only detects movement toward or away from its surface. If a vessel is lying parallel to the probe then the Doppler signal will not be picked up.

8.3.1.2 Ovary on Ultrasound The ovaries will be variably visible on transabdominal ultrasound. They are easier to identify in thin patients with a full bladder (Figures 8.3 and 8.4). Transvaginal scanning may be required if they cannot be identified through the abdominal wall.

8.4 Review of the Clinical Case

- What is your differential diagnosis?
- Why is US indicated?
- What is your final diagnosis and immediate management?

(a)   (b)

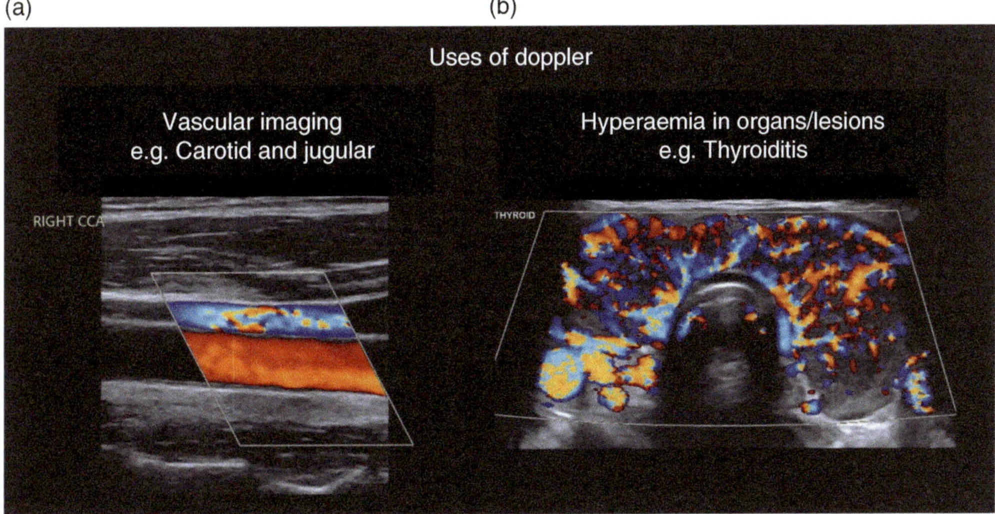

FIGURE 8.2 Examples of Doppler ultrasound use. (a) Doppler is excellent for vascular imaging. Carotid Doppler is shown here. The orange colour is blood flowing toward the probe (carotid artery) and blue is travelling away (jugular vein). (b) Hyperaemia is a useful sign which suggests inflammation. The example of thyroiditis is shown here. Other examples include tendinopathy, synovitis and tumours with vascularity.

8.4.1 **Differential Diagnosis**

- *Ovarian torsion*: most common in women of child-bearing age, with increased incidence in pregnancy. Ovulation induction is also a risk factor. In most cases there is an underlying adnexal lesion which predisposes to torsion. Common symptoms are lower abdominal pain, nausea and vomiting. It is possible for a torsion to cause low-grade pyrexia. Signs of infection (fever and raised WBC) with torsion should raise concerns for adnexal necrosis.
- *Tubo-ovarian abscess*: occurs as an end complication of pelvic inflammatory disease, so there may be a history of repeated sexually transmitted infections.
- *Ectopic pregnancy*: a pregnancy test is vital when dealing with lower abdominal pain in women of child-bearing age. Symptoms of ectopic generally present 6–8 weeks after the last menstrual period (but may be later in non-tubal ectopics).
- *Appendicitis*: incidence of appendicitis decreases with age but remains an important differential. Careful history taking and physical examination can help but ultimately imaging will be needed.
- *Ruptured ovarian cyst*: precipitating history of recent activity is present for both a ruptured cyst and torsion. An ovarian cyst rupture is more common around the time of ovulation, midcycle, while torsion can occur at any point during the menstrual cycle.

8.4.2 **Ultrasound**

Ultrasound is the best first-line test to assess for acute gynaecological pathology. Transvaginal scanning improves sensitivity but is often more difficult to arrange as a matter of urgency. Ultrasound can also be used to assess for appendicitis; however, it lacks sensitivity, especially when the appendix is retrocaecal.

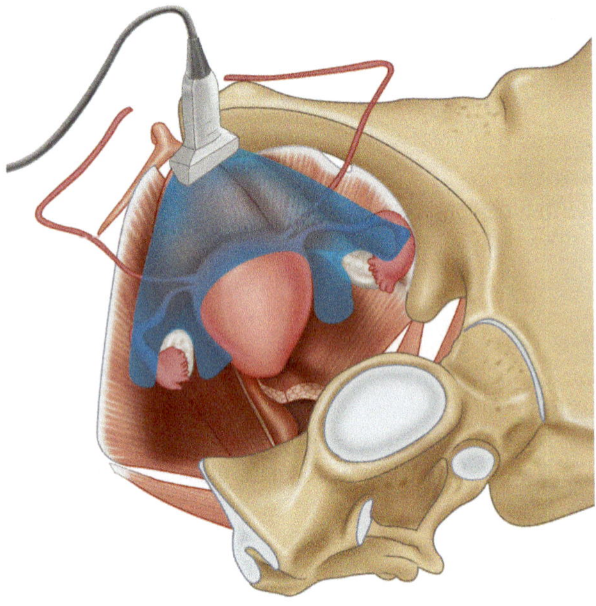

FIGURE 8.3 Female pelvic organs from above, showing the transverse suprapubic ultrasound view through the uterus and ovaries.

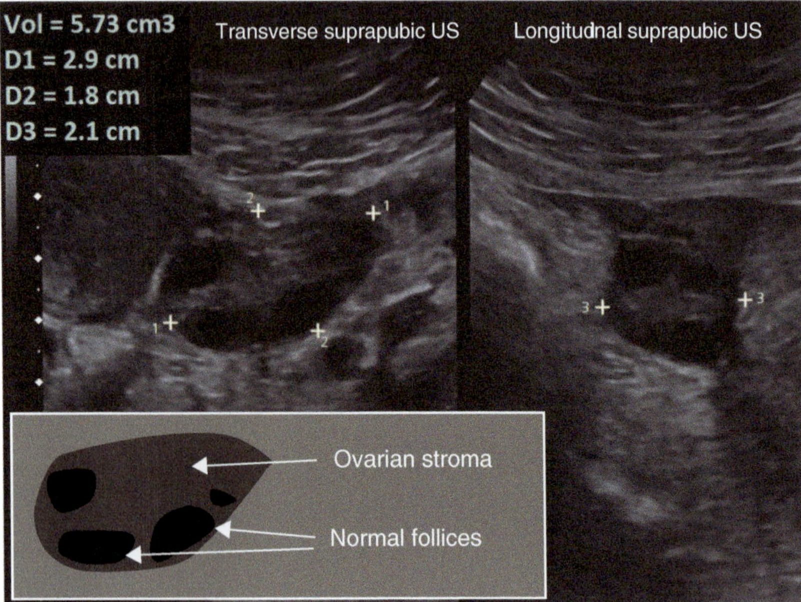

FIGURE 8.4 Transabdominal ultrasound of a normal ovary. Transverse and longitudinal suprapubic views. The ovaries are small and oval in shape, usually near the cornu of the uterus. These images are zoomed in to show the internal ovarian echotexture. The stroma is hypoechoic and the follicles anechoic. A normal ovary will have 6–10 follicles. If there are over 12 follicles then suspect a polycystic ovarian syndrome. Postmenopausal women will have reduced ovary volume with fewer follicles. The fallopian tubes are not visible on ultrasound, unless pathological (e.g. pyosalpinx or ectopic pregnancy).

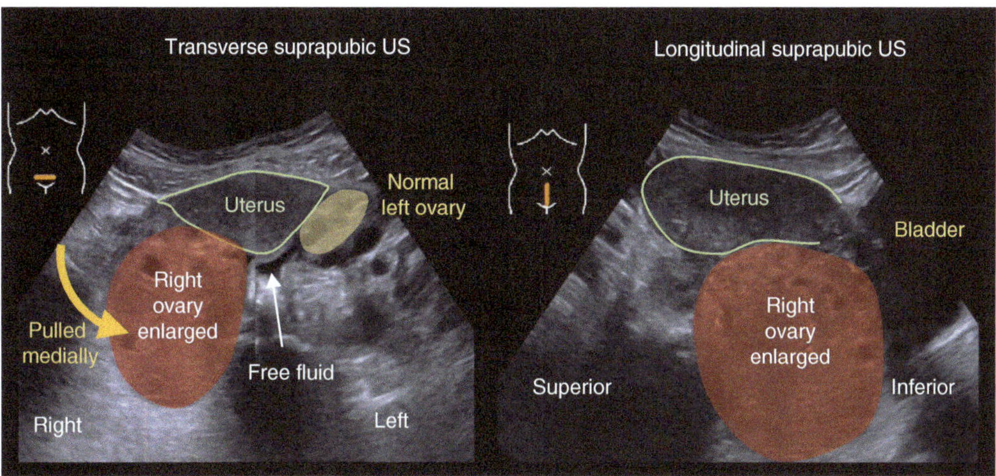

FIGURE 8.5 Patient A. Transabdominal ultrasound pelvis in transverse (right) and sagittal (left). The right ovary is enlarged and pulled medially into the pouch of Douglas. There is free fluid behind the uterus in the pouch of Douglas.

In torsion, the ovary will be enlarged with peripherally lying follicles. The twisting of the pedicle draws the ovary medially into the pouch of Douglas (Figure 8.5). Loss of colour Doppler flow is a late sign in torsion (Figure 8.6), hence preserved Doppler flow does not exclude the diagnosis.

Ovarian torsion will often result in free intraperitoneal fluid. This commonly pools in the pouch of Douglas (rectouterine pouch) and Morison's pouch (hepatorenal space) (Figure 8.7).

8.5 Final Diagnosis

Right ovarian torsion.

All ovarian torsion should be managed surgically. There may be an underlying adnexal lesion which has precipitated the torsion. Therefore, careful histological assessment of the torted lesion is required to exclude malignancy.

8.5.1 CT in Gynaecology

Computed tomography is inferior to ultrasound, due to the high radiation burden and limited assessment of the pelvic soft tissues. However, it may be the first investigation performed when it is unclear if the symptoms are due to a gynaecological pathology. Figure 8.8 highlights how it can be difficult to distinguish between the gynaecological causes on CT.

8.6 Take-home Message – Imaging of Acute Gynaecology Pathology

- Transabdominal ultrasound is the first-line test and may identify ovarian pathology, free fluid and appendicitis.

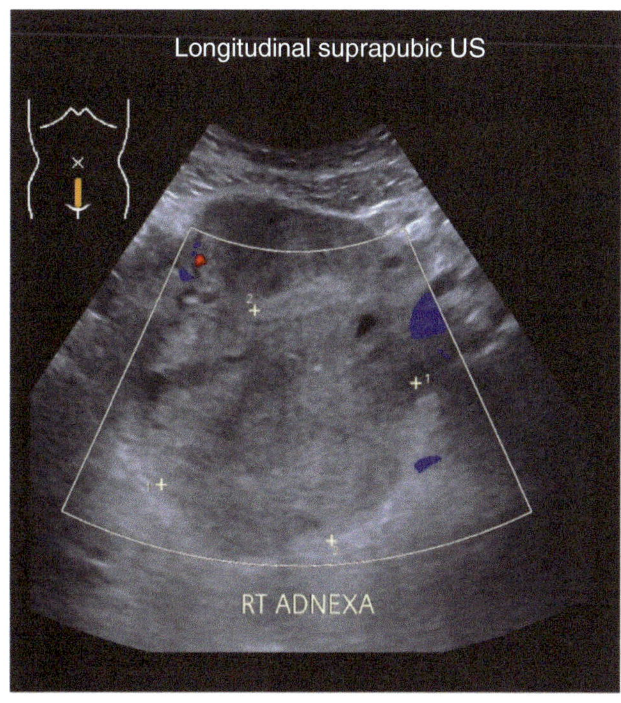

FIGURE 8.6 Patient A. Transabdominal ultrasound of right ovary with Doppler. There is no colour Doppler flow inside the right ovary, suggesting a lack of blood supply. This provides further evidence of an ovarian torsion.

- However, if there are limited views (e.g. bowel gas or body habitus) then these conditions cannot be excluded.
- Transvaginal ultrasound improves sensitivity for adnexal pathology.
- CT abdomen and pelvis with contrast may be appropriate in unwell patients with vague symptoms which cannot be localised to gynaecology pathology.

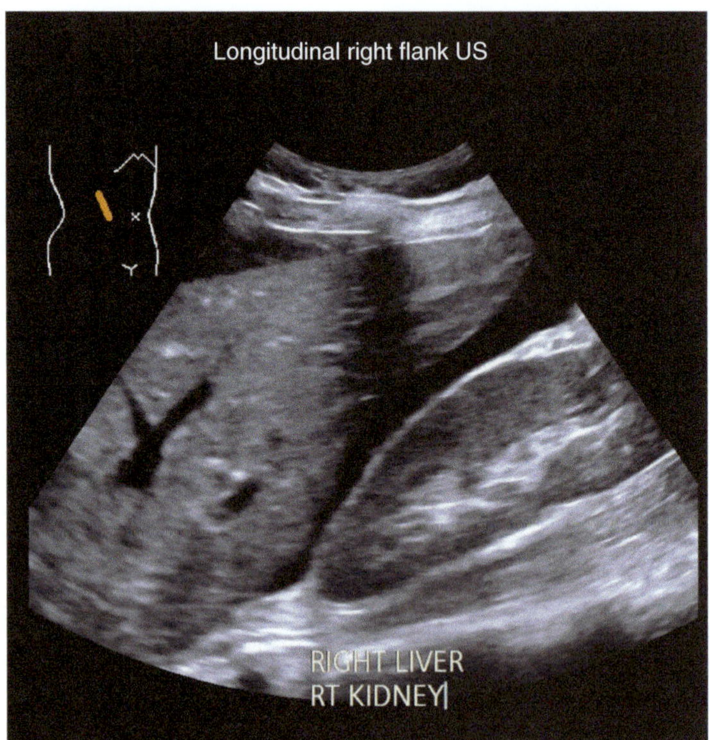

FIGURE 8.7 Patient A. Transabdominal ultrasound longitudinal view of hepatorenal space (Morison's pouch). There is free fluid between the liver and kidney, suggesting intraperitoneal pathology (GI Chapter 18). Ovarian torsion will often be associated with free peritoneal fluid. It is important to be aware that a small volume of free fluid in the pelvic can be physiologically normal in women of child-bearing age.

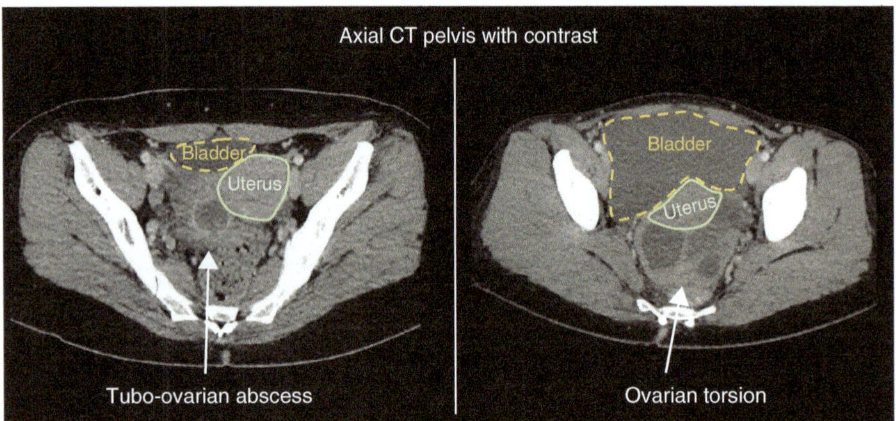

FIGURE 8.8 CT pelvis with contrast, axial slices. Tubo-ovarian abscess (left). Ovarian torsion (right). There are similarities in the appearances of adnexal pathology on CT and it is not always easy to differentiate differing pathologies. Tubo-ovarian abscess usually has a central fluid collection with an enhancing wall and surrounding fat stranding (see Abdo Chapter 19 – Figure 19.10 for a description of fat stranding); ovarian torsion usually shows a medialised adnexal mass with internal follicles/cysts. It may be possible to see the vascular pedicle twisting around. Be aware that surrounding fat stranding is possible when there is necrosis.

Further Resources

Balen, A.H., Laven, J.S., Tan, S.L., and Dewailly, D. (2003). Ultrasound assessment of the polycystic ovary: international consensus definitions. *Hum Reprod Update* 9 (6): 505–514.

Battaglia, C., Artini, P.G., Genazzani, A.D. et al. (1997). Color Doppler analysis in oligo- and amenorrheic women with polycystic ovary syndrome. *Gynecol Endocrinol* 11 (2): 105–110.

Huang, C., Hong, M.K., and Ding, D.C. (2017). A review of ovary torsion. *Ci Ji Yi Xue Za Zhi* 29 (3): 143–147.

Peña, J.E., Ufberg, D., Cooney, N., and Denis, A.L. (2000). Usefulness of Doppler sonography in the diagnosis of ovarian torsion. *Fertil Steril* 73 (5): 1047–1050.

White, M. and Stella, J. (2005). Ovarian torsion: 10-year perspective. *Emerg Med Australas* 17: 231–237.

CHAPTER 9

Testicle Pain

Joshua Lauder[1], Patrick Green[2], and Peter Driscoll[3]

[1] East Lancashire Hospitals NHS Trust, University of Central Lancashire and University of Manchester, UK
[2] Alder Hey Children's NHS Foundation Trust, Liverpool, UK
[3] School of Medicine and Dentistry, University of Central Lancashire, Preston, UK

9.1 Primary Case

9.1.1 Presentation

A 14-year-old male presents with severe left testicular pain.

9.1.1.1 History of Presenting Complaint

The symptoms started 48 hours ago and have progressively worsened. He was reluctant to tell his parents initially. The pain has not woken him up at night but gets worse when he moves and he is walking with a wide gait. He has not had any trauma and he has not vomited. He has not had any dysuria.

PMH: fit and well. Not sexually active.
SH: nil of note.
DH: nil of note.

9.1.2 Examination

He walked into the cubicle with a slightly wide-based gait. The left hemiscrotum was erythematous, swollen and uniformly tender. The swelling did not extend onto the perineum or into the groins. He had a minimally reduced cremasteric reflex on that side compared to the right and no blue dot could be appreciated. His TWIST score was 2 (Swelling (2)).

9.1.3 Ultrasound

Due to the duration of symptoms, an urgent ultrasound (US) of the testicle was arranged (Figure 9.1).

Clinical Case Questions

- What is your differential diagnosis?
- Why is US indicated?
- What is your final diagnosis and immediate management?

9.2 Radiology Self-assessment

9.2.1 Technical

- What is edge artefact on ultrasound?
- What is posterior acoustic enhancement on ultrasound?

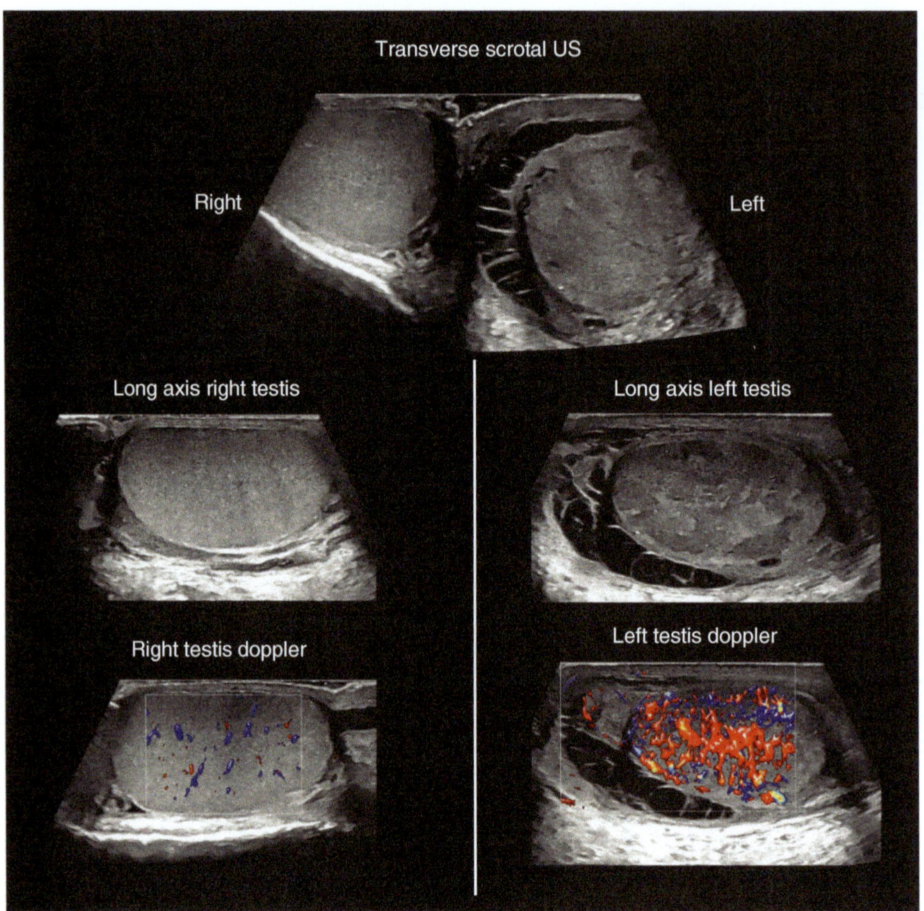

FIGURE 9.1 Patient A. Scrotal ultrasound.

9.2.2 Correlating Gross Anatomy to US

- What are the key anatomical landmarks in the scrotum (Figure 9.2)?
- What do the scrotal contents look like on ultrasound?

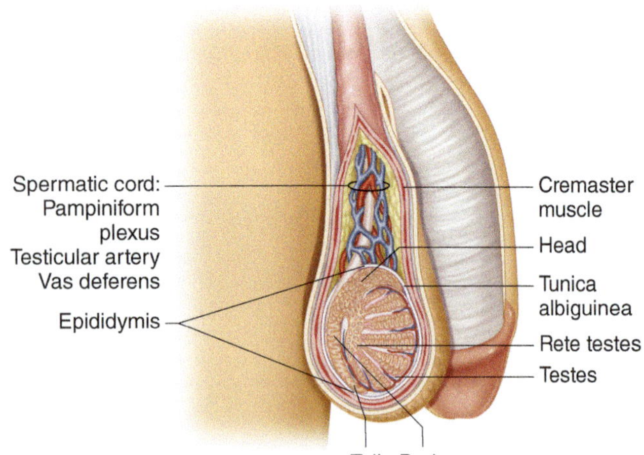

FIGURE 9.2 Diagram showing scrotal anatomy.

9.3 Key Radiology Review

9.3.1 Technical Aspects

9.3.1.1 Edge Artefact and Posterior Acoustic Enhancement Awareness of ultrasound artefacts is important, firstly so they are not mistaken for pathology and secondly to help with problem solving in difficult cases. For example, if a lesion is cystic then it will usually demonstrate posterior acoustic enhancement (Figure 9.3).

We use posterior acoustic enhancement to our advantage when scanning pelvic organs through the full urinary bladder (Pelvic Chapter 7 – Figure 7.4).

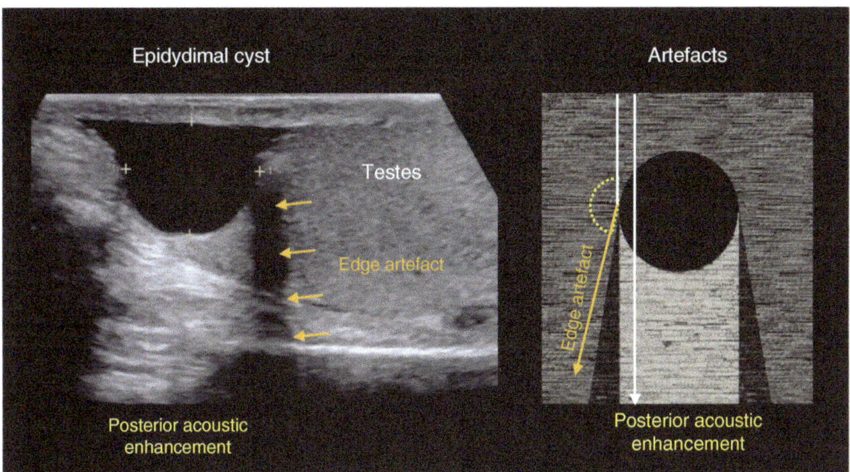

FIGURE 9.3 Ultrasound artefacts, using an epidydimal cyst as an example. *Edge artefact*: occurs when viewing a round object, for example a cyst. The ultrasound wave reflects off the edge into the deeper tissues, resulting in reduced signal return to the probe. This creates a shadow on the edge of round objects. Edge effect can also occur when viewing vessels in the short axis. This is one of the reasons why aorta measurement should be taken from anterior to posterior, rather than transversely (Abdo Chapter 22 – Figure 22.3). *Posterior acoustic enhancement*: this can be thought of as the opposite effect to posterior acoustic *shadowing* (Abdo Chapter 19 – Figure 19.9 gallstones). When the sound waves pass through a fluid-filled lesion (e.g. cyst or bladder), they are readily transmitted with no reflection and thus no attenuation of the wave. This improves the signal from the deeper tissues, making them appear brighter than the surrounding regions.

9.3.2 **Testicle on Ultrasound** (Figure 9.4)

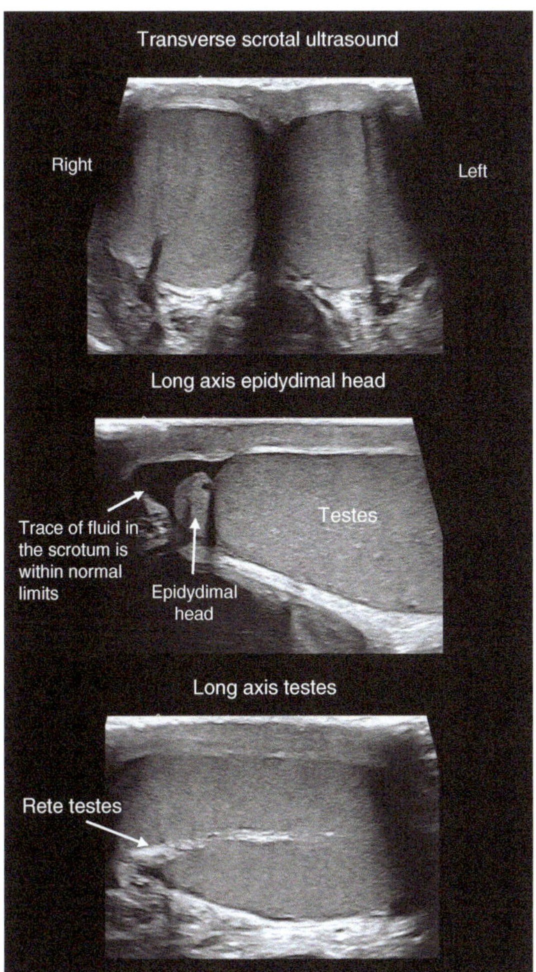

FIGURE 9.4 Normal testicular ultrasound. Both testes should be symmetrical in size and echotexture. The normal testis is of uniform echotexture with no focal lesions. The rete testes may be visible as a linear hyperechoic region. The epididymal head lies at the upper pole of the testes, the body wraps around the lateral margin of the testicle and the tail sits inferiorly. It is very common to encounter epidydimal cysts (see Figure 9.3). A trace of fluid in the scrotal sac is within normal limits (1–2 ml). A larger volume of fluid is termed a hydrocoele and may be secondary to epididymal or testicular pathology.

9.4 Review of the Clinical Case

- What is your differential diagnosis?
- Why is US indicated?
- What is your final diagnosis and immediate management?

9.4.1 Differential Diagnosis

- Testicular torsion.
  - TWIST score (Box 9.1): a TWIST score is recommended by the recent national testicular torsion pathway. While a low score does not completely exclude torsion, it helps guide decision making for those needing emergent exploration.
  - An ultrasound scan is indicated if there is pain for more than 48 hours, or in neonates.
  - While torsion can happen at any age, the two peaks in incidence are around birth and in teenage years. Neonates suspected of antenatal torsion are recommended to have an utrasound scan.
- Epididymo-orchitis.
  - Most are viral in origin but can result from bacterial infections or be a presenting sign of urinary tract anomalies.
- Trauma.
  - Severe trauma can cause scrotal haematomas which tend to be managed conservatively. However, trauma can also cause rupture of the tunica albuginea for which some centres will offer surgical repair.
- Torsion of the hydatid of Morgagni.
  - Müllerian remnants are typically located at the upper pole of the testicle/epididymis and are often multiple. They can undergo torsion and may be identifiable by the 'blue dot sign' on clinical examination. This is a focal blue discolouration to one hemiscrotum, usually in the superior aspect.
- Idiopathic scrotal oedema.
  - Ultrasound is not usually required to make this diagnosis but it can look very striking if performed! There is often severe oedema in the scrotal skin, and if this extends across into the next hemiscrotum, into the groin and onto the perineum, it gives you the clinical diagnosis. The skin is often so oedematous you lose the ability to palpate the testicle.
- Tumours.
  - Although rare, testicular tumours can present with scrotal swelling. Any hydrocoele in which you cannot palpate the testicle should undergo an ultrasound evaluation to assess the testicle for masses.

9.4.2 Ultrasound

If testicular torsion is strongly suspected, then emergency surgical exploration is required. It is not appropriate to delay active intervention while waiting for an ultrasound as the chance of salvaging the testicle reduces significantly with time.

If there is a strong suspicion of an alternative diagnosis which changes management, then ultrasound is indicated. Ultrasound is also appropriate if the symptoms have been present for longer than 48 hours, or in neonates with suspected antenatal torsion.

9.5 Final Diagnosis

Acute epididymo-orchitis (Figure 9.5).

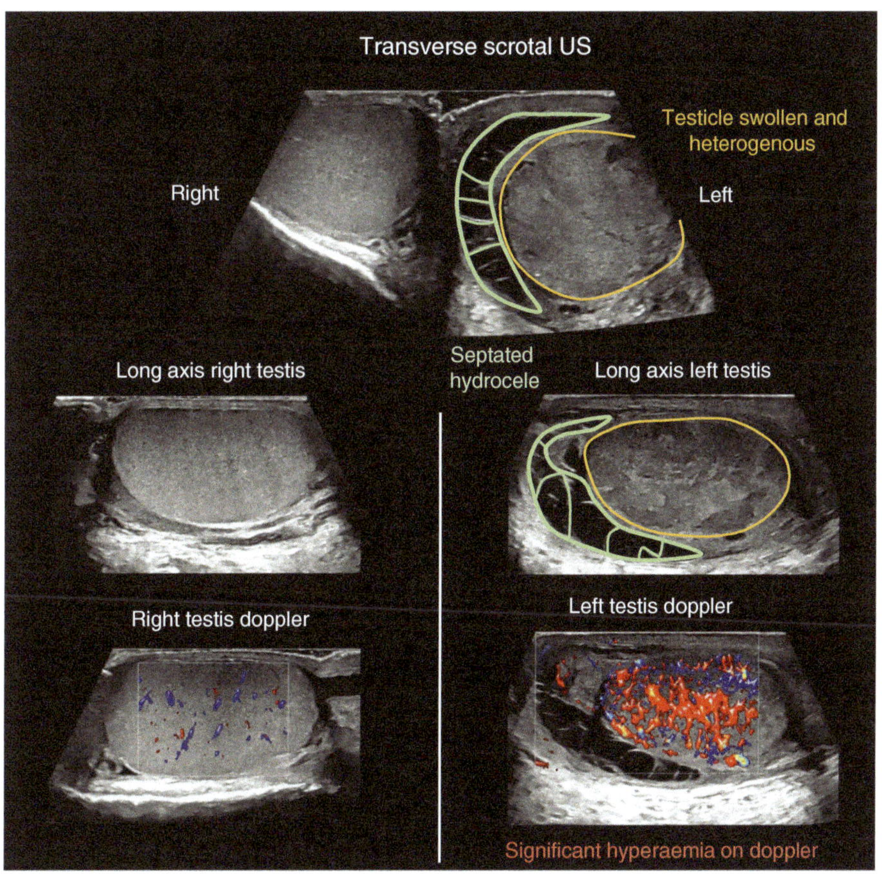

FIGURE 9.5 Patient A. Scrotal ultrasound showing epididymo-orchitis. The left testicle is swollen and heterogenous (the echotexture is no longer uniform). Doppler shows increased blood flow in the testicle (hyperaemia). There is also increased blood flow in the epididymis, to a lesser extent. There is a reactive hydrocoele which demonstrates septation due to the inflammatory response.

9.5.1 Ultrasound in Torsion (Figure 9.6)

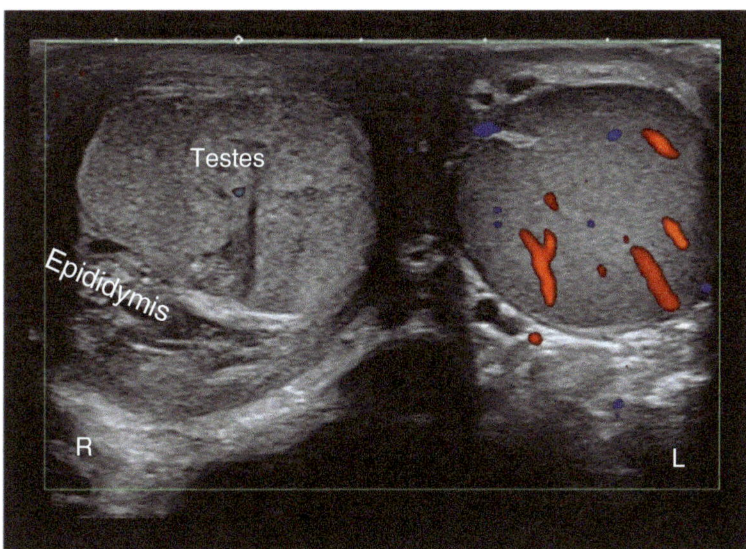

FIGURE 9.6 Ultrasound in a missed right testicular torsion. This patient presented three days after onset of pain. There is absent Doppler flow in the right testicle. The testicle and epididymis are swollen and heterogenous, representing necrosis.

9.6 Take-home Message – Testicular Pain

- Torsion is a clinical diagnosis. If the history and clinical examination favour this diagnosis then urgent surgical exploration is required.

- Ultrasound can be used if the diagnosis is uncertain or the pain is present for over 48 hours.

Further Resources

https://gettingitrightfirsttime.co.uk/wp-content/uploads/2024/02/ Paediatric-testicular-torsion-pathway-guide-FINAL-V1-February-2024.pdf

SECTION 3

Respiratory Section

CHAPTER 10

Thoracic Stabbing

Joshua Lauder[1], Aleksandr Valkov[2], Kris Philips[3], and Peter Driscoll[3]

[1] *East Lancashire Hospitals NHS Trust, University of Central Lancashire and University of Manchester, UK*
[2] *Salford Royal Hospital and University of Central Lancashire, Salford, UK*
[3] *School of Medicine and Dentistry, University of Central Lancashire, Preston, UK*

10.1 Primary Case

10.1.1 Presentation

A 25-year old male is brought by ambulance to the ED.

10.1.1.1 History of Presenting Complaint One hour ago he was involved in a street fight and sustained a stab wound to the left posterior chest. He complains of pain in his back, adjacent the wound. This increases when he takes a deep breath.

PMH: NAD.
SH: NAD.
DH: nil and no allergies.

10.1.2 Examination

- No dyspnoea at rest.
- A 2 cm stab wound to the left posterior chest. Surgical emphysema palpable.
- There are reduced breath sounds on the left side.
- The trachea is central and the patient is haemodynamically stable

Modified early warning signs (MEWS):

- Respiratory rate 24 bpm.
- SpO_2 98% (15 lpm oxygen via a facemask with a reservoir).
- HR 100 bt/min.
- BP 110/80 mmHg.
- Alert.
- Temp 36.9 °C.

10.1.3 CT

An urgent major trauma CT was performed (Figure 10.1).

Clinical Case Questions

- What is your differential diagnosis?
- Why is CT indicated?
- Why is contrast required?
- What is your system for interpreting these images?
- What is your final diagnosis and immediate management?

10.2 Radiology Self-assessment

10.2.1 Technical

- What is a lung window and when should it be used?
- What is the benefit of IV contrast in trauma?

10.2.2 Correlating Gross Anatomy to CT

- What does the pleural space look like on CT?
- How many lung lobes are there?
- What are the fissures and how do they appear on CT?

Diagnostic Imaging and Anatomy in Acute Care, First Edition. Edited by Joshua Lauder and Peter Driscoll.
© 2025 John Wiley & Sons Ltd. Published 2025 by John Wiley & Sons Ltd.
Companion website: www.wiley.com/go/DiagnosticImaginginAcuteCare

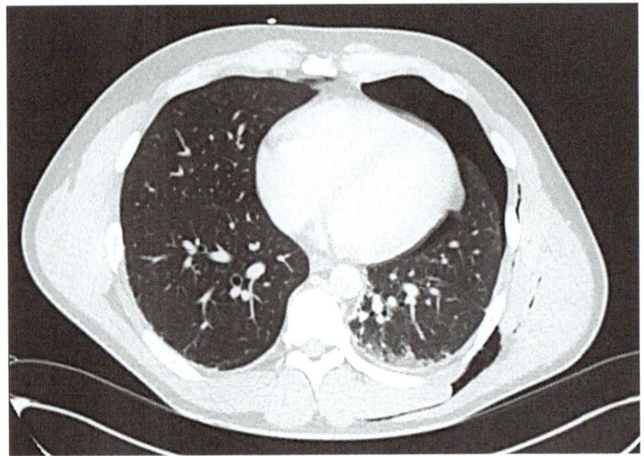

FIGURE 10.1 Patient A. Axial CT thorax on lung windows. Review the scan, paying attention to the gas-filled structures.

10.3 Key Radiology Review

10.3.1 Technical Aspects

10.3.1.1 Windowing It is vital to choose the correct window when viewing CT. Figure 10.2 shows the three main windows used in the thorax. The lung window should be used when assessing airways.

10.3.1.2 IV Contrast Intravenous contrast is always administered in trauma CT to identify active bleeding. As the contrast should normally remain inside the vessels, its leaking into the surrounding tissues is a sign of active haemorrhage. This is termed extravasation (Abdo Chapter 18 – blunt trauma). Contrast also provides a clearer view of the vessels and heart chambers (Figure 10.3).

10.4 Correlating the Anatomy with the CT Image

10.4.1 Pleura

The normal CT appearances of the pleural membranes, lung parenchyma and fissures are demonstrated in Figures 10.4–10.6.

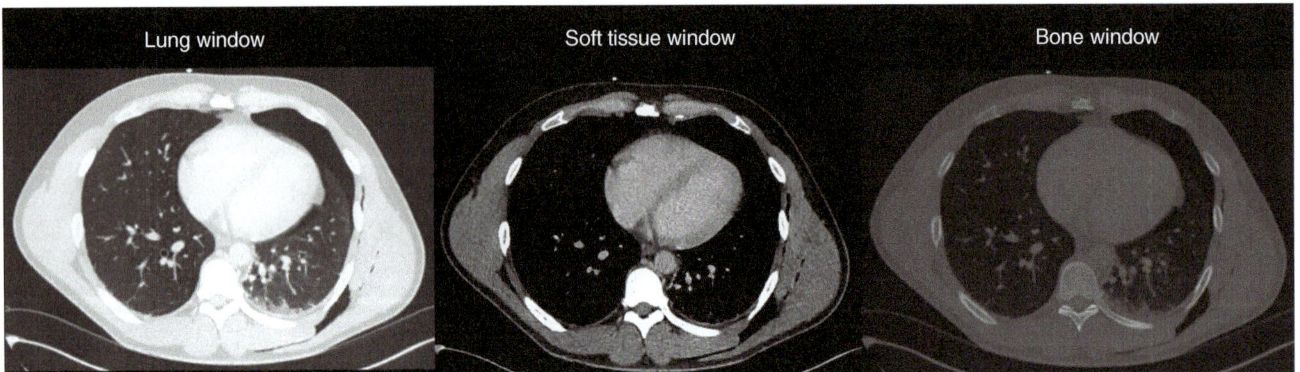

FIGURE 10.2 Patient A. Axial CT on lung window, soft tissue window and bone window. The lungs show much more intrinsic detail on the lung window, and it is possible to see pulmonary vasculature, bronchi and fissures. It is also easier to spot gas in abnormal locations, including the pleural space (pneumothorax) and subcutaneous tissue (surgical emphysema).

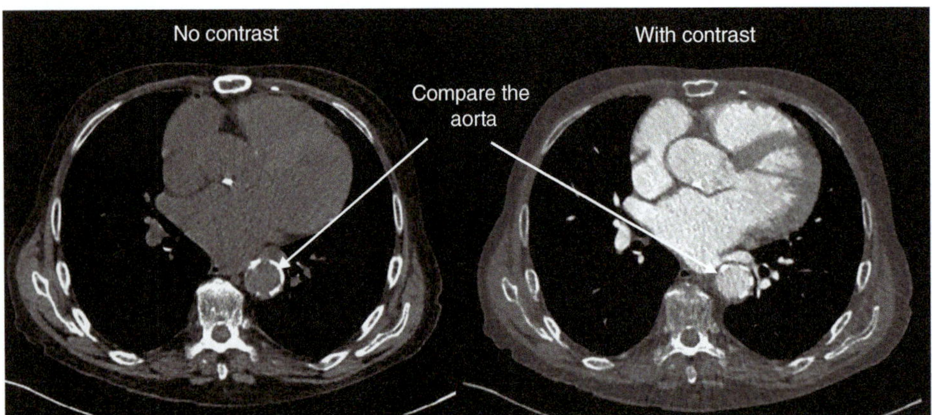

FIGURE 10.3 Axial CT on soft tissue windows, demonstrating the effect of IV contrast. The vessels and heart chambers are brighter after IV contrast.

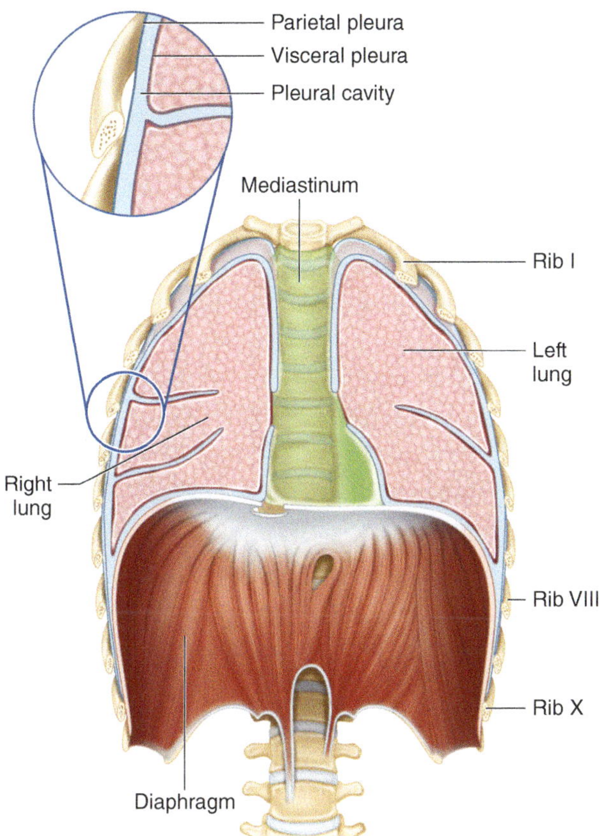

FIGURE 10.4 Anatomical diagram showing the pleura. Note how the parietal pleura adheres to the thoracic wall, while the visceral pleura adheres to the lungs, extending along the fissures. The pleural space extends significantly inferiorly in the costophrenic grooves. This is clinically important as upper abdominal injuries can involve the pleural space.

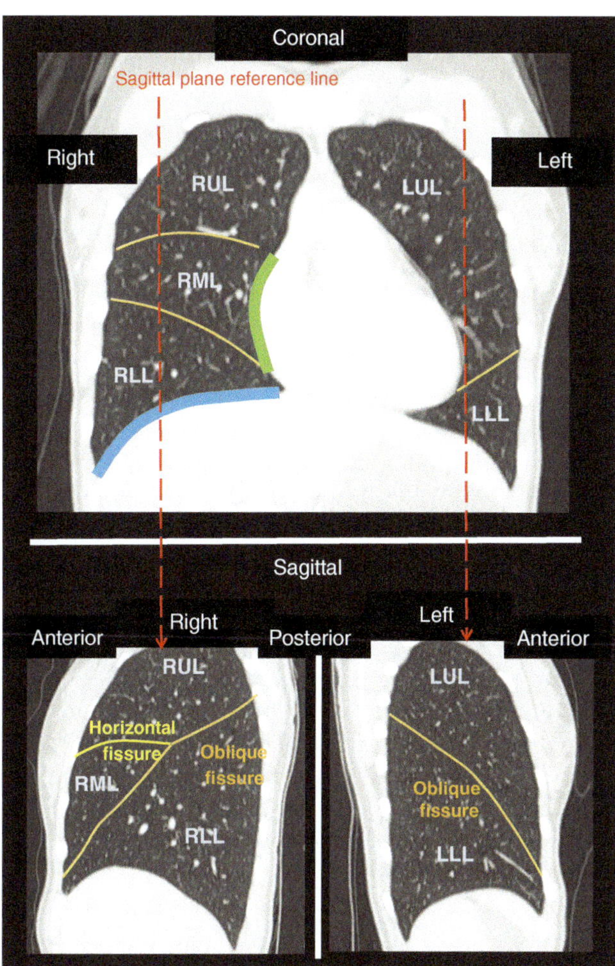

FIGURE 10.6 Coronal and sagittal CT thorax on lung windows. The fissures separate the lobes of the lungs as shown above. Note that the right middle lobe borders the right heart (green line) and the right lower lobe borders the diaphragm (blue line). This will become important in Respiratory Chapter 13 when we look at lobar collapse.

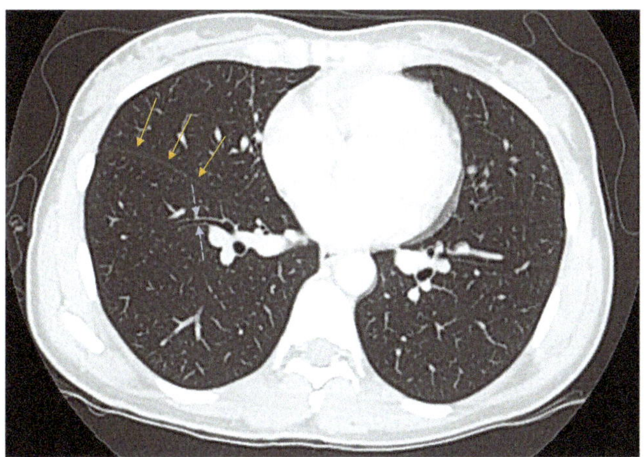

FIGURE 10.5 Axial CT thorax on lung windows. The parietal pleura is not visible on CT as it is adherent to the chest wall. Likewise, the visceral pleura is generally not visible, except in the fissures where a thin white line is observed (orange arrows show the right oblique fissure). It is possible to see the bronchi down to a very small calibre when lung windows are used (blue dashed arrows).

10.5 Review of the Clinical Case

- What is your differential diagnosis?
- Why is CT indicated?
- Why is contrast required?
- What is your final diagnosis and immediate management?

10.5.1 Differential Diagnosis

Any stab wound in the thorax, back or upper abdomen has a risk of piercing the pleural space. As this patient has unilateral reduced breath sounds, the main differential is between a pneumothorax, haemothorax or combination of these two. It is therefore vital to check for signs of decompensation during initial assessment. In this case the patient is tachycardic but maintaining saturations with no clinical evidence of mediastinal shift.

10.5.2 Indications for Imaging

Major trauma is defined as an injury, or combination of injuries, that are life-threatening and could be life changing due to long-term disability. In these cases, rapid diagnosis is the first step towards life-saving intervention. CT is the definitive investigation in trauma to the thorax as it not only allows the diagnosis of pneumothorax/haemothorax but also identifies areas of active bleeding which may warrant interventional radiology or surgical management.

Ultrasound is more accessible than CT, so may be performed in the prehospital or emergency department setting. Ultrasound can identify pneumothorax (see below), haemothorax and cardiac tamponade (Cardiac Chapter 14) as well as free fluid in the abdomen (Abdo Chapter 18). Despite this, ultrasound has limitations, particularly when looking at the thoracic aorta and retroperitoneum. For this reason, trauma CT should not be delayed.

If a patient is stable with low suspicion of major trauma then a chest X-ray would be the appropriate first-line investigation.

10.5.2.1 IV Contrast in Trauma CT Intravenous contrast is always necessary in trauma CT, as it allows detection of active haemorrhage (Abdo Chapter 18 – blunt trauma).

10.5.3 Pneumothorax on X-ray

You will probably be familiar with the appearance of pneumothorax on chest X-ray; the free gas ascends to the apex, as the patient is usually standing/sitting upright (Figure 10.7).

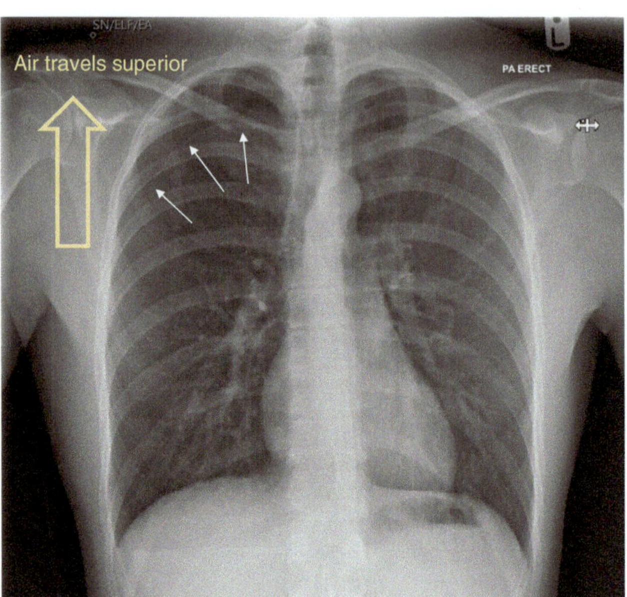

FIGURE 10.7 Erect PA CXR. There is a small right apical pneumothorax. These are best identified by looking for the lung edge (visceral pleura) as it falls away from the chest wall.

10.5.4 Pneumothorax on CT

The patient lies supine in a CT scanner, so the gas instead ascends to lie in the anterior inferior recess. This is demonstrated in the CT scan of Patient A (Figure 10.8).

Surgical emphysema (gas in the soft tissues) can help to identify the site of injury, whether the cause is a stabbing or rib fractures. In this case there is surgical emphysema in the left posterior chest wall (Figure 10.9).

10.5.5 Pneumothorax on Ultrasound

We have already described how ultrasound struggles to assess gas-filled structures due to complete reflection of the waves by the gas interface (Pelvis Chapter 7 – Figure 7.2). Despite this, ultrasound can diagnose pneumothorax. This

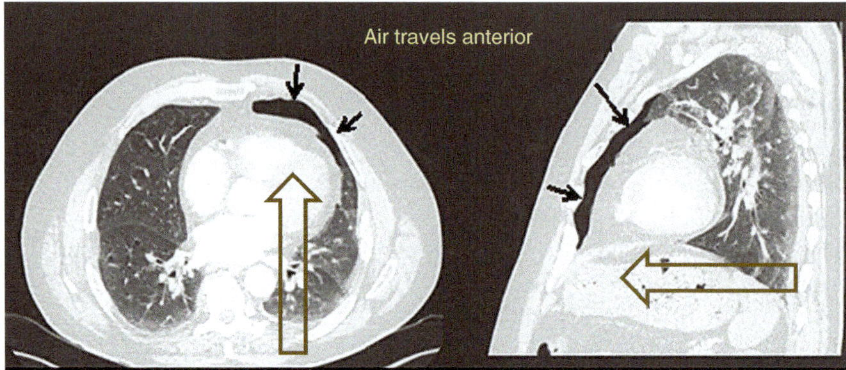

FIGURE 10.8 Axial and sagittal CT thorax on lung windows. There is a small-volume left-sided pneumothorax which gathers in the anterior inferior recess, in front of the heart. The sagittal plane can be used to aid in detection.

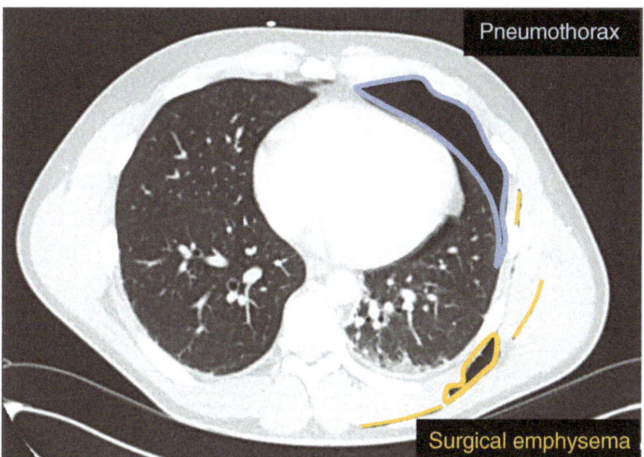

FIGURE 10.9 Patient A. Axial CT thorax on lung windows, annotated. There is a left-sided pneumothorax which gathers anteriorly. The left lung is slightly reduced in volume (collapse). There is subcutaneous gas (surgical emphysema) in the left posterior chest wall, indicating the stab wound location and suggesting that this is an open pneumothorax.

is possible because the visceral pleura pulls away from the parietal pleura and the normal movement between these layers is lost (Figure 10.10).

10.6 Final Diagnosis

Left pneumothorax and surgical emphysema.

10.6.1 Mediastinal Shift

If the pneumothorax progresses to tension, then the pressure causes the mediastinum to move to the contralateral side (mediastinal shift). The easiest way to assess for this is checking whether the trachea is central (Figure 10.11).

10.7 Take-home Message – Imaging in Trauma

- Ultrasound is a useful tool in trauma, able to diagnose life-threatening injuries including pneumothorax, haemothorax and cardiac tamponade, as well as identify free fluid in the abdomen. It can also be used to guide procedures.

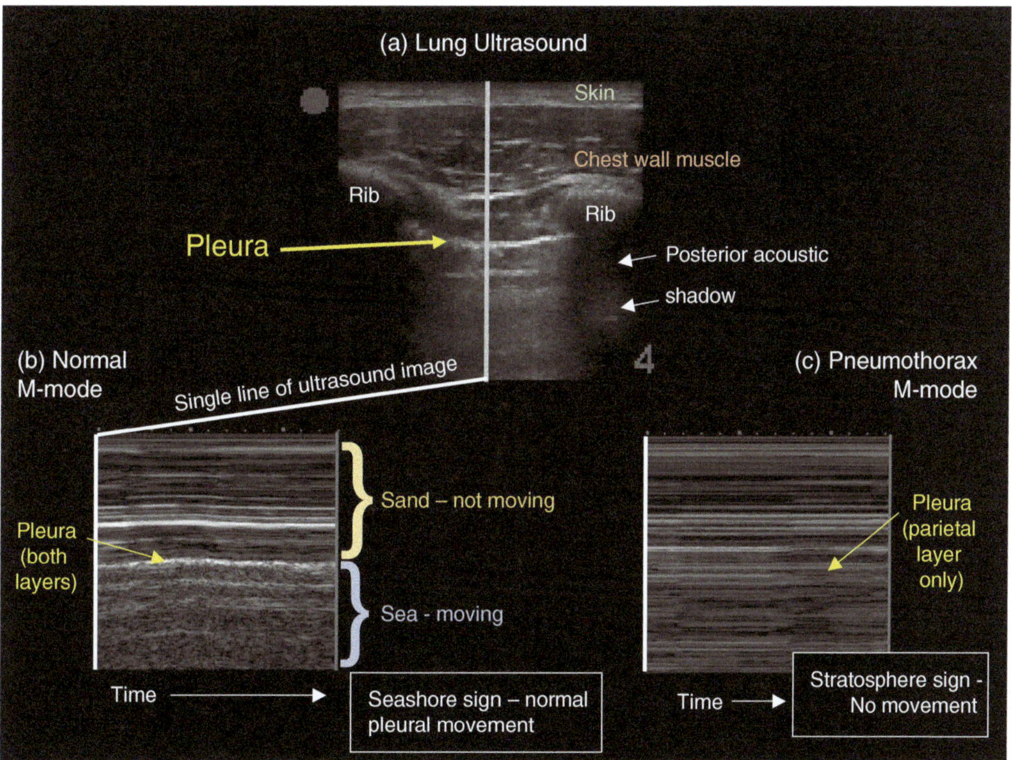

FIGURE 10.10 Chest ultrasound showing pneumothorax. (a) A conventional ultrasound image of the pleura is obtained, looking through the intercostal space. At this time the pleura should be moving with respiration. (b) M-mode ultrasound is then activated. This traces one line of the ultrasound image along the Y axis and time is traced along the X axis. Using this mode, it is more obvious that the pleura is moving as the image becomes blurred below the level of the pleura. This is called the seashore sign and is normal. (c) In pneumothorax, there is no movement of the pleural layers against each other, because the visceral pleura has become separated and is no longer visible due to the air gap. This results in a completely static M-mode image. This is also called the stratosphere sign (the stillness of outer space). Driscoll et al., (2023) / John Wiley & Sons.

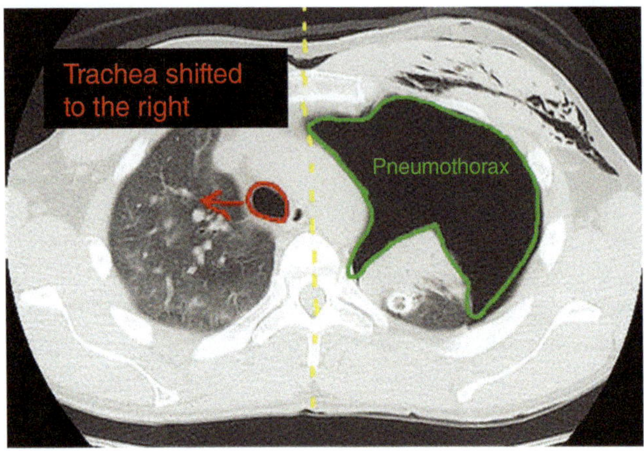

FIGURE 10.11 Axial CT thorax on lung windows. There is a large left-sided pneumothorax with mediastinal shift to the right. Draw a straight line from the spinous process through the middle of the sternum. The trachea should sit on this line all the way to the carina. *Source:* Driscoll et al. (2023)/John Wiley & Sons.

- Whole-body CT (head, neck, thorax, abdomen and pelvis) with IV contrast is the definitive imaging modality in major trauma. This has greater sensitivity than ultrasound and can identify active bleeding.
- If a patient has chest pain after minor injury and is clinically stable then CXR is an appropriate first-line investigation.

Further Resources

Driscoll, P.A., Goode, P.N. and Skinner, D.B. (2023) ABC of major trauma: Rescue, resuscitation with imaging, and rehabilitation. Hoboken, NJ, USA: Wiley Blackwell.

eFAST scanning guide – www.pocus101.com/efast-ultrasound-exam-made-easy-step-by-step-guide

CHAPTER 11

Blunt Chest Trauma

Joshua Lauder[1], Aleksandr Valkov[2], and Peter Driscoll[3]

[1] *East Lancashire Hospitals NHS Trust, University of Central Lancashire and University of Manchester, UK*
[2] *Salford Royal Hospital and University of Central Lancashire, Salford, UK*
[3] *School of Medicine and Dentistry, University of Central Lancashire, Preston, UK*

11.1 Primary Case

11.1.1 Presentation

A 70-old-male is brought by ambulance to the Emergency Department (ED).

11.1.1.1 History of Presenting Complaint He has a six-hour history of gradual increase in dyspnoea and pain over the left side of his chest.

Three days previously he had fallen on the stairs at home, hitting the left side of his chest. This was immediately painful and exacerbated by taking a deep breath. There was no haemoptysis. He is the sole carer of his demented wife and so decided not to seek medical care. He assumed he had fractured a rib and felt he could manage the pain with simple analgesics (paracetamol and a non-steroidal anti-inflammatory medication).

Today he noticed he was becoming more breathless on mild exertion and had resorted to sitting upright in a chair. He was concerned about his wife so called his GP. The latter, in addition to dealing with his wife, also called an ambulance so he could be assessed in the ED.

PMH:

- Atrial fibrillation; taking apixaban 5mg bd.
- Osteoporosis.

SH: lives with his wife who has dementia.

11.1.2 Examination

- Dyspnoea at rest.
- Significant tenderness to palpation of left ribs.
- Dull percussion left lower chest and reduced air entry.
- No mediastinal shift.

Modified early warning signs (MEWS):

- Respiratory rate 20 bpm.
- SpO_2 90% on room air.
- Temp 36.9 °C.
- HR 100 bt/min.
- BP 110/80 mmHg.
- Alert.

11.1.3 CT

An urgent major trauma CT was performed (Figure 11.1).

Clinical Case Questions

- What is your differential diagnosis?
- Why is CT indicated?
- Why is contrast required?
- What is your system for interpreting these images?
- What is your final diagnosis and immediate management?

Diagnostic Imaging and Anatomy in Acute Care, First Edition. Edited by Joshua Lauder and Peter Driscoll.
© 2025 John Wiley & Sons Ltd. Published 2025 by John Wiley & Sons Ltd.
Companion website: www.wiley.com/go/DiagnosticImaginginAcuteCare

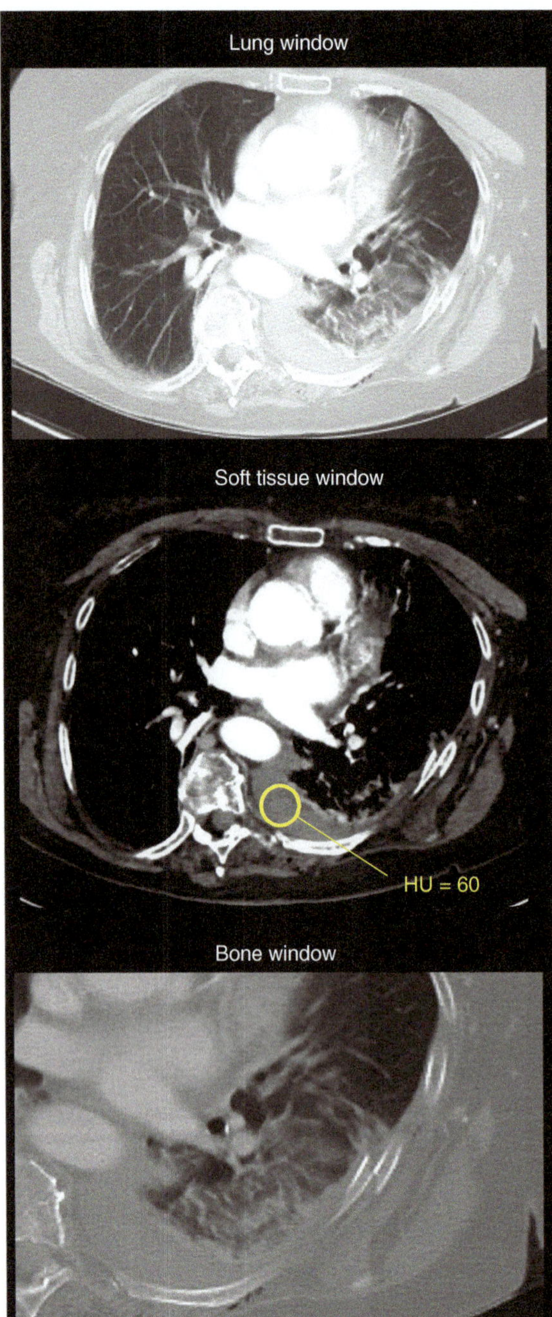

FIGURE 11.1 Patient A. Axial CT thorax, lung window, soft tissue window and bone window. HU, Hounsfield unit.

11.2 Radiology Self-assessment

11.2.1 Technical

- What do Hounsfield units measure?
- What does blood look like on CT?

11.2.2 Correlating Gross Anatomy to CT

- Where is the dependent region of the pleural space during CT?
- What do ribs look like on CT?

11.3 Key Radiology Review

11.3.1 Technical Aspects

Hounsfield units (HU) are a measure of density. For a recap of how the value is obtained, refer to Chapter 1. Water has a HU = 0; this value is found in normal anatomical fluids such as bile (gallbladder), urine (bladder) and CSF (ventricles). When manipulating a CT, a region of interest can be traced out. The software will then display the average HU in that region (Figure 11.2). This is a useful tool as it provides clues as to the cause of the lesions and fluid collections.

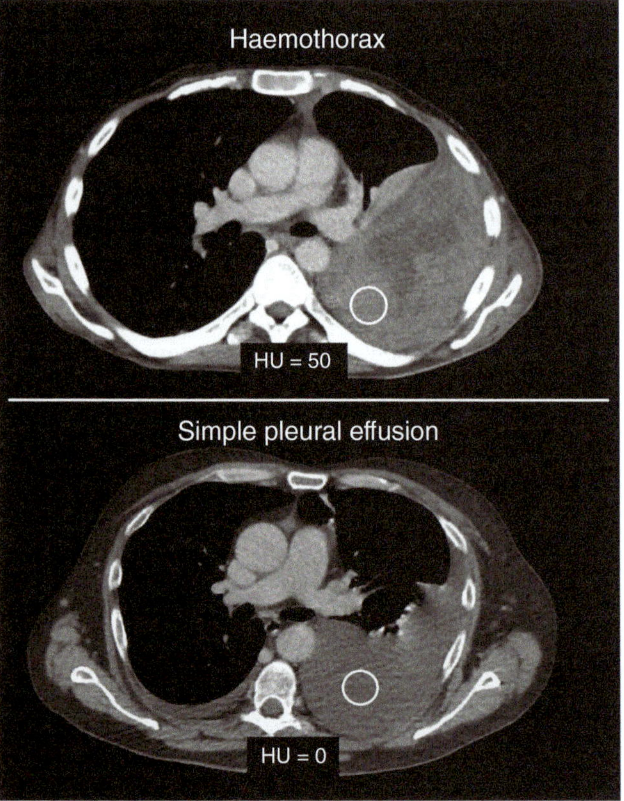

FIGURE 11.2 Axial CT of the thorax on soft tissue windows. Both of these patients have fluid in the pleural space which to the naked eye seem similar. However, the top example has a HU of 50, indicating it is blood or pus. The bottom example has a HU of 0 indicating simple pleural effusion.

11.3.2 Blood on CT

The density of blood on CT changes depending on its state. Flowing blood has the same density as soft tissues in the body, such as the muscles and unenhanced liver (30–40 HU). As the blood clots, it increases in density to a maximum of around 90 HU. Over time, the density declines as the haematoma is broken down and is either resorbed or becomes a seroma with the density of water (HU = 0). These chances are depicted graphically in Chapter 1.

A simple pleural effusion (e.g. resulting from heart failure) will have the same density as water (HU = 0). If pleural fluid is more dense, it suggests more complex constituents such as blood clots or pus (Figure 11.2).

11.4 Correlating the Anatomy with the CT Image

11.4.1 Ribs

Due to the angulated nature of the ribs, there will always be multiple different ribs on each slice through the thorax. The only way to be sure of which rib you are on is to count down from the first rib (Figure 11.3).

11.5 Review of the Clinical Case

- What is your differential diagnosis?
- Why is CT indicated?
- Why is contrast required?
- What is your system for interpreting these images?
- What is your final diagnosis and immediate management?

11.5.1 Differential Diagnosis

- Pleural effusion.
  - *Haemothorax*: the presence of trauma suggests a haemorrhagic cause for the pleural fluid. Accompanying rib fractures would also support this diagnosis. The HU of the pleural fluid is 60, indicating haemorrhage.
  - *Empyema*: an empyema may also be relatively dense on CT but the history would be different, with progressive deterioration over several days and accompanying pyrexia.
  - *Simple fluid*: this is less likely due to the history of acute trauma and density of pleural fluid on CT.

11.5.2 CT in Trauma

It is important to appreciate the key role CT has in cases of major trauma (e.g. high energy transfer, hypoxia, dyspnoea, tachypnoea, altered mental status, distracting injuries and anticoagulation). This should always be performed with IV contrast to look for active bleeding (Abdo Chapter 18 – Blunt Trauma, Figure 18.6).

In cases of minor trauma in a stable patient, CXR would be the first-line investigation. CT thorax should not

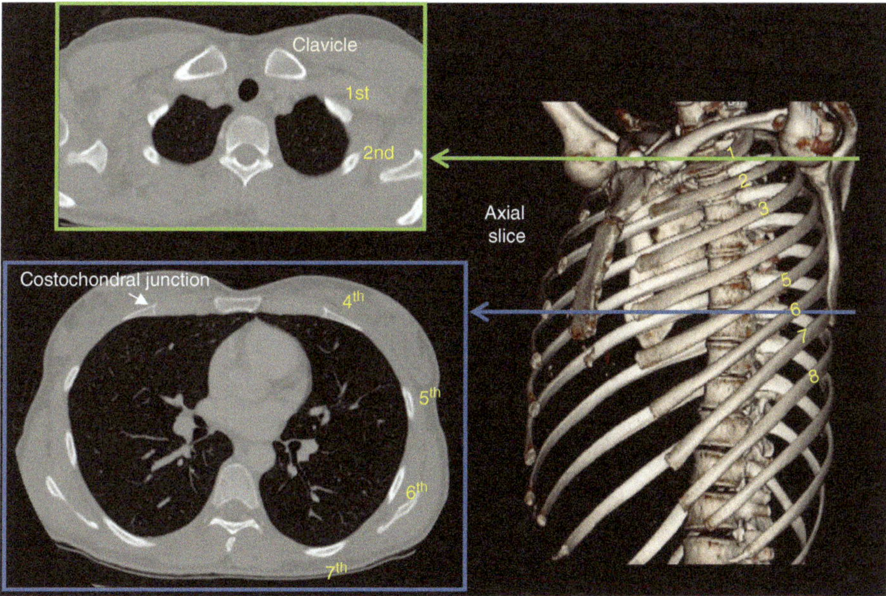

FIGURE 11.3 Axial CT of the thorax on bone windows at the level of the thoracic inlet (green) and lower sternum (blue). The anterior rib becomes cartilaginous at the costochondral junction.

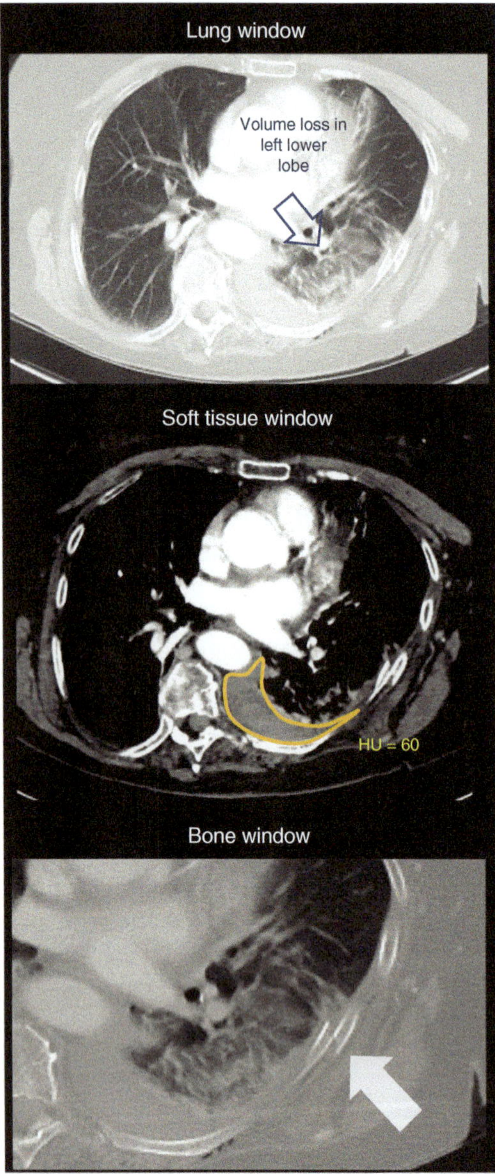

FIGURE 11.4 Patient A: the *lung window* is useful to check the airways and lungs. In this case the left lower lobe is increased in density and reduced in volume, suggesting partial collapse (hollow arrow). There is no pneumothorax anteriorly as in the previous case. There is the impression of something posterior to the left lung, but this is difficult to appreciate on this window. The *soft tissue window* is useful to look at fluid and the mediastinum. Now we can see there is fluid in the left pleural space posteriorly (orange). Measuring the Hounsfield units reveals a value of 60. This suggests it is more dense than simple fluid (HU = 0) and, given the history of trauma, represents a haemothorax. The *bone window* makes the causative rib fracture more obvious (white arrow). The fracture is slightly displaced, resulting in more damage to the underlying lung.

be overused in these patients as it does not improve clinical outcomes.

Review the CT of Patient A (Figure 11.4).

11.6 Final Diagnosis

Left rib fractures with associated left-sided haemothorax. Partial compressive collapse of left lower lobe (Respiratory Chapter 13 – Chronic Cough and Dyspnoea).

11.7 Take-home Message – Imaging in Trauma

- Ultrasound is a useful tool in trauma, able to diagnose life-threatening injuries including pneumothorax, haemothorax and cardiac tamponade, as well as identify free fluid in the abdomen. It can also be used to guide procedures (Respiratory Chapter 10 – Thoracic Stabbing).
- Whole-body CT (head, neck, thorax, abdomen and pelvis) with IV contrast is the definitive imaging modality in major trauma. This has greater sensitivity than ultrasound and can identify active bleeding.
- If a patient has chest pain after minor injury, and is clinically stable, then CXR is an appropriate first-line investigation. CT thorax should not be overused in these patients as it does not improve clinical outcomes.

Further Resources

Chapman, B.C., Overbey, D.M., Tesfalidet, F. et al. (2016). Clinical utility of chest computed tomography in patients with rib fractures CT chest and rib fractures. *Arch Trauma Res* 5 (4): e37070.

Guerrero-López, F., Vázquez-Mata, G., Alcázar-Romero, P.P. et al. (2000). Evaluation of the utility of computed tomography in the initial assessment of the critical care patient with chest trauma. *Crit Care Med* 28 (5): 1370–1375.

CHAPTER 12

Acute Dyspnoea

Joshua Lauder[1], Aleksandr Valkov[2], and Peter Driscoll[3]

[1]*East Lancashire Hospitals NHS Trust, University of Central Lancashire and University of Manchester, UK*
[2]*Salford Royal Hospital and University of Central Lancashire, Salford, UK*
[3]*School of Medicine and Dentistry, University of Central Lancashire, Preston, UK*

12.1 Primary Case

12.1.1 Presentation

A 50-year-old man is brought to the Emergency Department by ambulance. He has become markedly dyspnoeic over the last day.

12.1.1.1 History of Presenting Complaint Five days previously he started to feel unwell, complaining of a temperature and general muscular aches. He put this down to having flu. However, the symptoms persisted and he started to cough. Initially this was dry but it is now producing green sputum.

Over the last two days he has noticed pain on the right side of his chest. This increases when taking a deep breath.

PMH: NAD.

SH: lives with his wife who is well.

DH: nil and no allergies.

12.1.2 Examination

- Looks flushed and dehydrated.
- Dyspnoea at rest.
- Right upper chest: inspiratory crackles and bronchial breathing.

Modified early warning signs (MEWS):

- Respiratory rate 26 bpm.
- SpO$_2$ 90% on room air.
- Temp 38.9 °C.
- HR 110 bt/min.
- BP 130/70 mmHg.
- Alert.

12.1.3 Chest X-ray (CXR)

A CXR was performed (Figure 12.1).

Clinical Case Questions

- What is your differential diagnosis?
- When is a CXR indicated?
- What pattern of lung disease is shown?

12.2 Radiology Self-assessment

12.2.1 System for Interpretation

- What is your system for interpreting a CXR?
- What lung patterns are you aware of on CXR?

12.3 Key Radiology Review

It is useful to have a system for interpreting CXR and CT scans. This provides a reliable way to pick up pathology which could be missed if relying on pattern

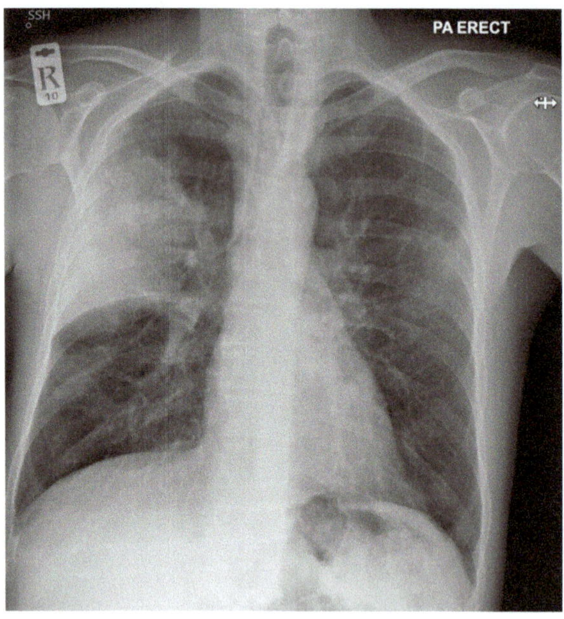

FIGURE 12.1 Patient A. CXR PA projection.

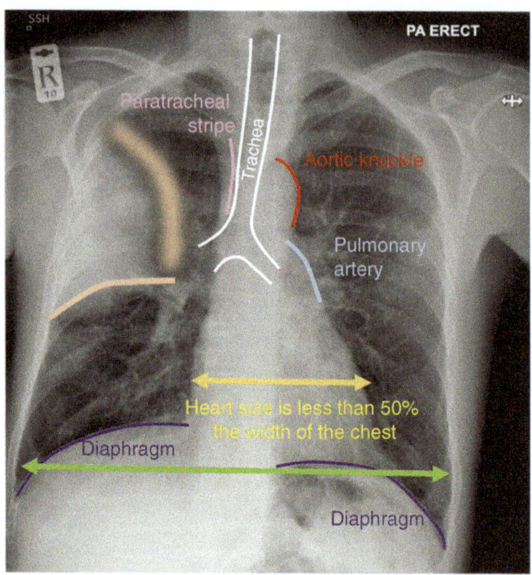

FIGURE 12.2 Patient A. CXR PA projection. Interpretation using the ABCDE system. (A) The airway is patent (white). (B) There is a large area of consolidation in the right upper lobe (light orange). The upper medial border is ill defined, fluffy and cloud-like, as we would expect with consolidation. However, the lower border is very well defined. This is because it abuts the horizontal fissure which acts as a barrier. (C) The heart size is normal (less than 50% the width of the chest). Normal appearance of the aortic knuckle (red), pulmonary artery (blue) and right paratracheal stripe (pink). (D) No free gas under the diaphragm (purple). (E) No fracture or bone lesion. Normal soft tissues.

recognition. In the case of the CXR, many different systems are used and they often follow a mnemonic. The ABCDE system is listed in Box 12.1. A demonstration of it being applied to interpreting Patient A's CXR is shown in Figure 12.2.

Box 12.1 | CXR Interpretation System

A – Airway and apparatus	Follow the trachea from the neck to the carina. Is it central? Are there any foreign bodies in the bronchi? The right lower lobe bronchus is the most vertical, so most aspirated objects end up here. If there is an endotracheal tube, is it correctly sited 5 cm above the carina? Check for other lines including nasogastric tube, chest drain and central lines.
B – Breathing	Check both lungs for symmetry. Are there any specific lung patterns? (See next section.) Look for pleural effusion by checking the costophrenic angles.
C – Circulation	Is the heart enlarged? Can you see the aortic knuckle and pulmonary artery? Check the hilar regions and right paratracheal stripe for lymphadenopathy.
D – Diaphragm	Look under the diaphragm for free gas.
E – Everything else	Check the bones for lesions and fractures. Look at the surrounding soft tissues, e.g. breast shadows

12.3.1 Lung Patterns

It is common to hear vague terms such as 'increased density' or 'opacification' when people are describing abnormalities on a CXR. These terms are very non-specific, essentially translating to 'there is a white blob'.

It is much more useful to characterise lung opacities according to the pattern. In addition to atelectasis (see Respiratory Chapter 13), there are three main patterns of lung disease described on CXR. These are defined by the pathological process which is occurring.

Pattern	Consolidation Synonyms: airspace opacification	Interstitial thickening Synonyms: reticulation, septal thickening	Nodule
Pathological process	This is when the alveolar sacs are filled with fluid, instead of air. There are five types of fluid which can cause this: pus (pneumonia), fluid (pulmonary oedema), blood (contusion), cells (cancer) and protein (proteinosis). **All will have the same appearance on CXR and CT** but can often be differentiated based on history and examination. 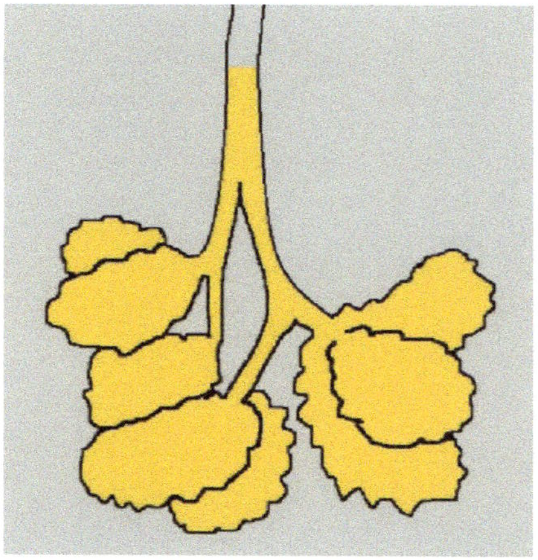	This is when the basement membrane becomes thickened. It occurs secondary to either fluid or fibrosis. Again, the history and examination will help to differentiate these two. 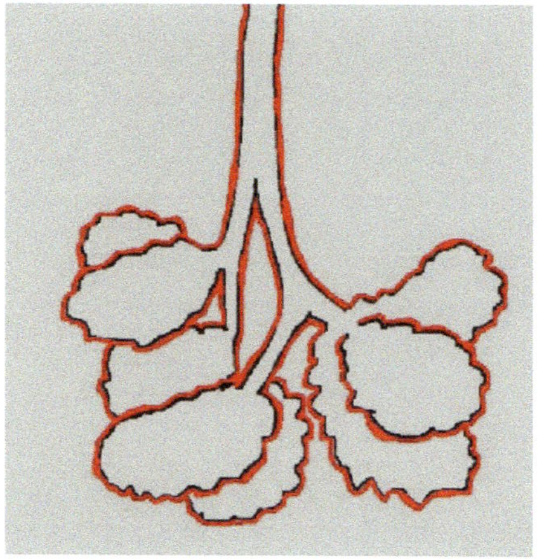	This is when extra tissue is added to the lung parenchyma. Lung cancer is a common cause for a nodule, but it is important to remember that there are also benign causes. 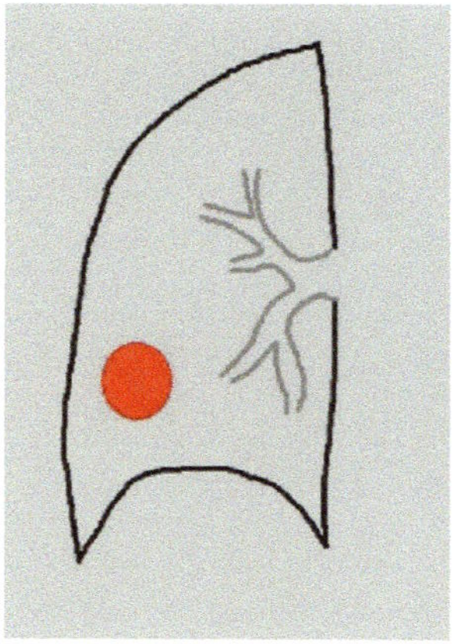

Appearance on imaging	This will usually appear as a fluffy cloud-like area of increased density. It could be very small and focal, or involve a whole lung. It may be possible to see the aerated bronchi travelling through the consolidation (air bronchogram sign). This can differentiate consolidation from a nodule, where the bronchi will be displaced or effaced.	This appears as multiple very thin lines. They will often be seen in the periphery of the lung, extending to the pleural surface in a perpendicular orientation. These are called Kerley B lines. Normal lungs don't have any lung markings visible within 2 cm of the pleura on a CXR.	This appears as a well-defined, rounded lesion. As the lesion is solid there will not be an air bronchogram sign.
CXR	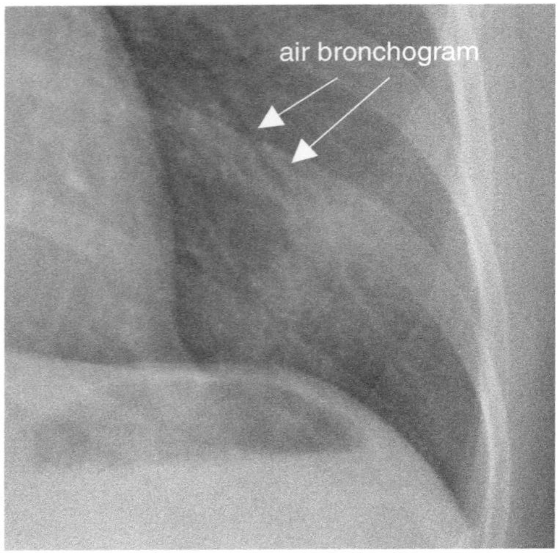	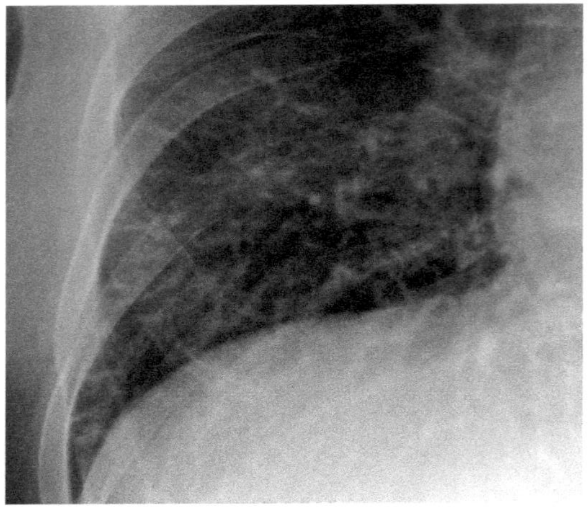	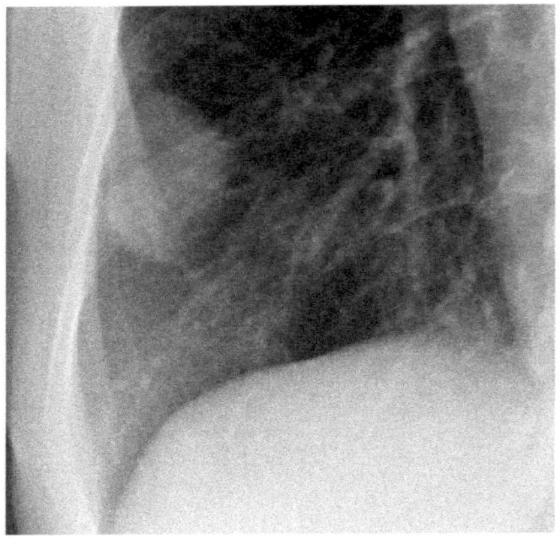
CT	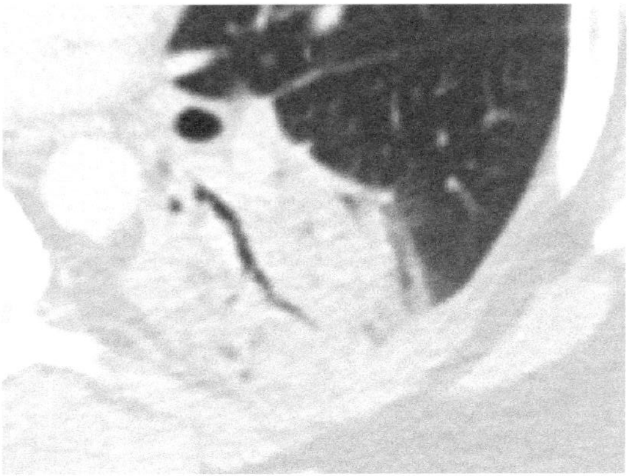	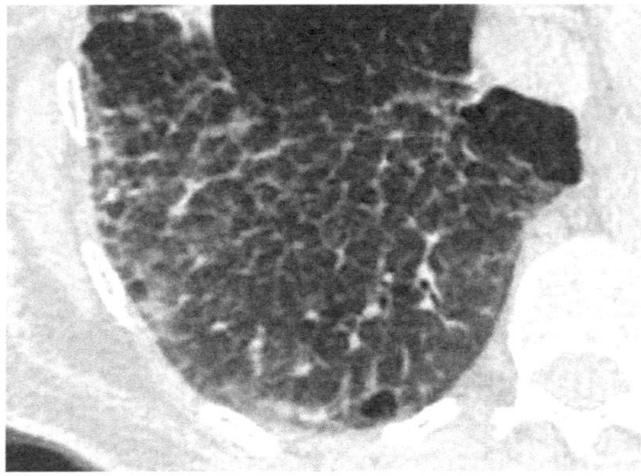	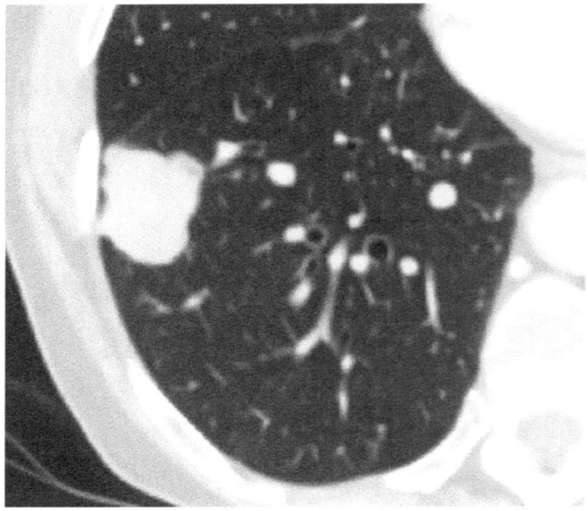

12.4 Review of the Clinical Case

- What is your differential diagnosis?
- When is a CXR indicated?
- What pattern of lung disease is shown?

12.4.1 Differential Diagnosis

Given the history of new-onset cough and fever, this is likely to be secondary to infective pneumonia. All patients attending hospital with suspected pneumonia should have a CXR.

If the CXR identifies lobar consolidation, it is not possible to differentiate viral or bacterial cause. Therefore sputum samples may be required if the patient is unwell.

Nevertheless, in certain cases the pattern of consolidation can help suggest types of infective causes. For example:

- COVID pneumonitis (and other viruses like influenza) classically have a bilateral peripheral consolidation pattern (Figure 12.3)
- active TB typically affects the upper lobes and may be unilateral or bilateral (Figure 12.4).

12.5 Final Diagnosis

Right upper lobe consolidation, representing infective pneumonia.

12.5.1 Other Types of Infective Pneumonia (Figures 12.3 and 12.4)

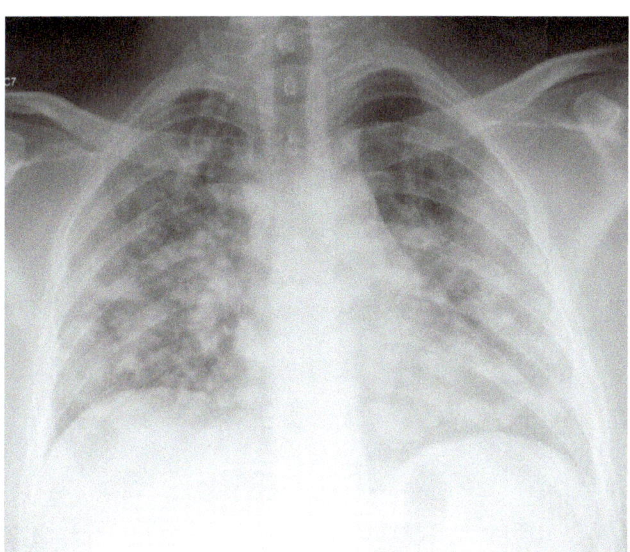

FIGURE 12.3 CXR AP projection of a patient with acute COVID pneumonitis. This results in bilateral multiple areas of consolidation which are predominantly in the peripheral lungs. There is an oxygen mask and tubing projected over the right lung.

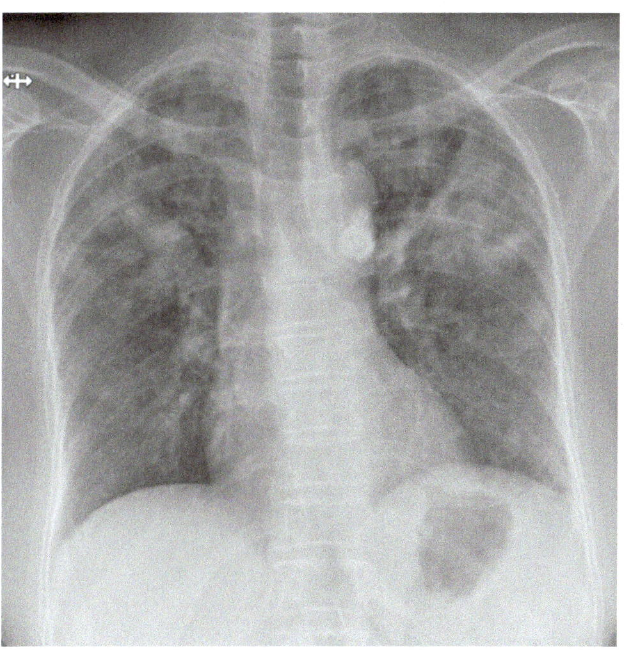

FIGURE 12.4 CXR PA projection of a patient with active TB. There is bilateral upper lobe consolidation.

12.6 Take-home Message – Imaging in Pneumonia

- Mild pneumonia may be managed in primary care without imaging.
- All patients attending hospital with suspected pneumonia should have a CXR. This is usually the only investigation required in suspected pneumonia.
- A CXR may be repeated if the patient fails to improve after treatment.
- If consolidation is persistent for more than six weeks then it could be masking an underlying malignancy. These patients will require a CT thorax, which is performed with no contrast as a low-dose protocol.

Further Resources

British Thoracic Society (2009). Guidelines for the management of community acquired pneumonia in adults: update 2009. *Thorax* 64 (Suppl. III): 1–55.

BTS Guideline for the Management of Community Acquired Pneumonia in Adults: update 2009. www.brit-thoracic.org.uk/quality-improvement/guidelines/pneumonia-adults/

CHAPTER 13

Chronic Cough and Dyspnoea

Joshua Lauder[1], Aleksandr Valkov[2], and Peter Driscoll[3]

[1]East Lancashire Hospitals NHS Trust, University of Central Lancashire and University of Manchester, UK
[2]Salford Royal Hospital and University of Central Lancashire, Salford, UK
[3]School of Medicine and Dentistry, University of Central Lancashire, Preston, UK

13.1 Primary Case

13.1.1 Presentation

A 70-year-old woman presents to her GP with a six-month history of worsening dyspnoea on exertion.

13.1.1.1 History of Presenting Complaint Her symptoms include a persistent, mainly dry, cough, diminished appetite, 2 kg weight loss and fatigue. In the last month she has noted specks of blood in her sputum.
PMH: mild COPD.
SH:

- smoker with a ⩾40 pack-per-year history.
- lives with her husband.

DH: nil and no allergies.

13.1.2 Examination

- Thin and pale.
- Trachea central.
- Right upper chest: reduced chest expansion and reduced breath sounds.

Modified early warning signs (MEWS):

- Respiratory rate 18 bpm.
- SpO$_2$ 92% on room air.
- Temp 36.9 °C.
- HR 80 bpm.
- BP 110/80 mmHg.
- Alert.

13.1.3 CXR and CT

An initial CXR was performed (Figure 13.1a). Based on the findings, an urgent CT was arranged (Figure 13.1b).

Clinical Case Questions

- What is your differential diagnosis?
- Why is CT indicated?
- What is your system for interpreting these images?
- What further imaging may be necessary?

13.2 Radiology Self-assessment

13.2.1 Technical

- What is positron emission tomography (PET)?
- Do you have a system for interpreting a CT thorax?

13.2.2 Correlating Gross Anatomy to CT

- What do the trachea and bronchi look like on CT?
- What does lung collapse look like on CT?

Diagnostic Imaging and Anatomy in Acute Care, First Edition. Edited by Joshua Lauder and Peter Driscoll.
© 2025 John Wiley & Sons Ltd. Published 2025 by John Wiley & Sons Ltd.
Companion website: www.wiley.com/go/DiagnosticImaginginAcuteCare

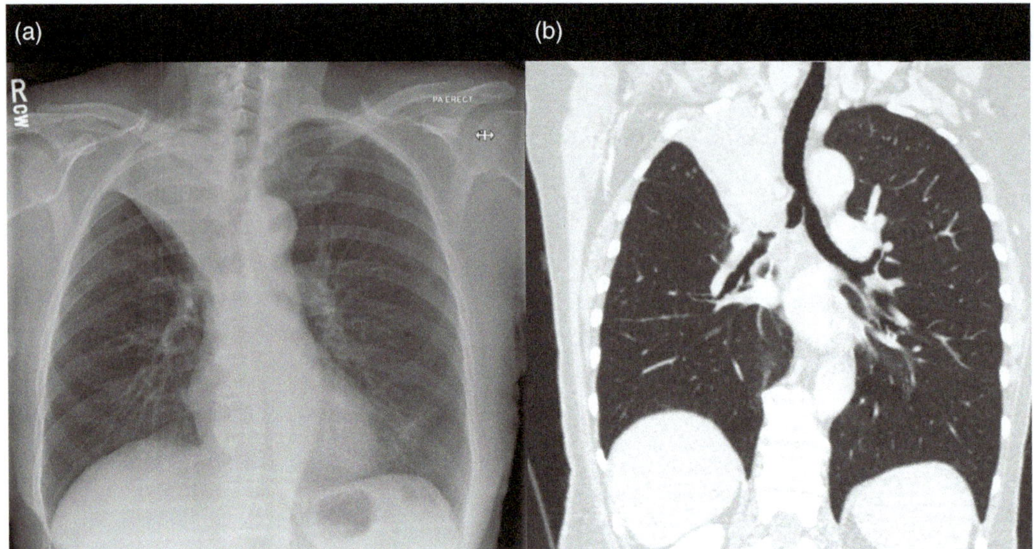

FIGURE 13.1 Patient A investigations. (a) CXR. (b) Coronal CT thorax on lung windows.

13.3 Key Radiology Review

13.3.1 Technical

Positron emission tomography is a branch of nuclear medicine. This modality differs from X-ray and CT, as a radioactive substance is introduced inside the patient, making them temporarily radioactive. The radiation emitted from the patient is detected by a scanner and this gives information about where the radioactive substance is collecting in the body.

In PET, glucose is labelled with a radioactive substance, creating (18)F-fluorodeoxyglucose (FDG). This acts in the body in the same way as regular glucose, travelling to areas of increased metabolic activity. The patient is then put in a scanner which detects the emitted radiation, allowing us to see areas of high metabolic activity. These are described as avid or 'hot' areas.

Highly metabolic organs like the brain and myocardium are avid on PET. Likewise, the kidneys and bladder will show avidity, as the FDG will be excreted by the urinary system.

Most cancers will also be avid, owing to their high metabolic rate. PET scanning improves the detection of malignancy, in the primary tumour, nodal metastasis and distant organ metastases.

In practice, the PET scan is usually combined with a CT, with the images being layered over one another. This gives metabolic information from the PET, combined with anatomical detail from the CT (Figure 13.2).

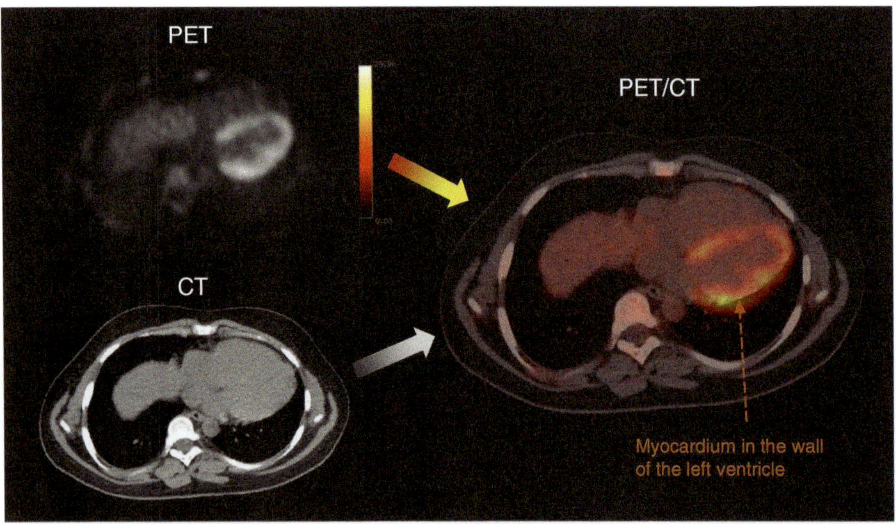

FIGURE 13.2 Axial PET, CT and PET/CT scan through the heart. The PET component shows areas of high metabolic activity, such as the myocardium of the left ventricle, but has relatively poor resolution. The CT scan has excellent resolution with exquisite anatomical detail. When these are combined, the CT scan remains as a grey scale and the PET component is given a colour scale (in this case dark red to bright yellow). The combined PET/CT has the benefit of excellent anatomical detail from the CT and metabolic information from the PET.

13.3.2 Correlating the Anatomy with the CT Image

13.3.2.1 Airway The trachea should be central in the neck and mediastinum with a rounded appearance on the axial slices. If the scan is taken in expiration then the trachea may have a flattened posterior surface (Figure 13.3).

13.3.2.2 CT Interpretation System Interpretation of a CT follows a similar system to that used for the CXR. However, there is the added complication of choosing the window level and anatomical plane for each step. Accurate lung assessment requires the use of the lung window. The anatomical plane use is more subjective, so experiment with looking at various parts of anatomy in the different planes and see which ones you prefer. Suggestions are given in Box 13.1.

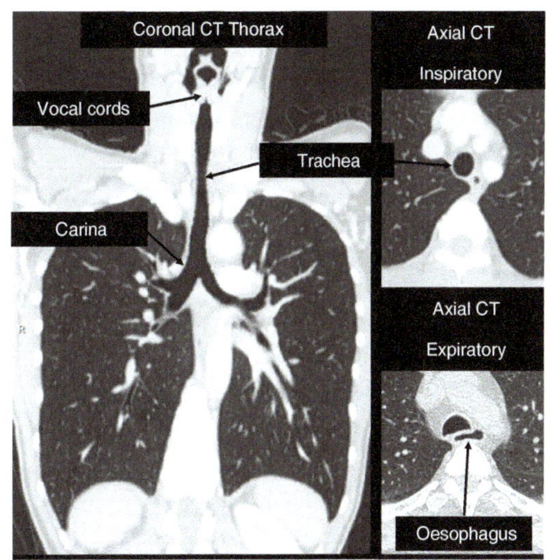

FIGURE 13.3 Coronal CT thorax and axial CT thorax on lung windows. Note the change in shape of the trachea on expiration.

Box 13.1 | AABCD Approach to Thoracic CT Interpretation

	Focus	Recommended CT window Anatomical plane notes	Comment
A	**Airway**	**Lung window** Axial plane is good to see the cross-section of the airways. Coronal plane can be used to check ET tube tip position (Figure 13.3).	Check the trachea and central airways down to the segmental bronchi. These should contain air with no foreign bodies or mucous plugging. Check if the trachea is central.
	Apparatus	Various windows can be used, depending on the apparatus of interest and whether there is bright contrast in the vessels (Figure 13.4)	Check for lines and tubes (e.g. endotracheal, nasogastric, chest drains, central lines). Confirm correct positioning and check for associated iatrogenic complications.
B	**Breathing**	**Lung window** Look for a pneumothorax (Respiratory Chapter 10 – Thoracic Stabbing) and lung pathology. **Mediastinal window** for a haemothorax/pleural effusion (Respiratory Chapter 11 – Blunt Chest Trauma) *Coronal plane* can give an overview of both lungs, mimicking the CXR view.	Check the lungs and pleural spaces for anything which will impair oxygenation. If there is opacification in the lung, try to decide what lung pattern is seen (Respiratory Chapter 12 – Acute Dyspnoea).
C	**Circulation**	**Soft tissue window** **(also called the mediastinal window)**	Check the heart and mediastinal vessels. If there is IV contrast, the vessels will be bright (white). Pulmonary embolus will appear as a filling defect (Cardiac Chapter 17 – Acute Shortness f Breath). Check for pericardial effusion (Cardiac Chapter 14 – Penetrating Trauma).
D	**Dense tissue**	**Bone window** *Coronal plane* gives an optimal view of the shoulders and ribs. *Sagittal plane* is best for reviewing the spine (see Spine Chapters 23 and 25).	Check the bones for fractures and bone lesions (Respiratory Chapter 11 – Blunt Chest Trauma). Check the line location when contrast is being used (Figure 13.4).

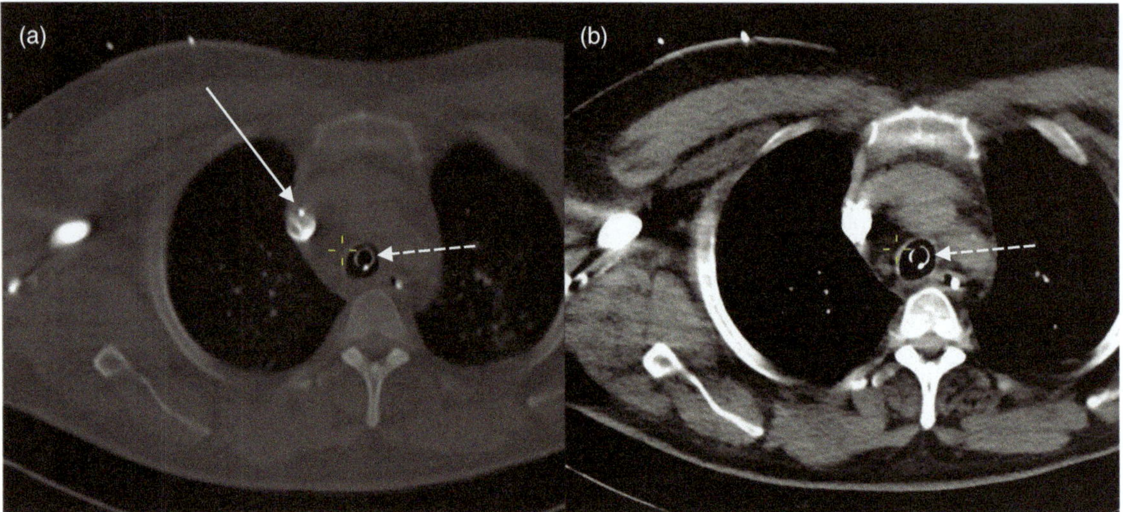

FIGURE 13.4 Axial CT thorax on bone windows (a) and mediastinal windows (b). The central line is obscured by the dense contrast on the mediastinal windows. Bone windows allow differentiation between the line (white arrow) and the contrast. Both images show the endotracheal tube (dashed arrow) lying in the trachea. *Source:* Driscoll et al. (2023)/John Wiley & Sons.

13.4 Review of the Clinical Case

- How does lung collapse present?
- What are the clinical features of lung collapse?
- What are the red flags for lung cancer?
- What secondary features can cancer patients exhibit?
- What is your differential diagnosis?

13.5 Review of the Clinical Case

- Why is CT indicated?
- What is your system for interpreting these images?
- What further imaging may be necessary?

13.5.1 Differential Diagnosis

There are several red flags for lung cancer in this case.

- Smoker over 40 with:
  - unexplained cough
  - unexplained dyspnoea
  - unexplained weight loss
  - unexplained appetite loss
  - unexplained fatigue.

Others include unexplained haemoptysis and chest pain.

13.5.2 CXR

Given these red flags, an urgent CXR is indicated (Figure 13.5). This shows a right upper lobe collapse.

13.5.3 Lung Collapse

Lung collapse and atelectasis are interchangeable terms. They refer to the flattening of the alveoli following their air content being expelled. This is in contrast to consolidation, which is the addition of fluid into the alveolar sacs. Hence, with consolidation, the lung volume is maintained (Respiratory Chapter 12).

Lung collapse/atelectasis can occur in a small region of the lung (Figure 13.6) or an entire lobe (Figures 13.5 and 13.8–13.10). As these have different causative factors. they need to be differentiated.

Causes of lobar lung collapse/atelectasis.

- *Inadequate inspiration* (Figure 13.6): this is commonly seen in postsurgical patients as well as the obese and elderly who are relatively immobile.
- *Extrinsic compression*: by fluid or gas in the pleural space. See haemothorax (Respiratory Chapter 11) and pneumothorax (Respiratory Chapter 10).
- *Obstruction of the airway*: this could be a benign process such as mucous plug in asthmatics or aspirated foreign body. It could also be caused by an endobronchial tumour (Figures 13.5 and 13.7).

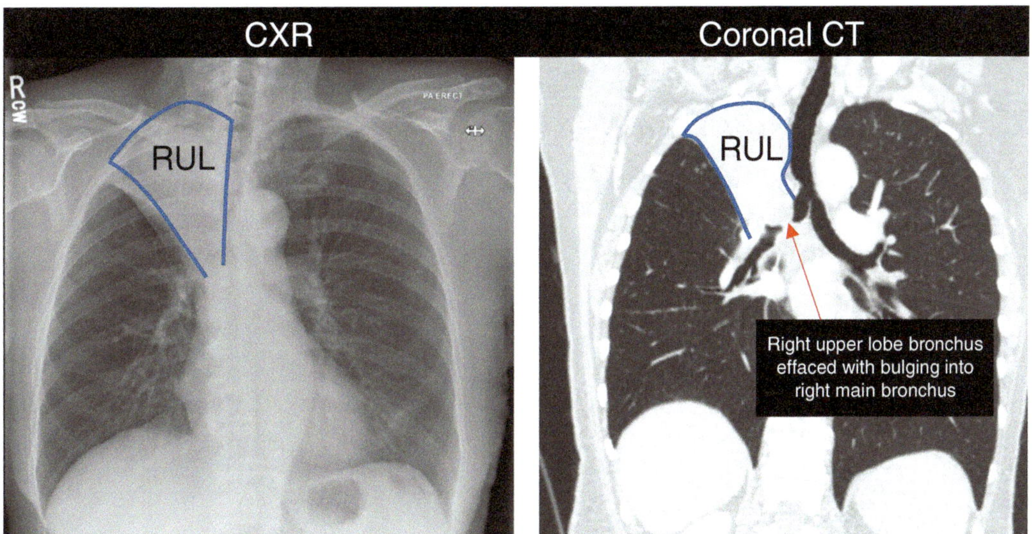

FIGURE 13.5 Patient A. CXR and coronal CT thorax on lung windows. There is complete collapse of the right upper lobe. On CXR this appears as a wedge-shaped area of increased density. Note also the deviation of the trachea due to the reduced lung volume pulling the mediastinum to the right. The central airways are better assessed on CT. The right upper lobe bronchus cannot be seen and there is bulging into the right main bronchus suspicious for a mass.

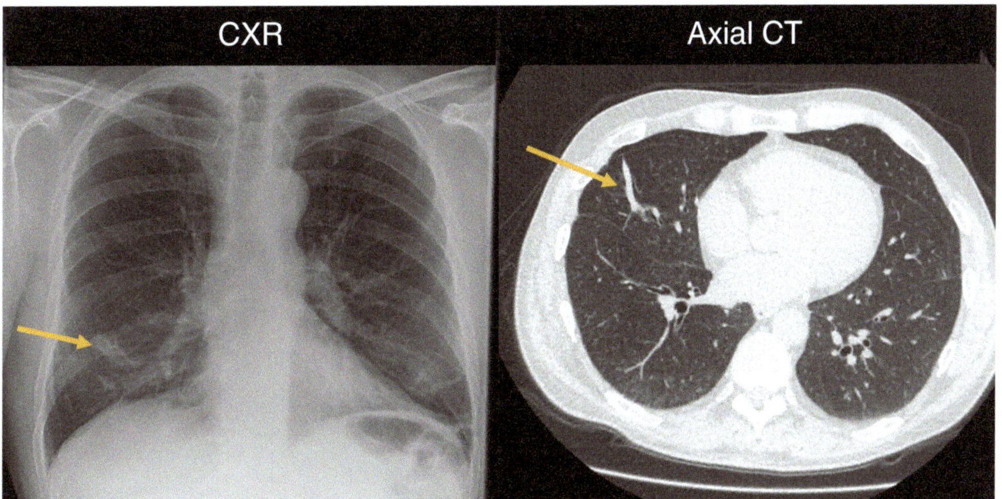

FIGURE 13.6 CXR and axial CT on lung windows. There is a small area of linear atelectasis in the right middle lobe (orange arrows). This is usually the result of poor inspiratory effort, rather than endobronchial obstruction.

- *Fibrosis of the lung parenchyma*: damage to the lung parenchyma can cause it to reduce in volume; this is usually a diffuse process affecting both lungs, rather than a focal lobar collapse.

In Chapters 10 and 11, we encountered lung collapse due to external compression by a haemothorax/pneumothorax. In this current case the lung collapse is caused by obstruction of the central airway. Given the concurrent red flags, the lesion is most likely to be a primary lung malignancy.

However, confirming this diagnosis on CT can be difficult because the tumour and collapsed lung can have similar densities. Therefore, a useful approach is to combine PET with CT to show areas of high glucose

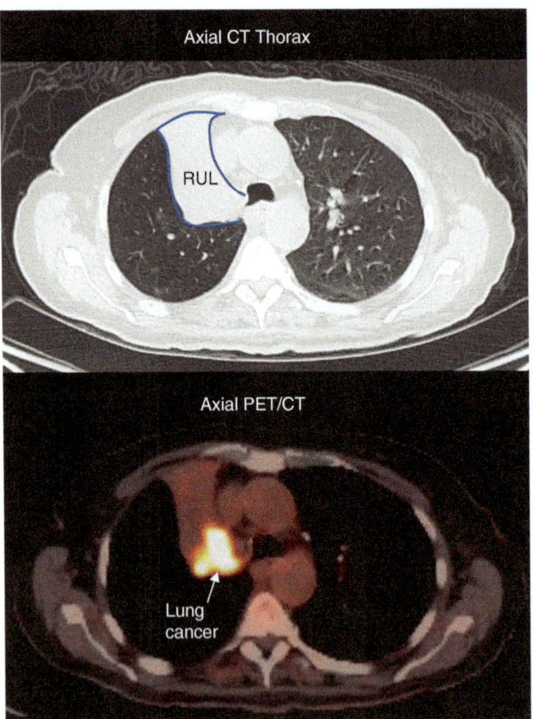

FIGURE 13.7 Patient A. Axial CT thorax on lung windows and axial PET/CT. The collapsed right upper lobe has a uniform density on the standard CT scan, making it difficult to ascertain whether the cause is an obstructing tumour or simple mucus. The PET shows avidity at the origin of the right upper lobe bronchus, confirming a tumour as the cause. This patient underwent endobronchial ultrasound biopsy to characterise the tumour histologically.

metabolism. This allows better delineation of the tumour (Figure 13.7) and increases sensitivity for metastases (not shown).

13.6 Final Diagnosis

Right upper lobe collapse secondary to endobronchial lung cancer.

13.6.1 Lung Collapse in Other Lobes

The appearance of lung collapse varies depending on the lobe involved. This is because each lobe will shrink in a unique way. There are two main features they all have in common. The first is an increase in density in the region of the collapse. The second is loss of silhouette in structures adjacent to the collapse.

There will also be secondary features of volume loss in the ipsilateral hemithorax. This could manifest as elevation of the diaphragm, crowding of the ribs or shift in the mediastinum to the affected side.

13.6.1.1 Right Middle Lobe Collapse (Figure 13.8)

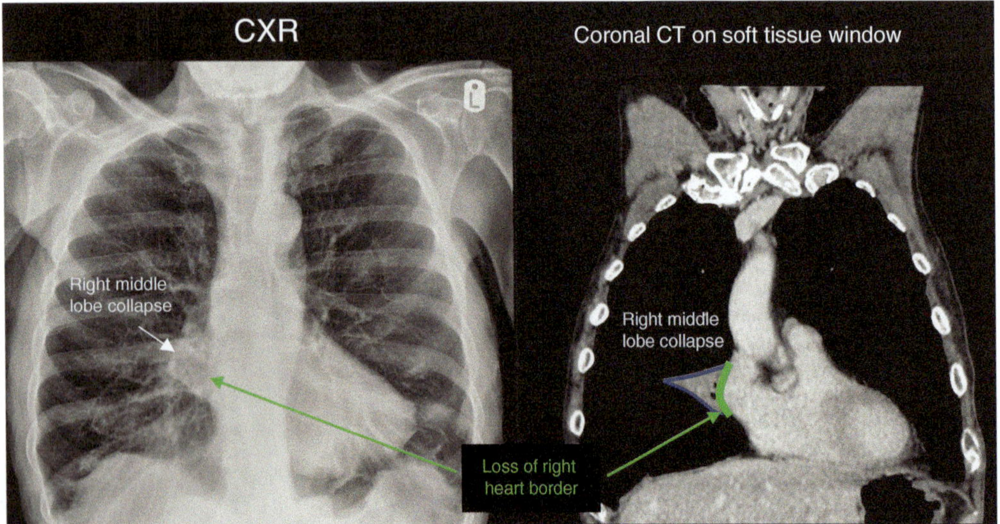

FIGURE 13.8 CXR and coronal CT thorax on soft tissue window. This shows a middle lobe collapse. The lobe is significantly reduced in volume with increased density. As the middle lobe abuts onto the right heart border, collapse results in a loss of the right heart border silhouette on CXR.

13.6.1.2 Left Upper Lobe Collapse (Figure 13.9)

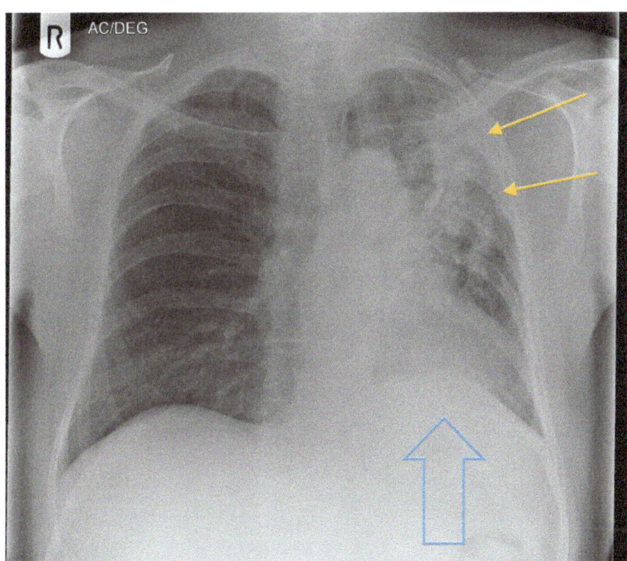

FIGURE 13.9 A CXR showing left upper lobe collapse. There is increased density in the left upper zone (orange arrows). Note the elevation of the left hemidiaphragm due to volume loss (hollow blue arrow).

13.6.1.3 Left Lower Lobe Collapse (Figure 13.10) The

left lower lobe is a notoriously difficult collapse to spot. This is because it collapses behind the heart. However, the above principles still apply.

13.7 Take-home Message – Imaging in Lung Cancer

- Urgent CXR is indicated if there are red flags for lung cancer.
- If CXR shows lung collapse then PET/CT may be required to look for an underlying malignancy.

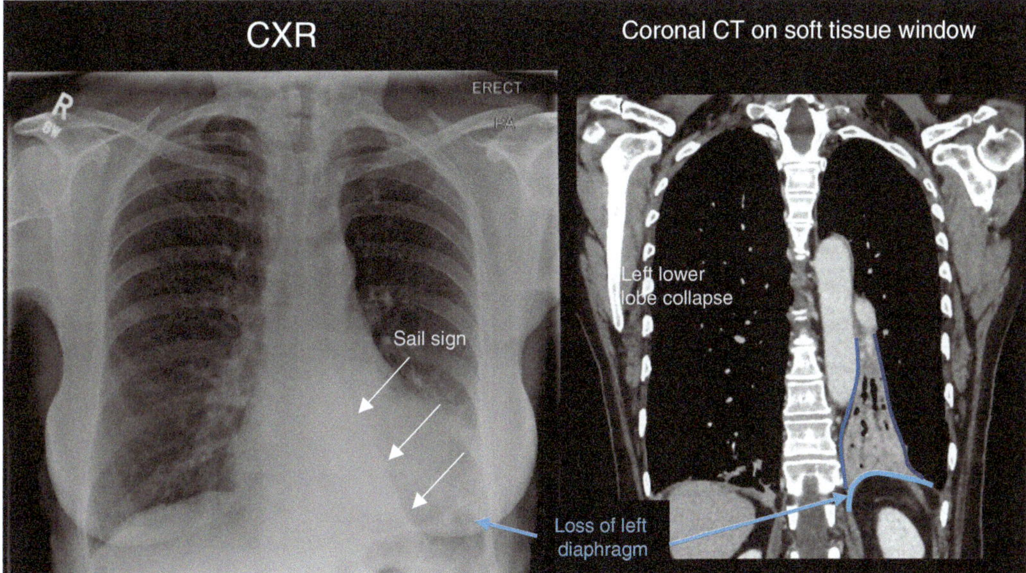

FIGURE 13.10 CXR, coronal CT thorax on soft tissue window. Left lower lobe collapse. There is increased density behind the heart with an apparent second left heart border line (white arrows). This is termed the 'sail sign'. As the left lower lobe abuts onto the diaphragm, collapse will result in loss of the diaphragm silhouette on CXR (compare to the right diaphragm).

Further Resources

NICE. Lung and pleural cancers – recognition and referral. https://cks.nice.org.uk/topics/lung-pleural-cancers-recognition-referral

Cardiac Section

CHAPTER 14

Penetrating Trauma

Joshua Lauder[1], Sanjay Banypersad[2], and Peter Driscoll[3]

[1] *East Lancashire Hospitals NHS Trust, University of Central Lancashire and University of Manchester, UK*
[2] *East Lancashire Hospitals NHS Trust, Blackburn, UK*
[3] *School of Medicine and Dentistry, University of Central Lancashire, Preston, UK*

14.1 Primary Case

14.1.1 Presentation

A 22-year-old male is brought to the Emergency Department by ambulance having been stabbed in the chest 60 minutes before. The knife was removed by a bystander at the scene.

14.1.2 Primary Survey

Airway:

- Clear.

Breathing:

- Respiratory rate 24 rpm.
- SpO_2 94% (10 l/min O_2).
- Left anterior chest wound.
- Dull percussion note on the left chest.
- Air entry on the right is greater than on the left side.
- Distended neck veins.

Circulation:

- No other wounds.
- HR 120 bpm.
- BP 90/50 mmHg.
- Difficult to hear the heart sounds.

Disability:

- Pupils equal and reacting to light and accommodation.
- Glasgow Coma Scale: Eye opening 4; Verbal response 5; Motor response M6.

PMH: nothing of note.

14.1.3 Point-of-care Ultrasound

In view of this presentation, a bedside ultrasound was performed (Figure 14.1).

14.1.4 CT

This was followed up with a major trauma CT with IV contrast (Figure 14.2).

> ### Clinical Case Questions
> - What structures are at risk?
> - What is your differential diagnosis? Why?
> - Why should an US be performed?
> - Why should a CT be performed?
> - What is your system for interpreting the imaging?

14.2 Radiology Self-assessment

14.2.1 Technical

- What is the role of ultrasound in trauma?
- When should a CT scan be performed in trauma?

Diagnostic Imaging and Anatomy in Acute Care, First Edition. Edited by Joshua Lauder and Peter Driscoll.
© 2025 John Wiley & Sons Ltd. Published 2025 by John Wiley & Sons Ltd.
Companion website: www.wiley.com/go/DiagnosticImaginginAcuteCare

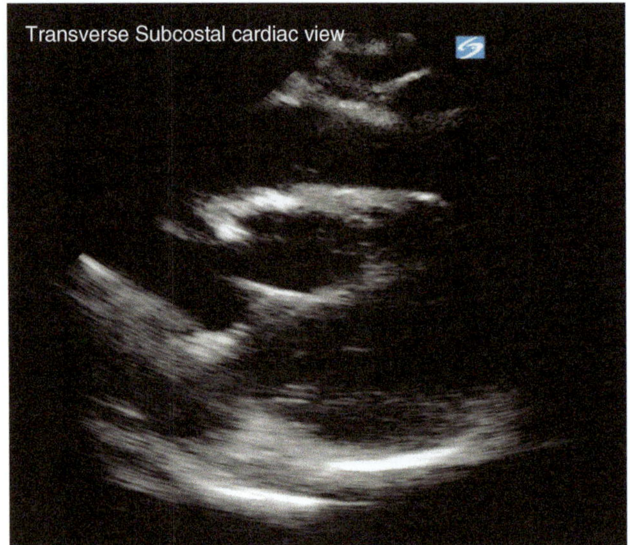

FIGURE 14.1 Subcostal ultrasound of the heart.

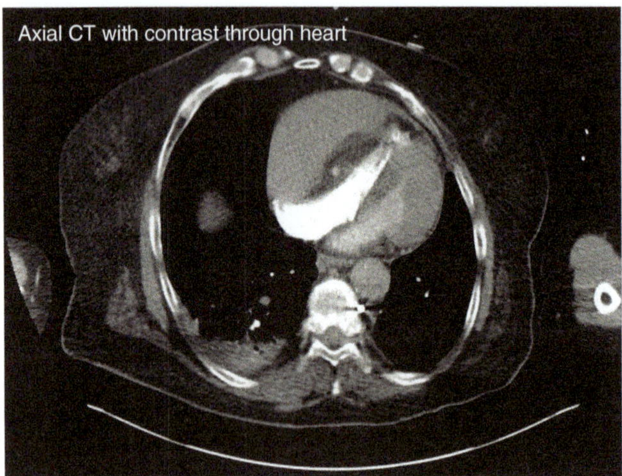

FIGURE 14.2 Axial CT, with contrast on soft tissue windows at the level of the heart.

14.2.2 Correlation to Anatomy on Ultrasound

- How is the subcostal ultrasound view obtained?

14.2.3 Correlating Anatomy to CT

- What does the pericardium look like on CT?
- Where are the pericardial recesses on CT?

14.3 Key Radiology Review

14.3.1 Technical Aspects

14.3.1.1 Ultrasound in Trauma As portable ultrasound is typically available in the Emergency Department or even prehospital setting, it is often the first imaging modality used in the trauma pathway. It is good for positively diagnosing conditions such as pneumothorax, haemothorax, pericardial effusions and haemoperitoneum so immediate management can begin.

However, ultrasound is operator dependent and has reduced sensitivity for certain traumatic conditions like retroperitoneal haemorrhage. Therefore, a normal ultrasound scan does not exclude a life-threatening injury. Furthermore, it is unlikely to locate the source of the bleeding in the chest or abdomen. For these reasons, it is not relied upon as a primary imaging modality in trauma.

14.3.1.2 CT in Trauma Computed tomography scans are the quickest and most comprehensive way to diagnose life-threatening and limb-threatening injuries. As traumatic injuries are time critical, it is important that the management pathway includes early CT scanning to guide further management. As some injuries can be hidden from physical examination and can cross different anatomical cavities (e.g. a penetrating abdominal injury can traverse the diaphragm and cause a pneumothorax), CT should include everything from the top of the head to mid-thighs.

In view of the area involved, the patient is exposed to significant ionising radiation, with known long-term cancer risk. This risk can be justified when there is a suspected life-threatening or limb-threatening,injury but should be avoided in minor trauma.

14.3.2 Rationale for IV Contrast

Intravenous contrast is always administered in trauma CT. This is discussed in Abdo Chapter 18.

14.3.3 Correlation to Anatomy on Ultrasound

14.3.3.1 Pericardium The pericardium surrounds the heart and has two layers (Figure 14.3). The tough fibrous outer layer prevents overexpansion of the cardiac chambers. In contrast, the slippery serous layer adheres to the fibrous layer (parietal) and the surface of the heart (visceral) and facilitates cardiac movement. These two serous layers have a potential cavity called the pericardial space. This usually contains 15–50 ml of ultrafiltrate plasma.

14.3.3.2 Subcostal View Ultrasound is usually the first-line investigation if pericardial abnormality is suspected, especially cardiac tamponade or pericardial effusion. This is because it is readily available and does not use ionising radiation. The downside is that the ribs and sternum limit the acoustic window, meaning that loculated pericardial effusions or lesions can be missed. Transoesophageal

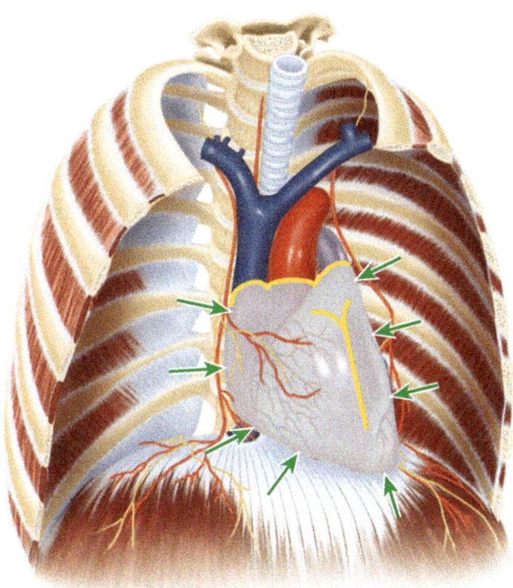

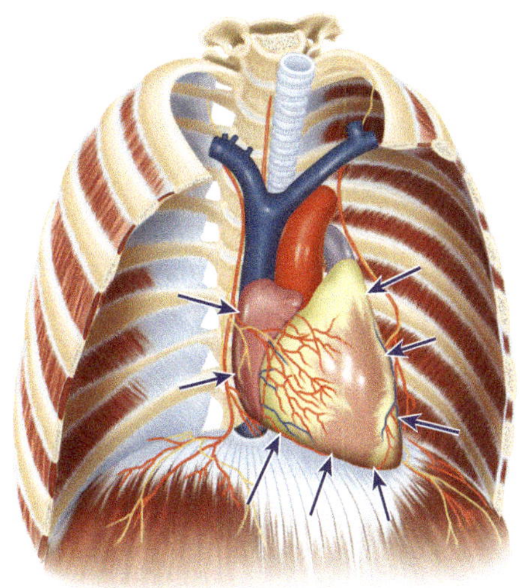

FIGURE 14.3 Anterior view of the mediastinum. The attachments of the fibrous pericardium are shown on the left image (green lines). In the right image the fibrous pericardium has been removed, revealing the heart covered with the visceral serous pericardium.

echocardiogram can overcome some of these limitations but is an invasive procedure.

There are four standard US views of the heart. As will be discussed in the next chapter, each has its own particular strengths in identifying cardiac features and functions. The subcostal (also called subxiphoid) view is considered in this chapter as it shows the dependent area of the pericardium where fluid collects initially.

The subcostal view is obtained with the patient lying supine (Figure 14.4).

(a)   Probe positioning

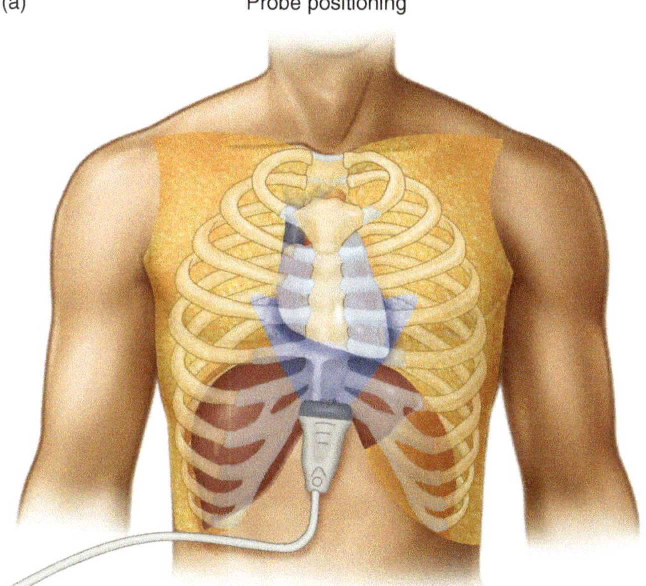

(b)   Subcostal view

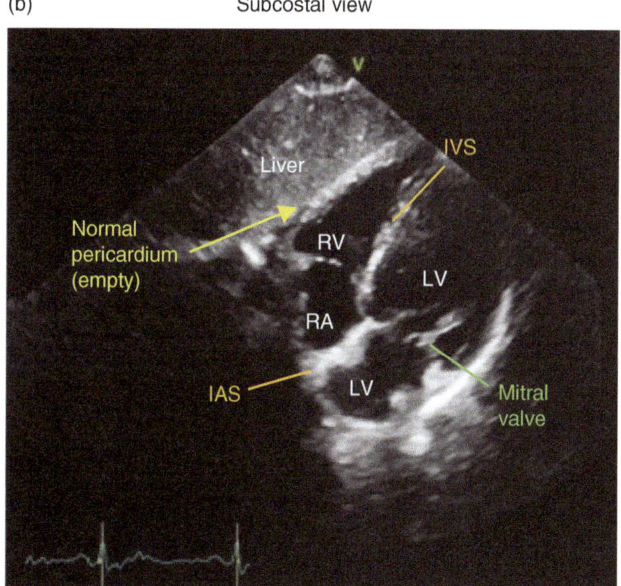

FIGURE 14.4 (a) Position of ultrasound probe when obtaining a subcostal view. (b) Transverse subcostal ultrasound image. RV, right ventricle; LV, left ventricle; RA, right atrium; LA, left atrium; IVS, interventricular septum; IAS, interatrial septum. The right ventricular myometrium and liver should be abutting each other. If there is a pericardial effusion, this space will fill with fluid (Figure 14.6).

14.4 Correlating the Anatomy with the CT Image

The normal pericardium is difficult to appreciate on CT (Figure 14.5). However, it becomes more obvious when an effusion is present (Figure 14.7).

14.5 Review of the Clinical Case

In light of the previous description, review this case again and try and answer the following questions.

- Why is US indicated?
- Why is CT indicated?
- What is your final diagnosis and definitive management?

14.5.1 Differential Diagnosis

A penetrating trauma patient could have injuries crossing multiple anatomical cavities. Therefore any stabbing in the central chest, upper abdomen or thoracic region may involve the pleural spaces, pericardiac space or peritoneum. Along with clinical examination, early imaging is necessary for rapid diagnosis to be made.

- eFAST (Extended Focused Assessment using Sonography in Trauma) is a standardised, effective approach for quickly checking for life-threatening trauma conditions.
- Trauma CT is the definitive investigation. This should not be delayed while trying to perform ultrasound.

14.5.2 Subcostal Ultrasound

Patient A has a large pericardial effusion. In the context of a penetrating trauma, this is likely to be haemopericardium (Figure 14.6).

14.5.3 Trauma CT

Computed tomography confirms the haemopericardium with significant compression of the ventricles resulting in

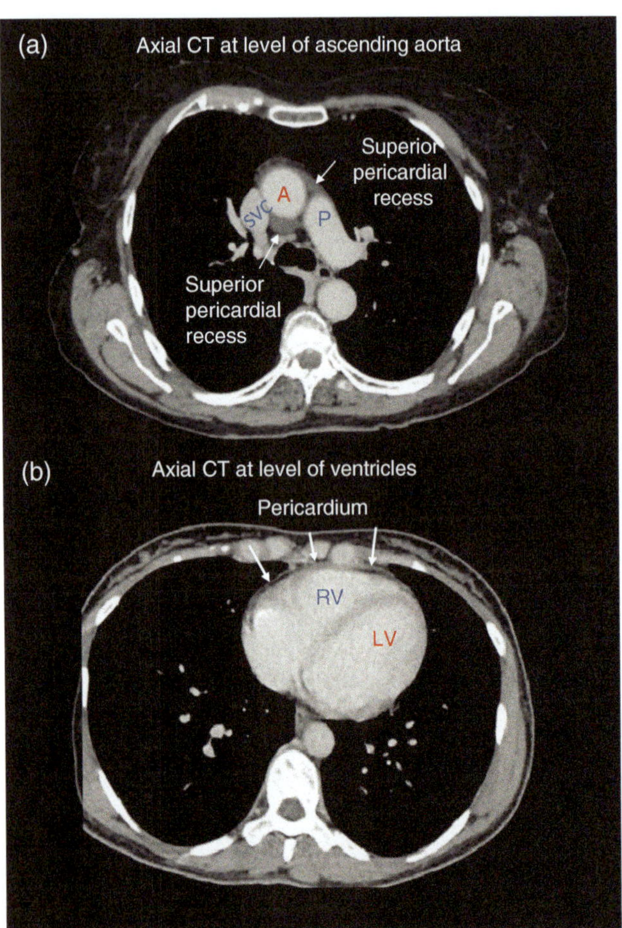

FIGURE 14.5 Axial CT with contrast, soft tissue windows. (a) Level of ascending aorta. A, aorta; P, pulmonary trunk; SVC, superior vena cava. The superior pericardial recess will be visible in almost all patients as it usually contains several millilitres of fluid. It surrounds the ascending aorta and pulmonary trunk and is also referred to as the transverse coronary sinus. (b) Level of ventricles. LV, left ventricle; RV, right ventricle. The normal pericardium is seen anterior to the heart as a pencil-thin white line. At the left heart border and posterior border, the pericardium is closely applied to the myocardium so it is more difficult to distinguish. The pericardium is easier to see on CT if patients have more visceral fat.

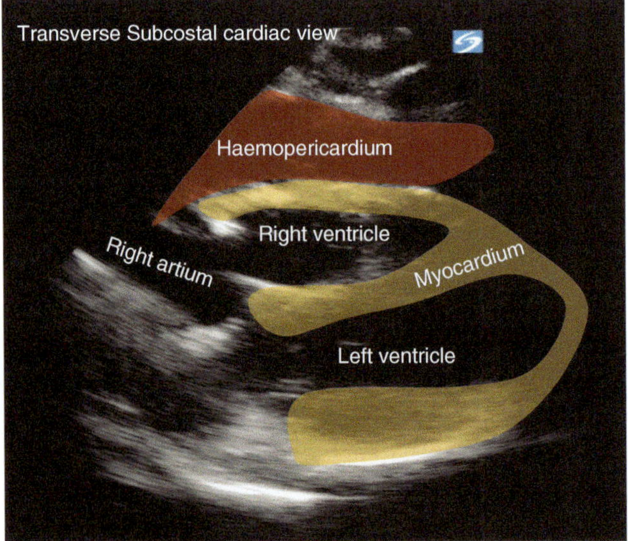

FIGURE 14.6 Patient A. Subcostal ultrasound of the heart. The ventricles are easily identified due to the thick-walled myocardium. The right atrium is also visible. Pericardial fluid can be identified surrounding the heart.

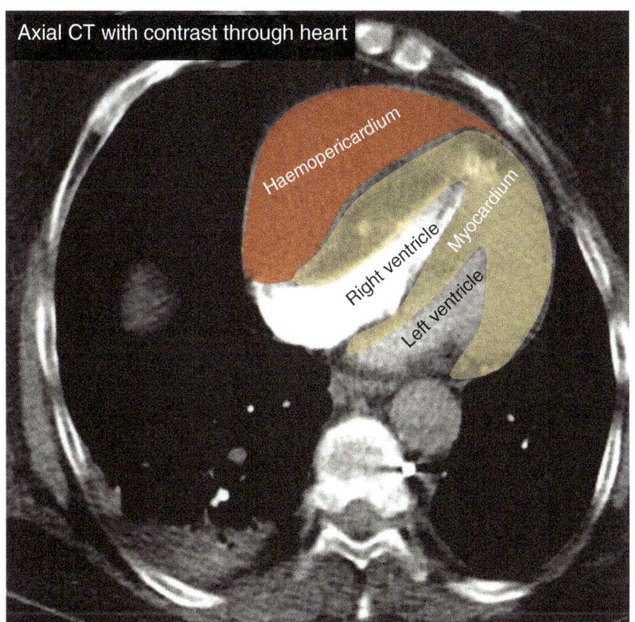

FIGURE 14.7 Patient A. Axial CT on soft tissue windows through the heart. There is a haemopericardium (red shading) resulting in cardiac tamponade. The right and left ventricles are compressed by the pericardial fluid. This reduces both preload and cardiac output. The stab injury is not visible on this CT slice.

cardiac tamponade (Figure 14.7). CT is important in this instance so that other injuries to the aorta and abdominal contents can be excluded.

14.5.4 Management

Cardiac tamponade requires urgent pericardiocentesis by an appropriately trained professional. This is usually performed with ultrasound guidance. Surgical drainage may be required if it is difficult to access or the blood clot cannot be evacuated with a needle.

14.6 Take-home Message – Pericardiac Imaging

- Echocardiography is the first-line investigation for the pericardium and has a high sensitivity for detecting pericardial effusions.
- In trauma an eFAST scan includes a subcostal view of the pericardium to exclude cardiac tamponade.
- CT is the definitive imaging modality in trauma.

Further Resources

Goldstein, J.A. (2004). Cardiac tamponade, constrictive pericarditis, and restrictive cardiomyopathy. *Curr Probl Cardiol* 29: 503–567.

Spodick, D.H. (2003). Acute cardiac tamponade. *N Engl J Med* 349 (7): 684–690.

CHAPTER 15

Chronic Shortness of Breath

Joshua Lauder[1], Sanjay Banypersad[2], Kris Phillips[3], and Peter Driscoll[3]

[1]East Lancashire Hospitals NHS Trust, University of Central Lancashire and University of Manchester, UK
[2]East Lancashire Hospitals NHS Trust, Blackburn, UK
[3]School of Medicine and Dentistry, University of Central Lancashire, Preston, UK

15.1 Primary Case

15.1.1 Presentation

A 65-year-old male presented to the Emergency Department.

15.1.1.1 History of Presenting Complaint He has been unwell for several months, feeling breathless on exertion. Today he suddenly became more breathless while walking to work. He is pale and coughing up pink froth.

PMH

- No relevant PMH.
- No regular medication.

OE

- Lips and fingertips are cyanosed.
- Ankles are swollen.
- Neck veins are swollen.
- Crackles over lower chest on auscultation.
- Pansystolic murmur in the axilla.

Modified early warning signs (MEWS):

- Respiratory rate 18 bpm.
- SpO_2 98% (15 l/min oxygen via a facemask with a reservoir).
- Temp 37.7 °C.
- HR 110 bt/min.
- BP 105/85 mmHg.
- Alert.

15.1.2 Echocardiogram

In view of this presentation, a dedicated echocardiogram was performed (Figure 15.1).

Clinical Case Questions

- What structures are at risk?
- What is your differential diagnosis? Why?
- Why should an US be performed?
- Why should a CT be performed?
- What is your system for interpreting the imaging?

15.2 Radiology Self-assessment

15.2.1 Technical

- How does echocardiography differ from standard ultrasound?
- What is colour Doppler?

15.2.2 Correlation to Anatomy on Echocardiography

- How is the four-chamber view obtained?
- How is the short axis parasternal view obtained?
- How is the long axis parasternal view obtained?

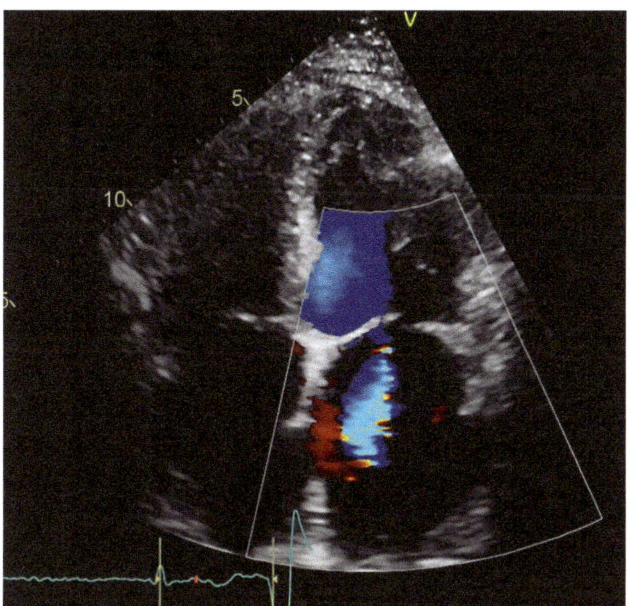

FIGURE 15.1 Echocardiogram. Four-chamber view. Still image in systole with colour Doppler.

15.3 Key Radiology Review

15.3.1 Technical Aspects

15.3.1.1 Echocardiogram   An echocardiogram is performed with a dedicated cardiac probe. Its small footprint makes it ideal for getting between the ribs to provide an unimpeded view of the heart. The frequency is relatively low (1.5–7.5 Hz) as 20 cm of depth is often required.

In contrast to ultrasound elsewhere in the body, echocardiograms are recorded as videos through the cardiac cycle, usually with a synchronous ECG trace. This allows for a functional assessment of the valves and cardiac output.

The four standard views are:

- Four-chamber view
- short axis parasternal view
- long axis parasternal view
- subcostal view (covered in the previous chapter).

15.3.1.2 Colour Doppler This is used as an adjunct to show blood flow through the heart and valves. Flow towards the probe appears orange, while flow away appears blue (Pelvis Chapter 8 – Figure 8.2).

15.4 Correlation to Anatomy on Echocardiography

For all views the patient is positioned so they are lying slightly on their left side with left upper limb elevated.

15.4.1 Four-chamber View

This provides an excellent view for the atrioventricular valves and ventricular contraction (Figure 15.2).

15.4.2 Short Axis Parasternal View

This view allows ventricular contraction to be assessed (Figure 15.3).

15.4.3 Long Axis Parasternal View

This is a good way to get an overview of heart function, particularly the left sided chambers and valves (Figure 15.4).

15.5 Review of the Clinical Case

- Why is echocardiography indicated?
- What is your final diagnosis and definitive management?

15.5.1 Differential Diagnosis

- A new murmur in the presence of cardiac or respiratory symptoms is an indication for an echocardiogram.
- Mitral regurgitation is the most common valve disease. Primary mitral regurgitation (also called degenerative or organic) occurs due to structural abnormality with the valve. Secondary mitral regurgitation (also called functional or ischemic) occurs due to left ventricular wall motion abnormalities.
- Patients with chronic mitral regurgitation develop left atrial enlargement which can trigger atrial fibrillation (AF).
- A history of rheumatic fever or untreated streptococcus infection may raise the possibility of mitral valve stenosis. This often occurs 20–40 years after the initial illness. In these patients mitral stenosis and regurgitation often co-exist as the valve becomes scarred and dysfunctional.
- Acute bacterial endocarditis should be excluded. These patients often have fever and septicaemia. There will usually be risk factors such as intravenous drug use or being immunocompromised.

(a) Probe positioning – four chamber view

(b) Anatomical four chamber view

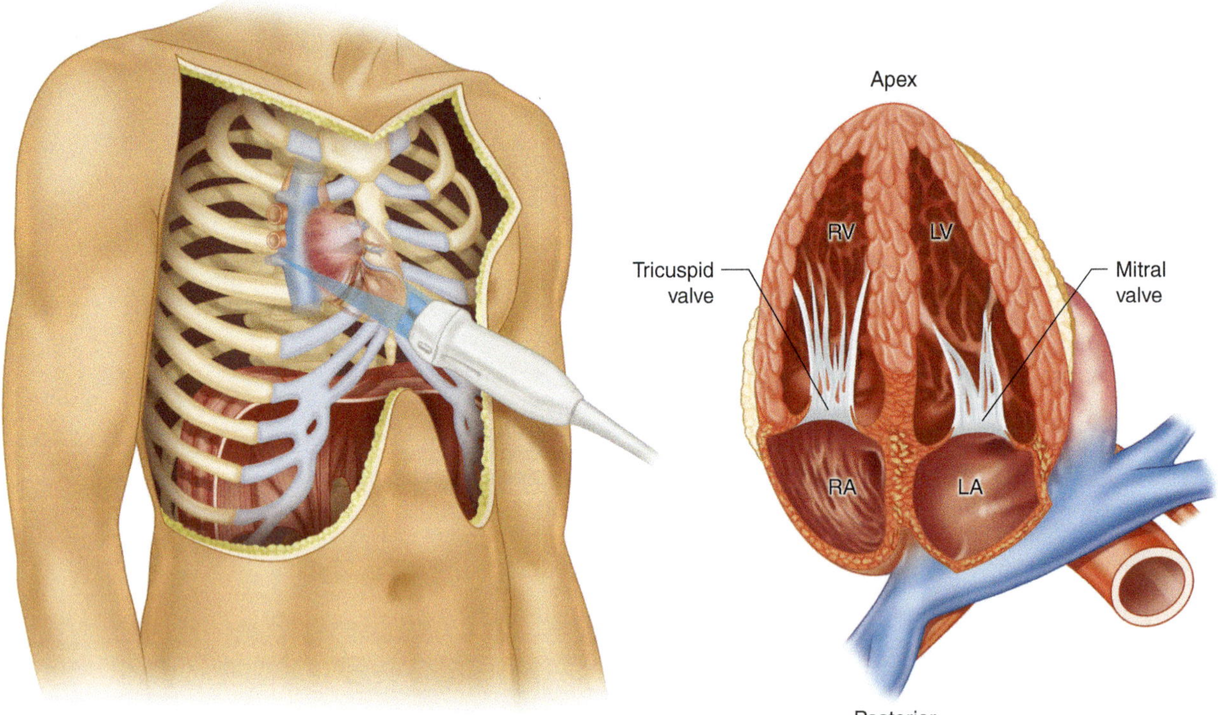

(c) Four chamber view (systole)

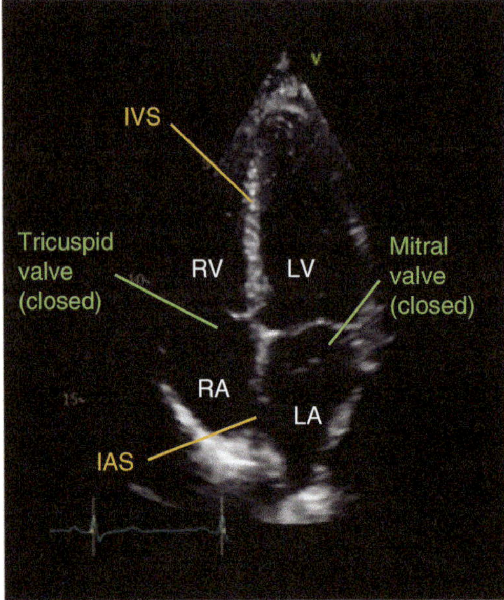

FIGURE 15.2 (a) Position of ultrasound probe when obtaining a four-chamber view. (b) Anatomical four-chamber view. (c) Four-chamber ultrasound view. The atrioventricular (tricuspid and mitral) valves are seen side on and need to be observed through the cardiac cycle. These valves should be closed during systole. RV, right ventricle; LV, left ventricle; RA, right atrium. LA, left atrium; IVS, interventricular septum; IAS, interatrial septum.

(a) Probe positioning – short axis parasternal

(b) Anatomical short axis parasternal view

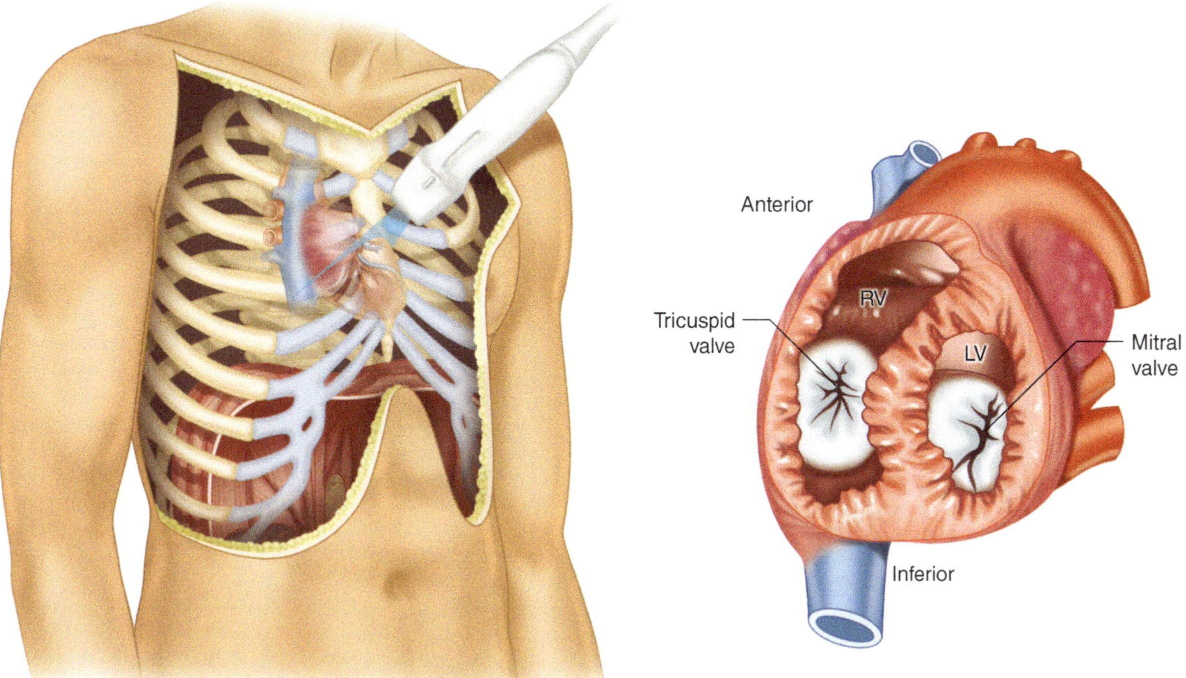

(c) Short axis parasternal view (diastole)

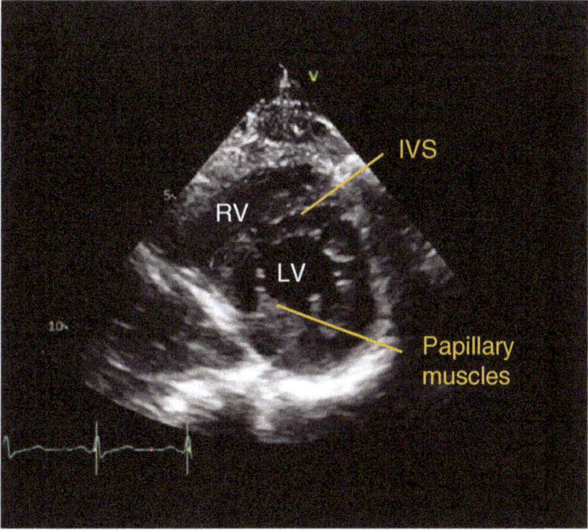

FIGURE 15.3 (a) Position of ultrasound probe when obtaining a short axis parasternal view. (b) Anatomical short axis parasternal view. (c) Short axis parasternal ultrasound view. The ventricles can be traced in the short axis from apex to base and should demonstrate circumferential contraction during the cardiac cycle. RV, right ventricle; LV, left ventricle; IVS, interventricular septum.

(a) Probe positioning – long axis parasternal view

(b) Anatomical parasternal long axis view

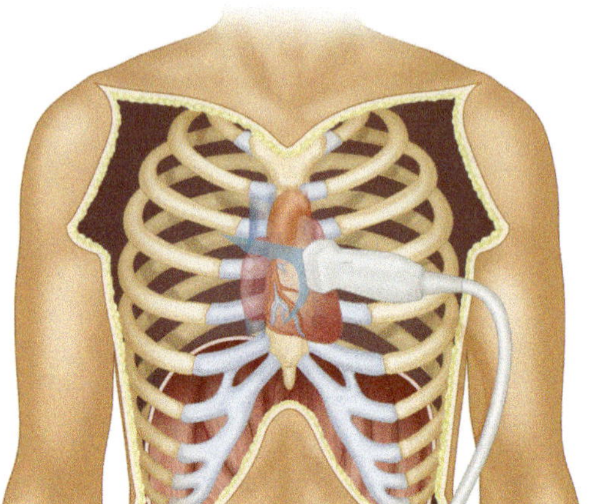

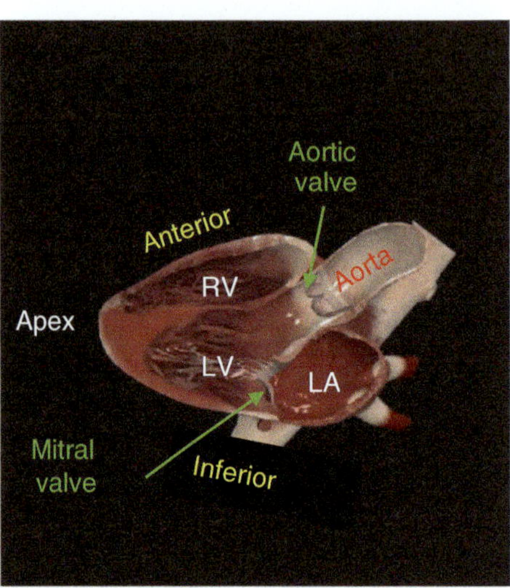

(c) Long axis parasternal view (diastole)

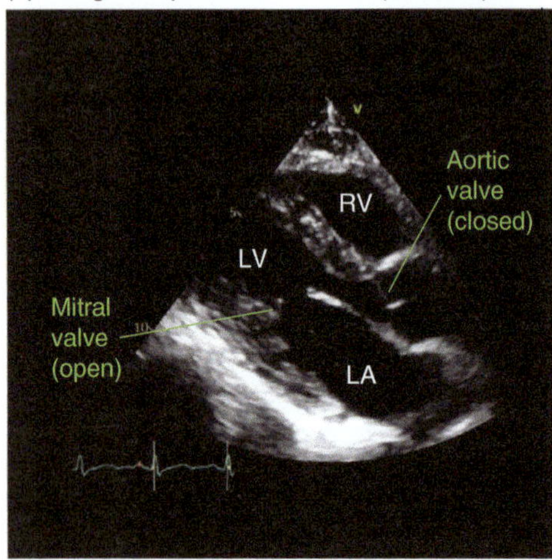

FIGURE 15.4 (a) Position of ultrasound probe when obtaining a long axis parasternal view. (b) Anatomical long axis parasternal view. (c) Long axis parasternal view. This view shows the relationship between the left-sided valves. During diastole the mitral valve is open and aortic valve is closed. This is reversed during systole. LV, left ventricle; LA, left atrium; RV, right ventricle.

15.5.2 Echocardiogram

Patient A has mitral regurgitation as demonstrated on the four-chamber view (Figure 15.5). This is best appreciated in systole in Doppler mode, where a regurgitative jet is shown flowing back into the left atrium.

15.5.3 Management

Patients with severe mitral regurgitation with associated symptoms or left ventricular dysfunction will be offered a valve replacement. If there is coexisting AF, this is also a relative indication for surgery.

15.6 Take-home Message – Valve Imaging

- Echocardiography is the gold standard for assessing the valves.
- Transoesophageal echocardiography shows the valve in more detail but is invasive. It is therefore usually reserved for overcoming artefacts (e.g. acoustic shadowing from mitral annulus calcification).
- Cardiac CT may be performed as part of the work-up for valve replacement, for example prior to transcatheter aortic valve implantation.
- In special cases cardiac MRI may be used to assess valve disease.

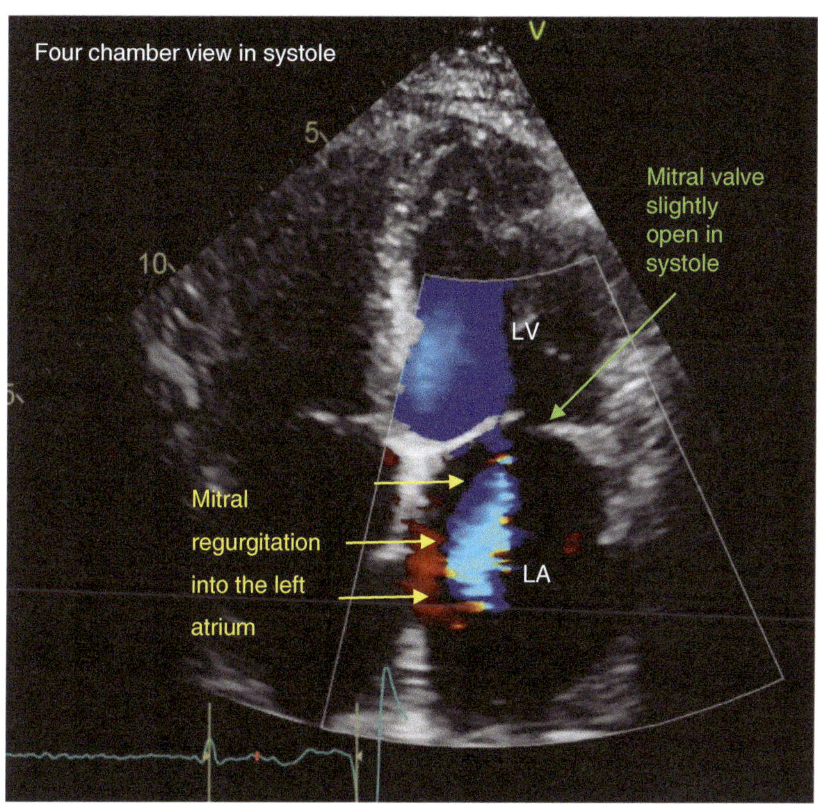

FIGURE 15.5 Patient A echocardiogram. Four-chamber view of the heart. Still image in systole with colour Doppler. There is mitral regurgitation.

Further Resources

Apostolidou, E., Maslow, A.D., and Poppas, A. (2017). Primary mitral valve regurgitation: update and review. *Glob Cardiol Sci Pract* 2017 (1): e201703.

CHAPTER 16

Chest Pain and Syncope

Joshua Lauder[1], Sanjay Banypersad[2], and Peter Driscoll[3]

[1] East Lancashire Hospitals NHS Trust, University of Central Lancashire and University of Manchester, UK
[2] East Lancashire Hospitals NHS Trust, Blackburn, UK
[3] School of Medicine and Dentistry, University of Central Lancashire, Preston, UK

16.1 Primary Case

16.1.1 Presentation

A 51-year-old male presents to the Emergency Department having fainted after going to the toilet. This was followed by constricting pain in the chest which lasted 30 minutes but has now resolved.

16.1.1.1 History of Presenting Complaint Upon further questioning, it emerges that these symptoms have been ongoing for several months prior to presentation and are worse during exertion.

PMH

- Hypertension, taking amlodipine 10 mg and ramipril 10 mg.
- Smokes 10 cigarettes a day.

OE

- Lungs clear.
- Normal capillary refill.

Modified early warning signs (MEWS):

- Respiratory rate 14 bpm.
- SpO_2 94% on room air.
- Temp 37.7 °C.
- HR 85 bt/min.
- BP 138/98 mmHg.
- Alert.

16.1.2 Resting 12-lead ECG

- Normal, no ST elevation or depression, no T wave inversion.

16.1.3 Bloods

- Full blood count – normal.
- Urea and electrolytes – normal.
- Liver function tests – normal.
- Troponin I – 15 ng/l (normal range 0–58).

16.1.4 CT Coronary Angiography

In view of this presentation an outpatient CT coronary angiography was performed (Figure 16.1).

Clinical Case Questions

- What is your differential diagnosis? Why?
- When is cardiac CT indicated?
- What is your system for interpreting the imaging?

Diagnostic Imaging and Anatomy in Acute Care, First Edition. Edited by Joshua Lauder and Peter Driscoll.
© 2025 John Wiley & Sons Ltd. Published 2025 by John Wiley & Sons Ltd.
Companion website: www.wiley.com/go/DiagnosticImaginginAcuteCare

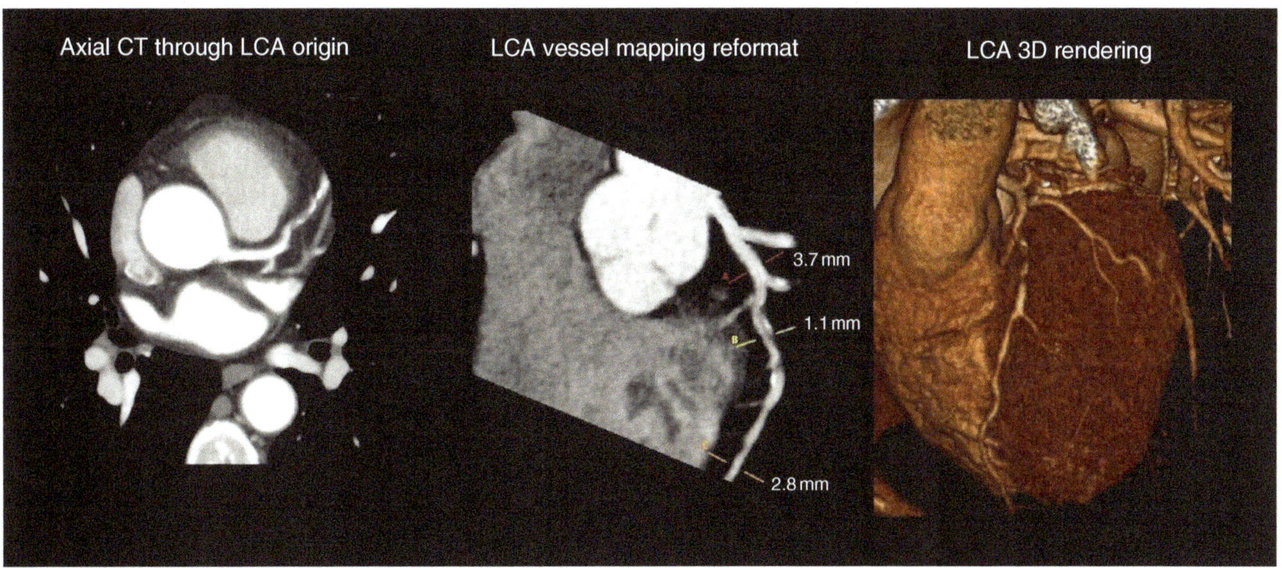

FIGURE 16.1 ECG-gated cardiac CT of the left coronary artery (LCA).

16.2 Radiology Self-assessment

16.2.1 Technical

- How is CT coronary angiography performed?
- What are the advantages of this technique compared to standard CT?

16.2.2 Correlation to Anatomy on Cardiac CT

- What does the coronary anatomy look like on cardiac CT?

16.3 Key Radiology Review

16.3.1 Technical Aspects

16.3.1.1 CT Coronary Angiography (ECG-gated Cardiac CT) Cardiac assessment is limited on standard CT by motion artefact of the beating heart (Figure 16.2). This is overcome on modern CT scanners by using ECG gating. This enables the scan to be performed during diastole so there is no movement of the coronary arteries, myometrium or valves. Contrast is also given in the angiographic phase to provide optimum opacification of the coronary arteries.

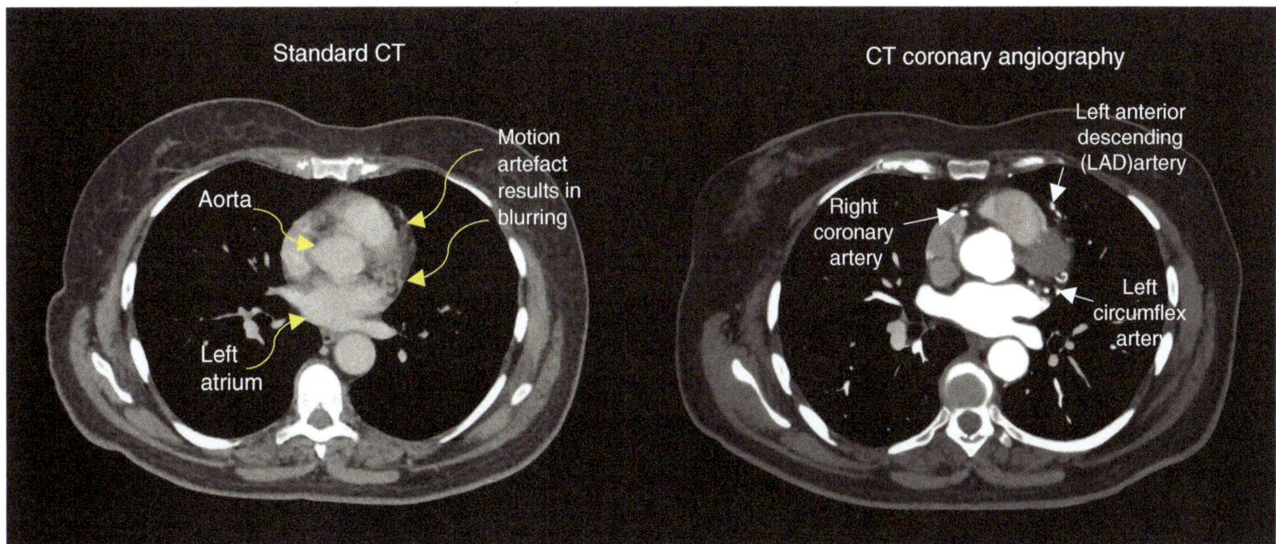

FIGURE 16.2 Axial CT thorax on soft tissue windows. Standard CT with portal venous phase contrast (left); there is blurring around the aorta and coronary vessels due to the beating of the heart. CT coronary angiography (right); ECG gating allows the scan to be performed in diastole while the heart is still. Note how crisp the cardiac chambers and coronary vessels appear.

16.4 Correlation to Anatomy on Cardiac CT

16.4.1 Coronary Circulation

The coronary arteries arise from the aortic root. The left coronary artery (LCA) splits into the left anterior descending (LAD) (also called the anterior interventricular artery) and circumflex. The right coronary artery (RCA) travels in the atrioventricular groove around the right side of the heart (Figure 16.3).

The most common coronary anatomy arrangement is **right heart dominance** (~85%) (Figure 16.4). This is when the posterior descending artery (PDA) (also termed posterior interventricular artery) is supplied by the RCA. In **left heart dominance** (~10%), the PDA is supplied by the circumflex artery (a branch of the LCA). A small proportion of people (~5%) have dual supply of PDA, termed **co-dominance**.

The heart dominance has relevance for ischaemic territories and implications for treatment.

16.4.2 Vessel Mapping

This is a software package which allows automatic tracing of the vessels on CT angiogram. It provides a 2D slice which follows the vessel, allowing accurate assessment of calibre changes and length of stenosis (Figure 16.7).

16.5 Review of the Clinical Case

- Why is cardiac CT indicated?
- What is your final diagnosis and definitive management?

16.5.1 Differential Diagnosis

- This patient presents with transient symptoms of cardiac sounding chest pain on exertion. There are no ECG changes or rise in cardiac enzymes. This suggests stable angina.
- All patients with stable angina should have outpatient cardiac CT.

(a) CT 3D Superior view

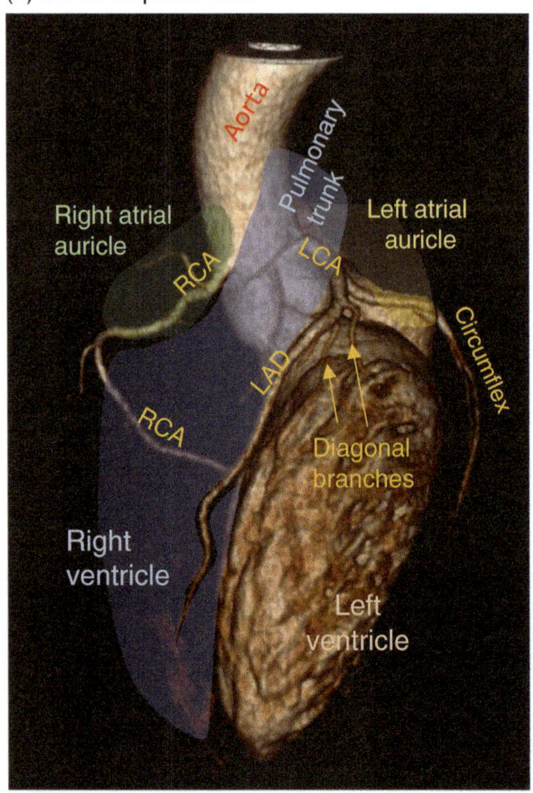

(b) 3D anatomy Superior view

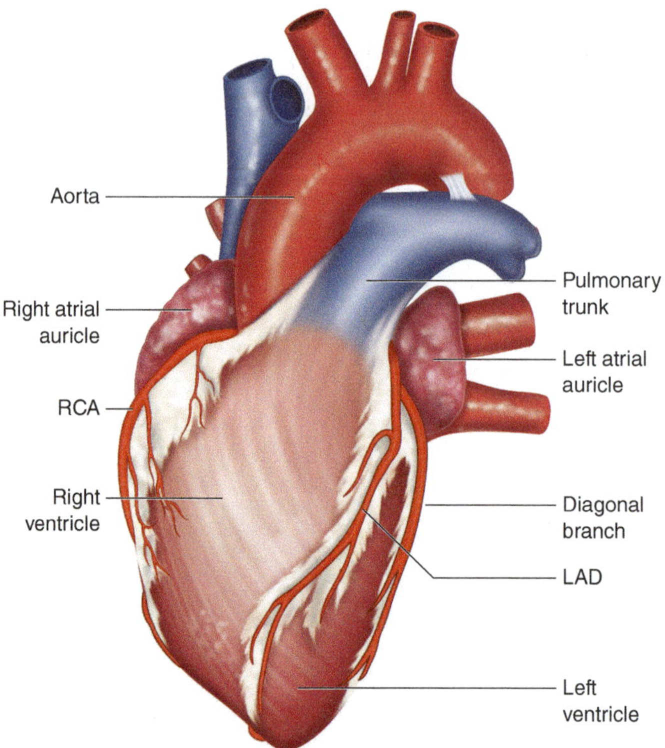

FIGURE 16.3 (a) 3D rendering of the cardiac CT. Superior view. Right ventricle, right atrial auricle and left atrial auricle have been superimposed. (b) 3D cardiac anatomy. Superior view. The origins of the left coronary artery and circumflex artery are hidden from view by the pulmonary trunk and left atrial auricle respectively. LCA, left coronary artery; LAD, left anterior descending artery; RCA, right coronary artery.

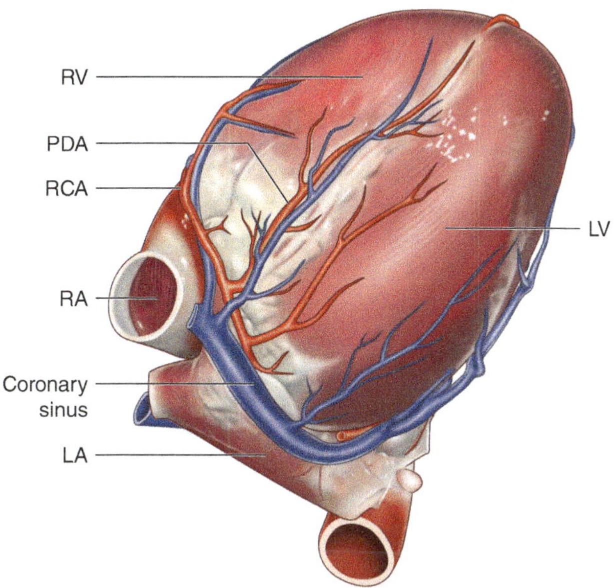

FIGURE 16.4 (a) 3D rendering of cardiac CT. Inferior view. This demonstrates a right heart dominance as the PDA originates from the RCA. In practice, however, the coronary arteries and cardiac valves are usually viewed using ECG-gated cardiac CT imaging (Figure 16.5). The coronary sinus collects most of the venous blood from the myocardium. It lies on the inferior surface of the atrioventricular groove and drains into the right atrium (see Figure 16.6). (b) 3D rendering of cardiac CT. Inferior view. The right atrium is seen through the IVC. RA, right atrium; RV, right ventricle; LV, left ventricle; LA, left atrium, PDA, posterior descending artery.

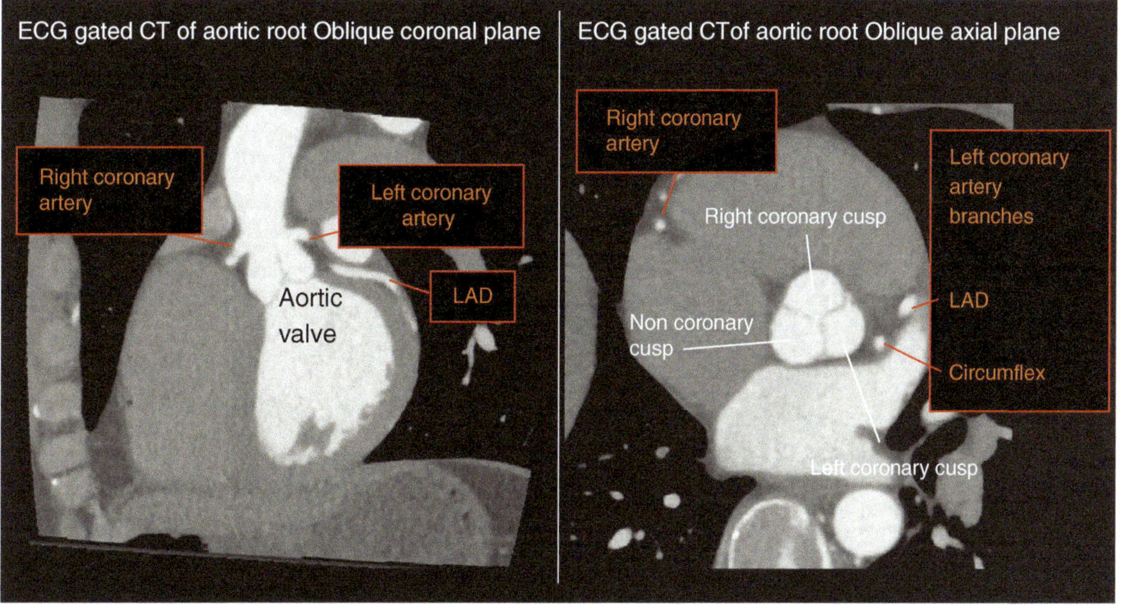

FIGURE 16.5 ECG-gated cardiac CT of aortic root, oblique coronal plane (left) and oblique axial plane (right). LAD, left anterior descending artery. The right and left coronary arteries arise from the right coronary cusp and left coronary cusp respectively.

- Acute coronary syndrome (ACS) should always be excluded before a diagnosis of stable angina is made. ACS comprises three conditions: ST elevation myocardial infarction (STEMI), non-ST elevation myocardial infarction (NSTEMI) and unstable angina.

  - STEMI – complete and persistent blockage of the coronary artery resulting in myocardial necrosis with ST elevation on ECG.
  - NSTEMI and unstable angina – partial or intermittent blockage of the coronary artery which usually results

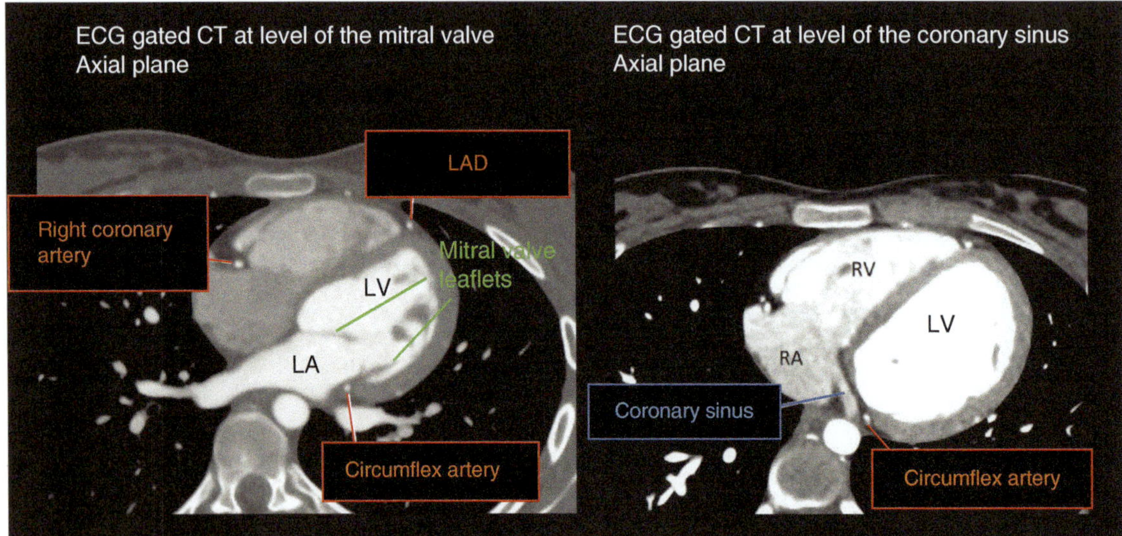

FIGURE 16.6 ECG-gated cardiac CT at the level of the mitral valve (left) and coronary sinus (right). Here the relative position of the major coronary arteries can be appreciated. The coronary sinus lies along a similar course to the circumflex artery before draining into the right atrium. LAD, left anterior descending artery; LV, left ventricle; LA, left atrium; RV, right ventricle; RA, right atrium.

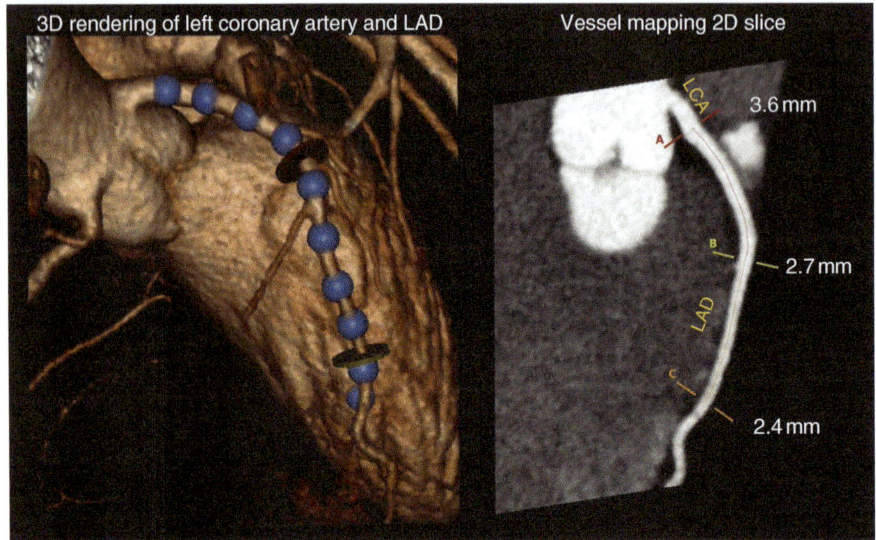

FIGURE 16.7 Vessel mapping on cardiac CT in a normal patient. This is the left coronary artery (LCA) continuing into the left anterior descending artery (LAD). The circumflex and diagonal artery branches are not visible in this plane. It is normal for arteries to narrow distally but there should be no focal stenosis.

in myocardial necrosis in NSTEMI but not in unstable angina. The ECG may show ST-segment depression and T-wave inversion, but can be normal. High-sensitivity blood tests for serum troponin are used to differentiate between NSTEMI and unstable angina.

16.5.2 Cardiac CT

This patient has a severe stenosis in the LAD. This involves the midportion, distal to the D1 diagonal branch origin (Figure 16.8).

16.5.3 Management

The finding of a severe proximal coronary artery stenosis with symptoms is an indication for catheter angiography. This allows flow/pressure studies across the stenosis to be performed.

Definitive management in this case involved percutaneous coronary intervention (PCI) with stenting (Figure 16.9).

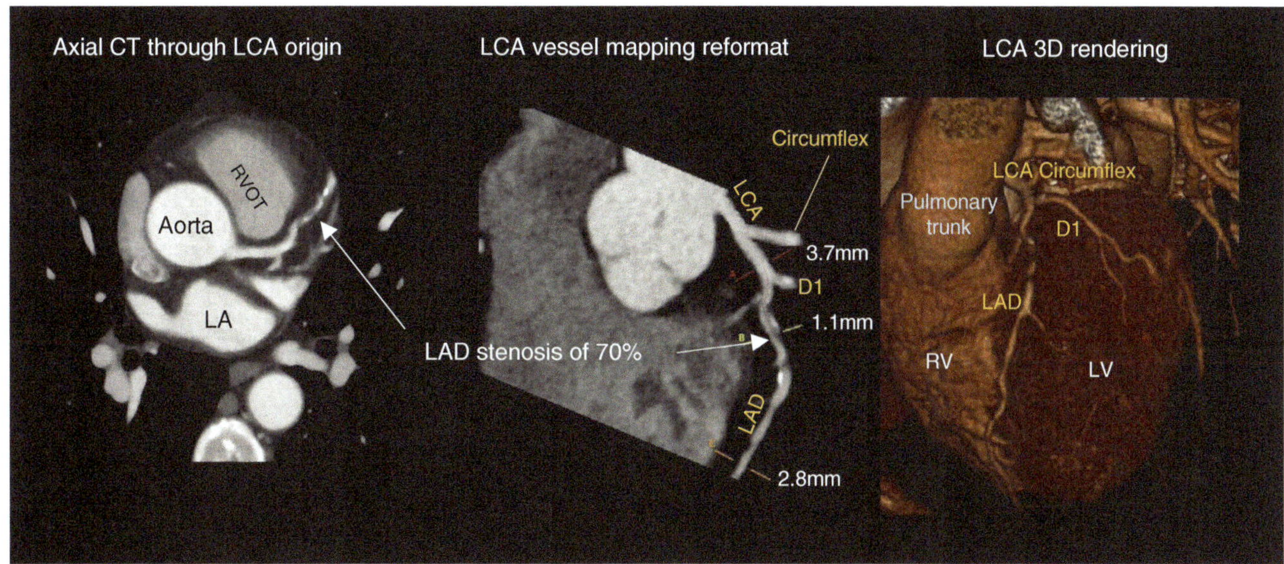

FIGURE 16.8 Patient A. ECG-gated cardiac CT of the left coronary artery (LCA). There is calcification in the wall of the LAD with a stenosis. The vessel mapping reformat allows measurement of the vessel calibre at different points. This can be used to calculate the relative stenosis and length of the affected segment. These values have implications for treatment. LA, left atrium; LV, left ventricle; RV, right ventricle; RVOT, right ventricular outflow tract; LAD, left anterior descending artery; D1, first diagonal branch artery.

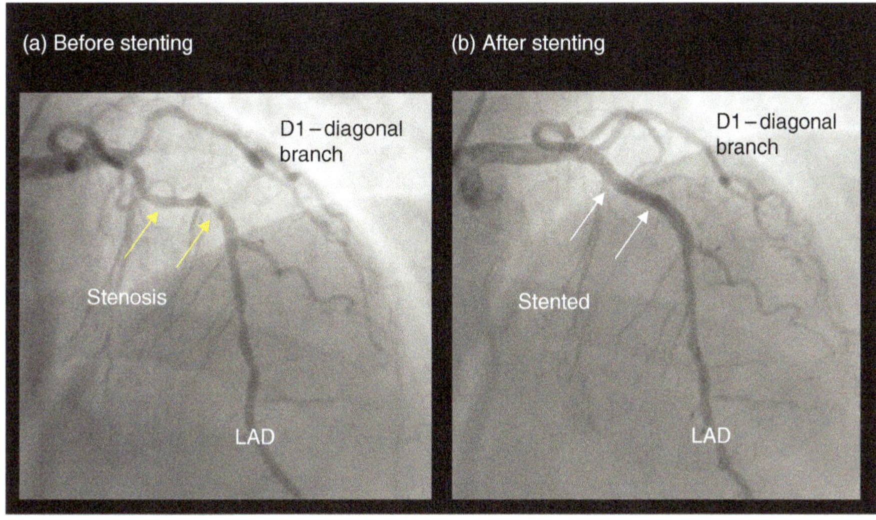

FIGURE 16.9 PCI images (a) before stenting (b) after stenting. Note the poor filling of the LAD, correlating with the CT scan. After stenting this segment of the artery has widened.

16.6 Take-home Message – Ischaemic Heart Disease Imaging

- Patients with acute coronary syndrome will tend to go for catheter angiography, as this allows immediate treatment with PCI.

- Cardiac CT is the first-line investigation in all patients with angina symptoms (both atypical or typical) or those who are asymptomatic with ECG changes suggestive for ischaemia.

Further Resources

Aricatt, D.P., Prabhu, A., Avadhani, R. et al. (2023). A study of coronary dominance and its clinical significance. *Folia Morphol* 82 (1): 102–107.

Moss, A.J., Williams, M.C., Newby, D.E., and Nicol, E.D. (2017). The updated NICE guidelines: cardiac CT as the first-line test for coronary artery disease. *Curr Cardiovasc Imaging Rep* 10 (5): 15.

National Institute for Health and Clinical Excellence (2016). Chest pain of recent onset: assessment and diagnosis of recent onset chest pain or discomfort of suspected cardiac origin (update). CG95. London: National Institute for Health and Clinical Excellence. The updated UK guideline that uses cost–utility analysis to recommend CTCA as the first-line investigation for suspected symptomatic coronary artery disease.

National Institute of Health and Care Excellence (2020). Acute coronary syndrome. NICE guideline 185. www.nice.org.uk/guidance/ng185.

CHAPTER 17

Acute Shortness of Breath

Joshua Lauder[1], Aleksandr Valkov[2], and Peter Driscoll[3]

[1] *East Lancashire Hospitals NHS Trust, University of Central Lancashire and University of Manchester, UK*
[2] *Salford Royal Hospital and University of Central Lancashire, Salford, UK*
[3] *School of Medicine and Dentistry, University of Central Lancashire, Preston, UK*

17.1 Primary Case

17.1.1 Presentation

A 54-year-old male presents to the Emergency Department with a one-day history of increasing shortness of breath and chest pain on breathing.

17.1.1.1 History of Presenting Complaint Upon questioning, he describes badly spraining his ankle five weeks ago and having to rest it. Ten days ago he did a six-hour drive for work and has noticed the ankle becoming increasingly painful over the last week.

PMH

- No past medical history.
- No regular medication.

OE

- Visibly breathless.
- Lungs clear.
- Right ankle and calf are swollen and hot to touch. There is pedal oedema and dilated superficial veins are present.
- No bony tenderness or deformity was detected.

Modified early warning signs (MEWS):

- Respiratory rate 24 bpm.
- SpO_2 93% on room air.
- Temp 36.7 °C.

- HR 112 bt/min.
- BP 115/85 mmHg.
- Alert.

17.1.2 Resting 12-lead ECG

- Sinus tachycardia, right bundle branch block (RBBB) and T-wave inversion V1–3.

17.1.3 Bloods

- WBC 9×10^9/l (3–11×10^9/l).
- CRP 4 mg/l (0–5 mg/l).

17.1.4 Chest X-ray

- Normal.

17.1.5 CTPA

Considering these findings, a CT pulmonary angiogram (CTPA) was arranged (Figure 17.1).

Clinical Case Questions
- What is your differential diagnosis? Why?
- When should CTPA be performed?
- What is your system for interpreting the imaging?

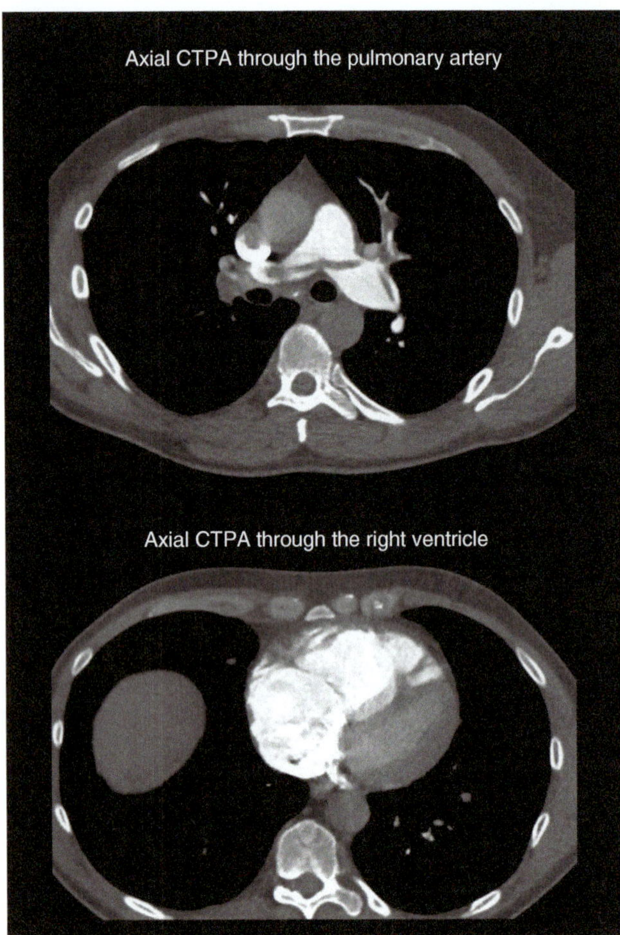

FIGURE 17.1 Patient A. CTPA. Axial on soft tissue windows. (Top) Level of the pulmonary artery. (Bottom) Level of the right ventricle.

17.2 Radiology Self-assessment

17.2.1 Technical

- How does CTPA differ from standard CT?
- What is V/Q scanning?

17.2.2 Correlation to Anatomy on CTPA

- What does the pulmonary artery look like on a CTPA?
- How can you assess for heart strain on a CTPA?

17.3 Key Radiology Review

17.3.1 Technical Aspects

17.3.1.1 CTPA CTPA is performed in the same way as a standard CT thorax with contrast, the only difference being that the contrast phase is relatively early (around 30 seconds after

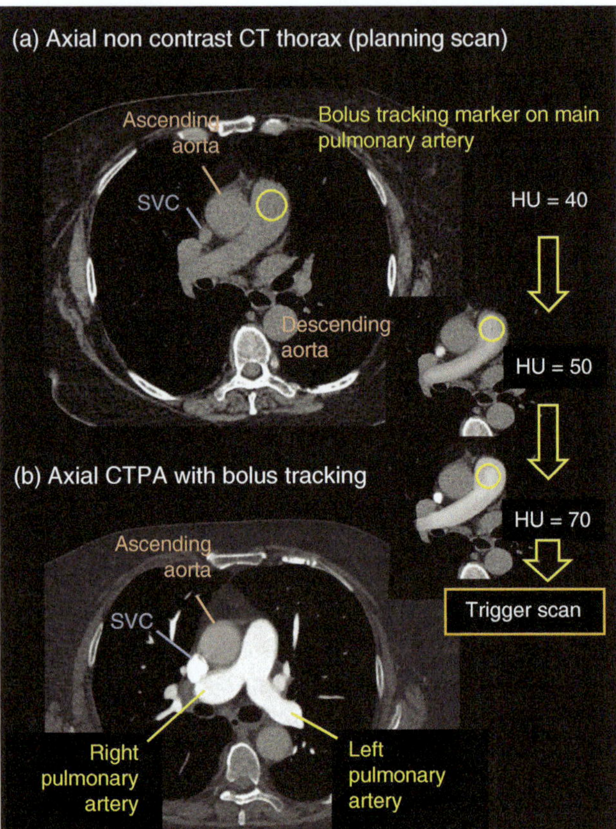

FIGURE 17.2 Bolus tracking. (a) Axial non-contrast CT thorax (planning scan). (b) Axial CTPA with bolus tracking. A planning scan is done to identify the pulmonary artery and draw a region of interest (yellow circle). The intravenous contrast is then given through a cannula. A screening CT slice is performed every few seconds through the region of interest and the Hounsfield units are recorded each time. The contrast travels from the arm via the SVC to the right heart, before filling the pulmonary trunk. When the Hounsfield units in the region of interest reach a trigger point, the full CT scan is performed. With this method, even if cardiac output is reduced, the scan will not be performed until there is adequate contrast opacification in the pulmonary arteries, thus improving quality.

injection). A challenge is that variations in cardiac output can significantly alter the contrast timing. To mitigate this a technique called bolus tracking is often used (Figure 17.2).

As opposed to the coronary arteries, the pulmonary arterial tree does not move much during the cardiac cycle, so no ECG gating is required (see Cardiac Chapter 16 – Chest Pain and Syncope – Figure 16.2).

17.3.2 Ventilation/Perfusion (V/Q) Scan

This is a branch of nuclear medicine (see Introduction Chapter 1). As with X-ray and CT, nuclear medicine exposes the patient to ionising radiation and so poses a long-term cancer risk. The difference is that during a nuclear medicine study, radioactive pharmaceuticals are introduced into the patient. This could be via intravenous injection, oral or inspiratory routes.

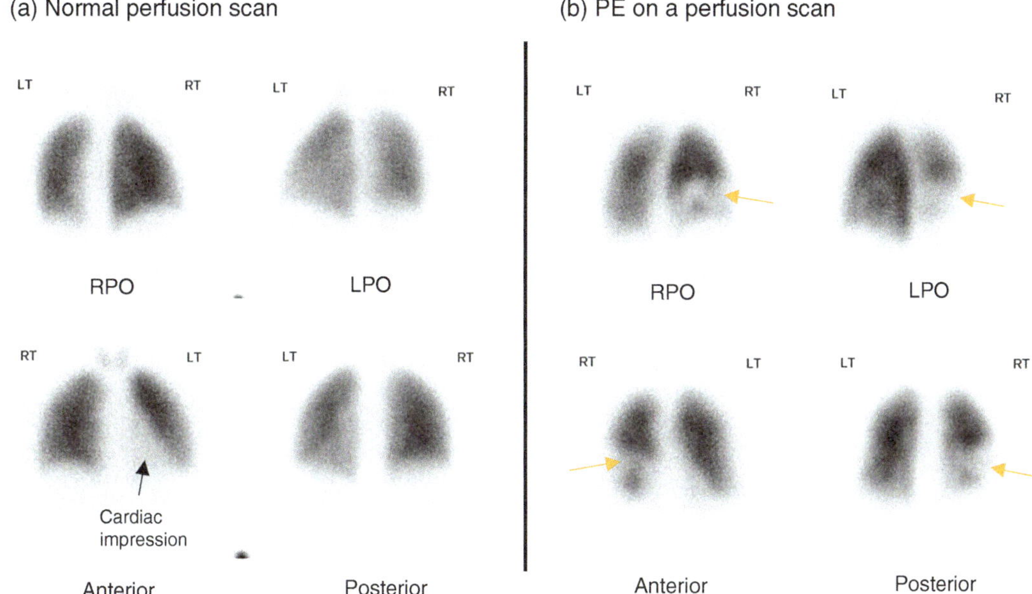

FIGURE 17.3 (a) Normal perfusion scan. (b) Pulmonary embolism on a V/Q scan. The perfused areas of the lungs appear black. A normal perfusion scan gives images from different angles. From the anterior view, the heart makes an impression on the left lung. This shows perfusion defects in the lower lobe of the right lung (orange arrows) and is highly suggestive of pulmonary embolism. If there is diagnostic uncertainty on a V/Q scan then a CTPA will be used to assess further. RPO, right posterior oblique; LPO, left posterior oblique.

The patient is then positioned inside a special detector called a gamma camera, which records the radiation emitted from the patient. Nuclear medicine studies provide functional information about the body but have much less anatomical definition compared to X-ray and CT.

Often, only the perfusion component of the study is performed (Figure 17.3). The patient has a radioactive pharmaceutical injected intravenously. This travels to the lungs via the pulmonary arteries and should fill the lung capillary bed equally.

The ventilation component of the study involves the patient inhaling radioactive gas and observing the aerated parts of the lung (not shown). This component is not always performed as ventilation is likely to be normal if the chest X-ray is normal.

17.4 Correlation to Anatomy

The heart should always be reviewed on CTPA. Normally the volumes of the left and right ventricles are similar. However, the walls of the left ventricle are thicker (Figure 17.4).

17.5 Review of the Clinical Case

- What is your differential diagnosis?
- Why is CTPA indicated?
- What is your final diagnosis and definitive management?

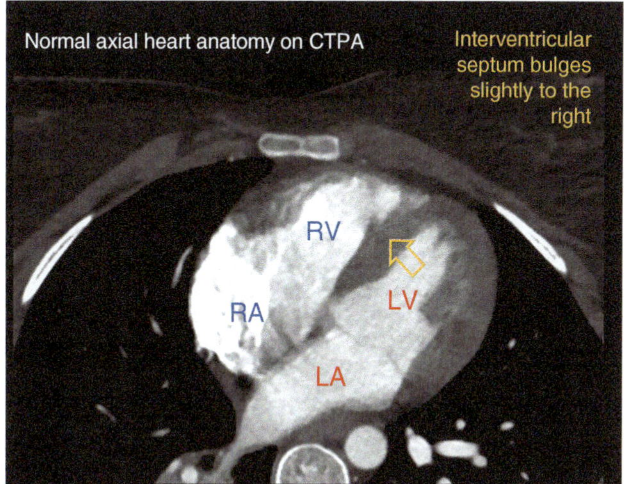

FIGURE 17.4 Normal axial CTPA through the heart. The interventricular septum bulges slightly to the right owing to higher pressures in the left side of heart. RV, right ventricle; RA, right atrium; LV, left ventricle; LA, left atrium.

17.5.1 Differential Diagnosis

- Patient A has a history of immobility in the lower limb, compounded by a long drive. This increases the risk for deep venous thrombosis (DVT) development. On clinical examination the ankle and calf are swollen.
- This, in combination with shortness of breath and tachycardia, are highly suspicious for a pulmonary embolism (PE).

- In patients with overall low probability of PE, the Pulmonary Embolism Rule out criteria (PERC) score can be used to assess likelihood of PE (Box 17.1). As the history is very suspicious for a PE, PERC should not be used for this patient.
- A Wells score for PE can be used to help with triage investigations (Box 17.2). Patient A has a Wells score of 9.
- Patients with a Wells score more than 4 should be worked up as follows.
  - Patient A is very likely to have a PE and needs definitive imaging, so D-dimer is not indicated.
  - CXR should be performed first to exclude other causes of breathlessness (e.g. pneumonia and pneumothorax). PE is not visible on CXR, but it may be possible to detect secondary effects such as right heart strain and pulmonary hypertension (Figure 17.5).
  - A treatment dose of factor Xa inhibitor (apixaban/rivaroxaban) should be given, or if not suitable/available, a low molecular weight heparin can be used.
  - If the patient has a contraindication to anticoagulation, CTPA should be arranged urgently.
  - CTPA is the modality of choice in patients over 40 years old, or those with an abnormal CXR.
  - V/Q scan is an option in patients under 40 years old with a normal CXR. This is advantageous as it exposes the patient to a lower dose of radiation.

Box 17.1 | PERC Score (Pulmonary Embolism Rule out Criteria)

1. Age > 50?
2. Heart rate > 100 bpm?
3. O_2 Sat on room air < 95%?
4. Prior history of venous thromboembolism?
5. Surgery or trauma in last four weeks?
6. Haemoptysis?
7. Exogenous oestrogen?
8. Unilateral leg swelling?

If answer is **yes** to any of these questions, the patient fails the PERC score and PE cannot be excluded.

Box 17.2 | Wells Criteria for PE

1. Clinical signs or symptoms of DVT
   a. Yes – 3
   b. No – 0
2. PE is the most likely diagnosis
   a. Yes – 3
   b. No – 0
3. Heart rate over 100
   a. Yes – 1.5
   b. No – 0
4. Immobilisation in last three days or surgery in previous four weeks
   a. Yes – 1.5
   b. No – 0
5. Previous diagnosis of PE or DVT
   a. Yes – 1.5
   b. No – 0
6. Haemoptysis
   a. Yes – 1
   b. No – 0
7. Malignancy with treatment within six months or palliative
   a. Yes – 1
   b. No – 0

Wells score over 4 – needs CTPA or V/Q scan
Wells score 4 or under – get D-dimer. If D-dimer is positive then needs CTPA or V/Q scan

- If there are signs of DVT and the expertise is available, then a Doppler ultrasound of the leg can be useful in patients with contraindications to chest imaging (e.g. contrast allergy or pregnancy).
- In haemodynamically unstable patients, a bedside echo could be used to assess for right heart strain. This can also help to decide which patients may require thrombolysis.
- Patients with a Wells score of 4 or less should have a D-dimer. If positive, then the above imaging pathway should be followed.

Other differential diagnoses to consider with this presentation are aortic dissection, atypical infection and heart failure.

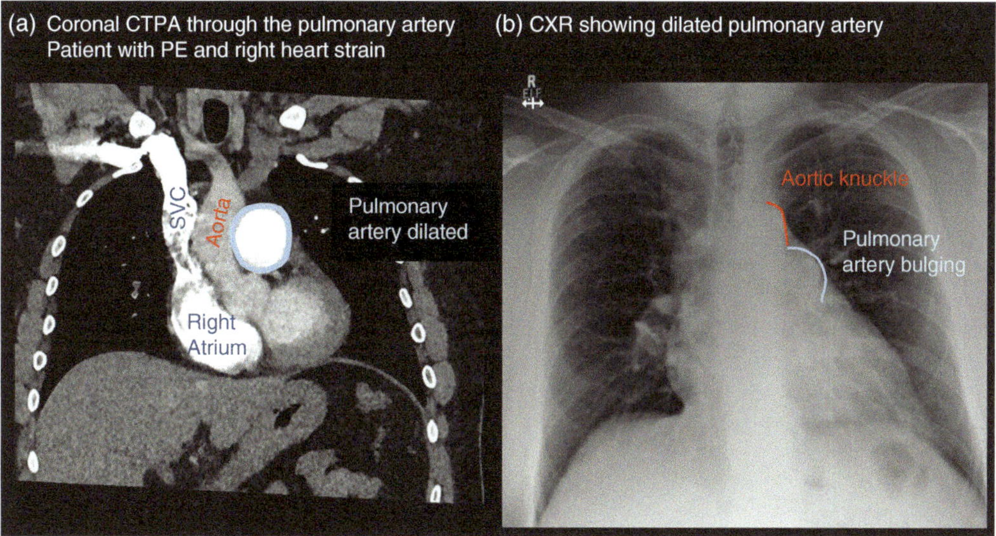

FIGURE 17.5 Different patient with pulmonary embolism, right heart strain and dilated pulmonary artery. (a) Coronal CTPA through pulmonary artery. (b) CXR showing dilated pulmonary artery. In some cases of severe right heart strain, the main pulmonary artery will dilate to such a degree it is visible on plain X-ray. (Compare this CXR with Respiratory Chapter 12 – Figure 12.2.)

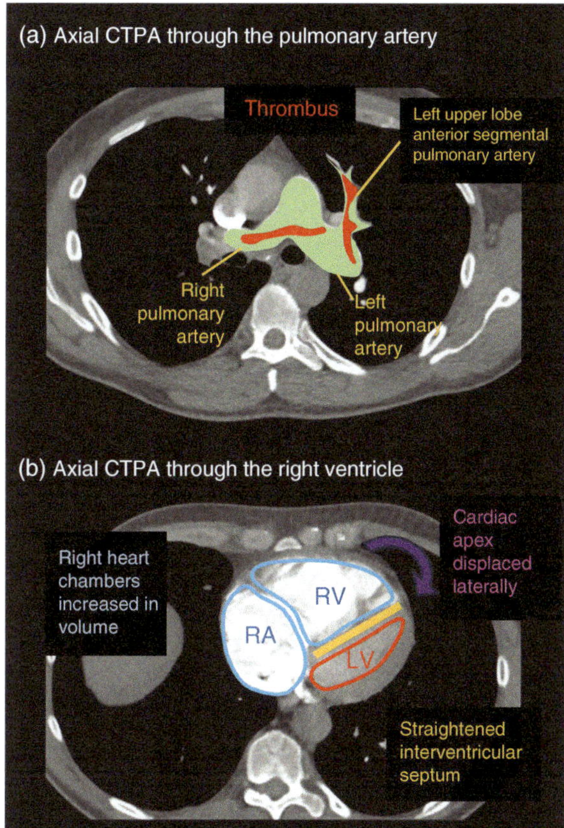

FIGURE 17.6 Patient A. CTPA. Axial on soft tissue windows. (a) Level of the pulmonary artery. (b) Level of the right ventricle. Pulmonary embolism manifests on CTPA as a filling defect. This means the vessel fills with contrast (green) but there are areas of non-filling which appear dark (shaded red here). This filling defect/thrombus is straddling the left and right main pulmonary arteries, as well as extending into the segmental pulmonary arteries. Note the greater volume of the right side of the heart compared to the left. This is a marker of right heart strain and implies that the output from the right ventricle is being impeded.

17.5.2 **CTPA**

Patient A has a saddle pulmonary embolus. There are also features of right heart strain (Figure 17.6).

17.5.3 **Final Diagnosis**

Acute pulmonary embolism causing right heart strain. As the patient is haemodynamically stable this was treated with rivaroxaban.

If patients are shocked, then thrombolysis may be indicated.

17.6 Take-home Message – Imaging in PE

- CXR is the first-line investigation, done to exclude other causes for symptoms.
- CTPA is preferred in patients over 40 or those with abnormal CXR.
- V/Q scan is an option in patients under 40 with a normal CXR.
- If there are signs of DVT then Doppler ultrasound of the leg can be useful.
- There is a role for bedside echocardiogram to assess for right heart strain in unwell patients.

Further Resources

NICE pulmonary embolism guidelines: https://cks.nice.org.uk/topics/pulmonary-embolism/#:~:text=For%20people%20with%20a%20Wells,offered%2C%20then%20hospital%20admission%20arranged

PERC: www.mdcalc.com/calc/347/perc-rule-pulmonary-embolism

Wells criteria for PE www.uptodate.com/contents/image?imageKey=PULM/54767

British Thoracic Society guidelines for the management of suspected acute pulmonary embolism: https://thorax.bmj.com/content/58/6/470

Abdominal Section

Blunt Trauma

Joshua Lauder[1], Benjamin Layton[2], and Peter Driscoll[3]

[1] East Lancashire Hospitals NHS Trust, University of Central Lancashire and University of Manchester, UK
[2] Morecambe Bay Hospitals Trust, Lancaster, UK
[3] School of Medicine and Dentistry, University of Central Lancashire, Preston, UK

18.1 Primary Case

18.1.1 Presentation

A 25-year old male is brought to the Emergency Department by ambulance. He had fallen 5 m from a roof while repairing a gutter.

18.1.1.1 History of Presenting Complaint During the fall he hit a wooden fence and is now complaining of upper abdominal pain.

PMH: NAD.
SH: NAD.
DH: nil and no allergies.

18.1.2 Examination

Airway and cervical spine:

- Airway – clear.
- Neck – immobilised.

Breathing:

- No wounds or marks on the neck, neck veins flat.
- Symmetrical chest movement.
- No wounds or abrasions on chest.
- Trachea central.
- Expansion equal but reduced both sides. No surgical emphysema.
- Percussion: equal both sides.
- Auscultate: symmetrical and shallow air entry right and left.

Circulation:

- Pale, cool skin. Capillary refill time over three seconds.
- Abrasion over epigastrium, tender upper abdomen with guarding.
- Bowel sounds absent.
- Pelvis clinically intact.
- Multiple contusions. No penetrating wounds.

Modified early warning signs (MEWS):

- Respiratory rate 30 rpm.
- SpO_2 poor signal, reading 94% (FIO_2 85%).
- Temp 36.9 °C.
- HR 128/min.
- BP 78/58 mmHg.
- Alert.

18.1.3 Investigation

In view of this presentation an urgent CT with contrast was arranged (Figure 18.1).

Clinical Case Questions

- What is your differential diagnosis?
- Why is CT indicated?
- Why is contrast required?
- What is your system for interpreting these images?
- What is your final diagnosis and definitive management?

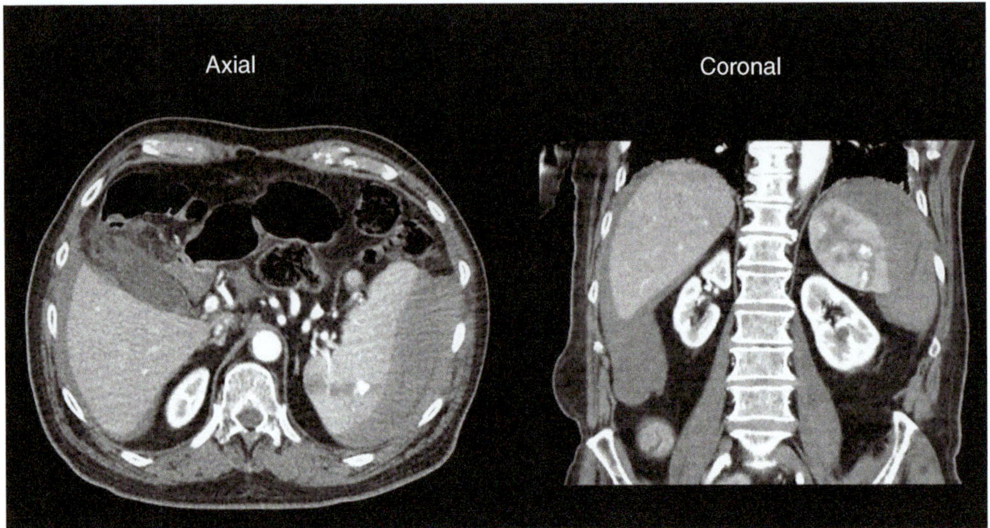

FIGURE 18.1 Patient A. CT with contrast. (Left) Axial view – upper abdominal level. (Right) Coronal view – lower thorax, abdomen and pelvis.

18.2 Radiology Self-assessment

18.2.1 Technical

- When should a CT scan be performed in trauma?
- What is the benefit of intravenous (IV) contrast in trauma CT scans?

18.2.2 Correlating Gross Anatomy to CT

- What does the spleen look like on postcontrast CT?
- Where are the dependent recesses of the peritoneal space?

18.3 Key Radiology Review

18.3.1 Technical Aspects

18.3.1.1 Rationale for CT in Trauma CT scans are the quickest and most comprehensive way to diagnose life-threatening and limb-threatening injuries. As traumatic injuries are time critical, it is important that the management pathway includes early CT scanning to guide further management. As some injuries can be hidden from physical examination and can cross different anatomical cavities (e.g. a penetrating abdominal injury can traverse the diaphragm and cause pneumothorax), CT should include everything from the top of the head to mid-thighs.

In view of the area involved, the patient is exposed to significant ionising radiation, with known long-term cancer risk. This risk can be justified with a suspected life-threatening or limb-threatening injury but should be avoided in minor trauma.

18.3.1.2 Rationale for IV Contrast Intravenous contrast is always administered in trauma CT to identify active bleeding. In the normal situation the contrast will remain intravascular, enhance the viscera and allow the parenchyma of organs to be seen (Figure 18.2). However, when there is active haemorrhage contrast leaks out into the surrounding tissues. This is termed extravasation (see Figure 18.6) and often requires further management, with either interventional radiology or surgery.

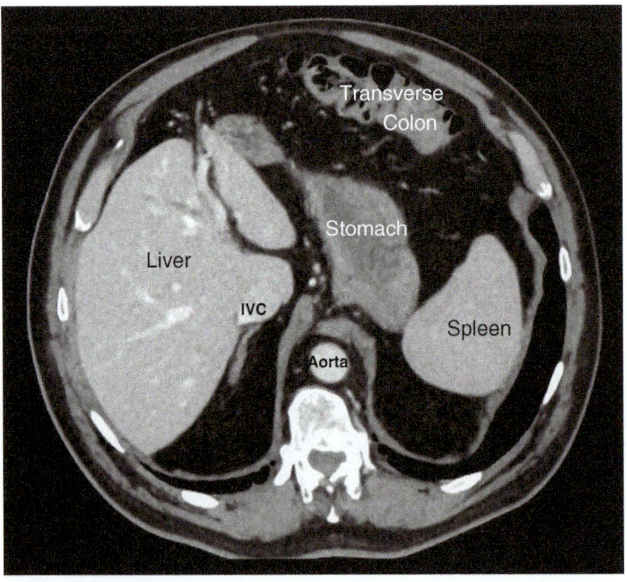

FIGURE 18.2 Axial CT of the upper abdomen with contrast. Normal case. The spleen and liver are both enhancing, and the parenchyma appears homogenous (i.e. the same shade of grey throughout). The bright lines going through the liver represent normal blood vessels.

18.3.1.3 Ultrasound in Trauma As portable ultrasound is typically available, it is often the first imaging modality available in the trauma pathway. It is good for positively diagnosing conditions such as pneumothorax, haemothorax, pericardial effusions and haemoperitoneum. Consequently, when identified, immediate management can begin before the patient arrives in the radiology department for CT.

However, ultrasound has reduced sensitivity for certain traumatic conditions like retroperitoneal haemorrhage and cannot see the thoracic aorta. Therefore, a normal ultrasound scan does not exclude a life-threatening injury. Furthermore, it is unlikely to locate the source of bleeding in the chest or abdomen. For these reasons, it is not relied upon as a primary imaging modality in trauma.

18.4 Correlating the Anatomy with the CT Image

18.4.1 Anatomy Images

As well as being aware of the organs in the abdomen, it is important to appreciate the extent of the peritoneal space and which organs lie within it.

An injury, or other pathology, to an intraperitoneal organ can result in free fluid which extends into the peritoneal space. The latter has certain areas in which fluid can pool because of gravity (Figure 18.3). These are termed the dependent spaces and should be specifically checked on CT or ultrasound (Figures 18.4, 18.5 and 18.7).

18.5 Review of the Clinical Case

- What is your differential diagnosis for the haemodynamic instability?

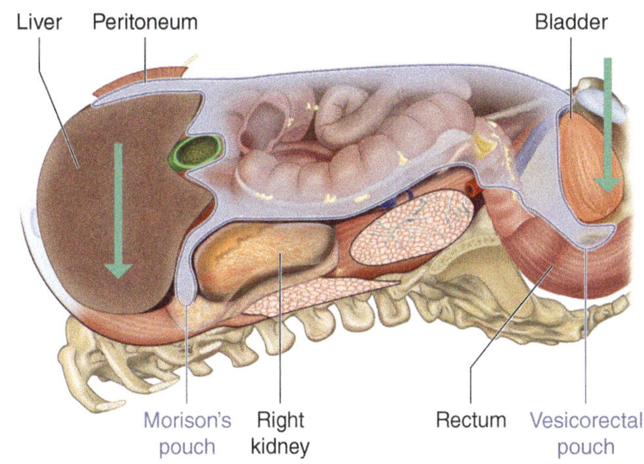

FIGURE 18.3 Sagittal anatomical cross-section through the right midclavicular line (male). When patients are lying supine, the most posterior areas of the peritoneal space are Morison's pouch, the vesicorectal pouch and, in females, the rectouterine pouch. These are therefore dependent areas where free fluid collects due to gravity (green arrows).

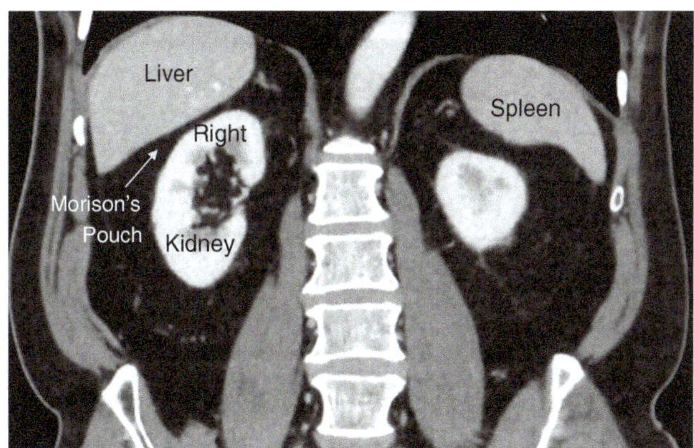

FIGURE 18.4 Coronal CT abdomen with contrast showing Morison's pouch (hepatorenal space). Normal case. There should only be fat (seen as a very dark band on CT) separating the liver from the kidney. There should also be a similar dark fat plane surrounding all the abdominal organs. When this is lost, or contains stranding of oedema, it is a sign of pathology (see next section).

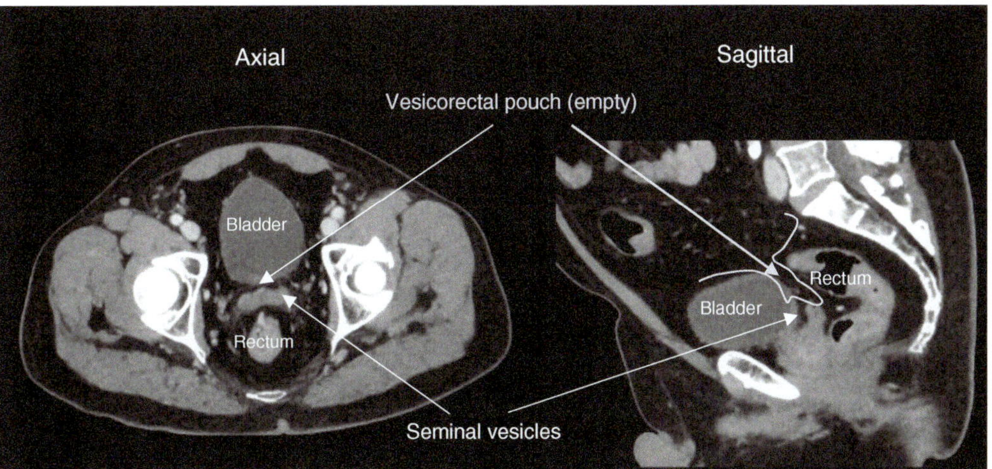

FIGURE 18.5 Axial and sagittal CT pelvis with contrast showing the vesicorectal pouch. Normal case (male). Note the seminal vesicles lying inferior to the pouch. Take care not to mistake these for free fluid lying in the pouch (see Figure 18.8).

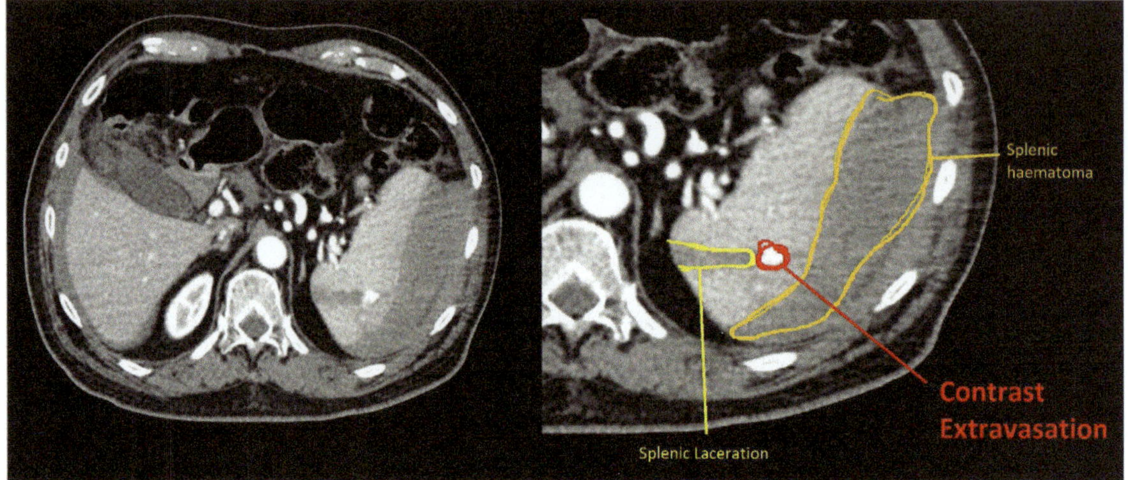

FIGURE 18.6 Patient A. Axial CT upper abdomen with contrast. The dark (hypodense) horizonal line through the spleen is the laceration (it has less contrast than the surrounding parenchyma). At the lateral margin of this there is a bright dot which represents contrast extravasation (active bleeding). There is also a hypodense haematoma surrounding the spleen laterally. This could be subcapsular or intraperitoneal. Further blood extends around the liver in the intraperitoneal space.

- Why is CT indicated?
- Why is contrast required?
- What is your final diagnosis and definitive management?

18.5.1 Differential Diagnosis

A trauma patient with abdominal injury and haemodynamic instability could have suffered a solid organ injury (e.g. liver/spleen/kidney), hollow viscus injury (e.g. gastrointestinal tract) or vascular injury (e.g. aortic haemorrhage). If there is bleeding into the peritoneal space, the patient can quickly lose their circulating blood volume and develop hypovolaemic shock.

From the perspective of time, feasibility and specificity, CT with contrast is the most effective way of identifying which of these possible injuries are present.

18.5.2 Imaging

Patient A has sustained a splenic laceration with haemoperitoneum. The blood lies in the peritoneal space around the liver and spleen (Figure 18.6), also extending into Morison's pouch. The latter may be visible on ultrasound (Figure 18.7). In patient A's case, the blood was also collecting in the vesicorectal pouch (Figure 18.8).

18.5.3 Management

Contrast extravasation means there is active bleeding and requires urgent discussion with the surgeons and interventional radiology.

In this case, patient A went for endovascular coiling of the bleeding splenic artery branch (Figure 18.9). In addition

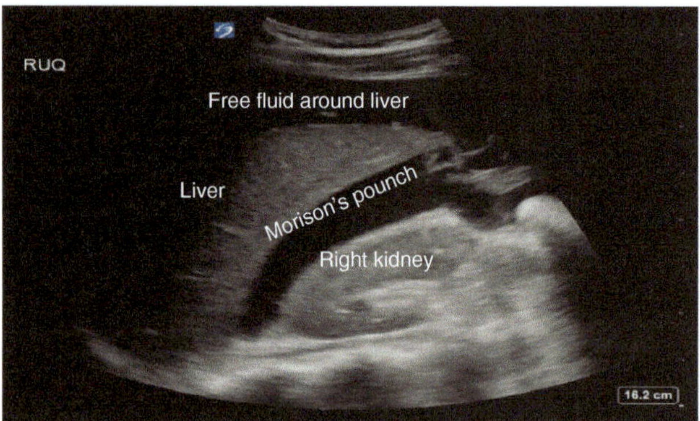

FIGURE 18.7 Abdominal ultrasound of the RUQ showing free fluid between the liver and right kidney (Morison's pouch).

to gaining haemostasis, this technique has the added benefit of retaining splenic function, as opposed to traditional surgery with splenectomy.

18.6 Take-home Message – Imaging in Trauma

- Ultrasound is a useful tool in trauma, able to diagnose life-threatening injuries including pneumothorax, haemothorax and cardiac tamponade, as well as identify free fluid in the abdomen. It can also be used to guide procedures.
- Whole-body CT (head, neck, thorax, abdomen and pelvis) with IV contrast is the definitive imaging modality in major trauma. This has greater sensitivity than ultrasound and can identify active bleeding.

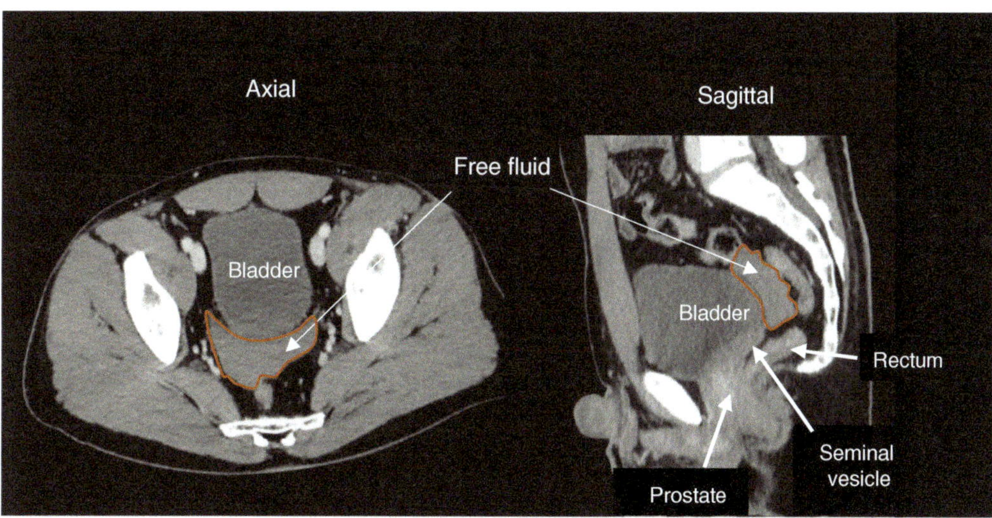

FIGURE 18.8 Patient A. Axial and sagittal CT pelvis with contrast showing free fluid in the pelvis (in this case blood). In a male patient, the fluid pools between the bladder and the rectum, filling the vesicorectal pouch. Compare this image to Figure 18.5, showing the normal anatomy. Do not confuse the seminal vesicles (which lie lower) with free fluid in the vesicorectal pouch.

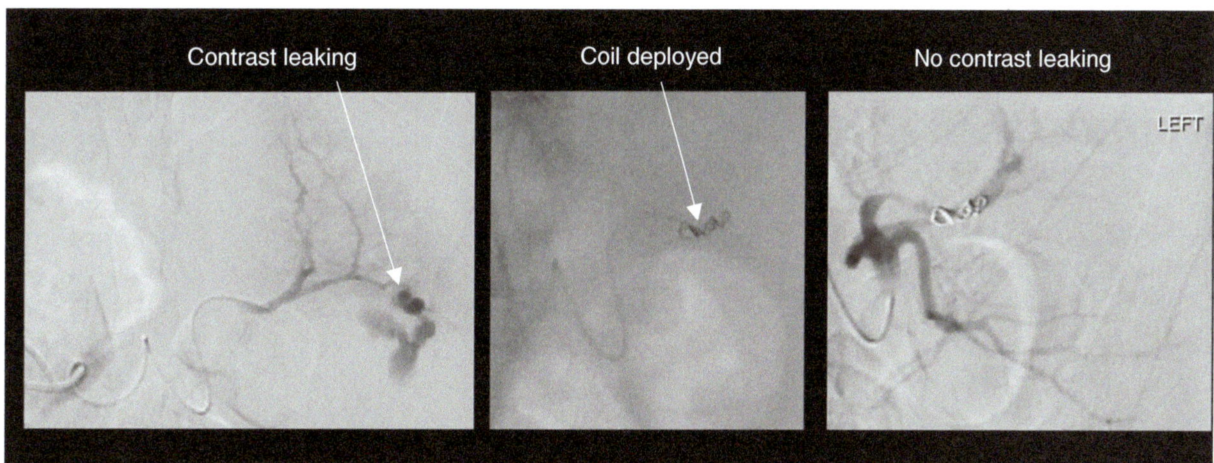

FIGURE 18.9 Fluoroscopic (X-ray) images from endovascular coiling. On the left image the contrast is leaking from the splenic laceration. In the middle image, an endovascular coil has been deployed. In the postprocedure image on the right, the contrast is no longer leaking, indicating that the bleeding has stopped.

Further Resources

National Institute for Health and Care Excellence. Major trauma: assessment and initial management. www.nice.org.uk/guidance/ng39

CHAPTER 19

Right Upper Quadrant Pain

Joshua Lauder[1], Benjamin Layton[2], and Peter Driscoll[3]

[1] East Lancashire Hospitals NHS Trust, University of Central Lancashire and University of Manchester, UK
[2] Morecambe Bay Hospitals Trust, Lancaster, UK
[3] School of Medicine and Dentistry, University of Central Lancashire, Preston, UK

19.1 Primary Case

19.1.1 Presentation

A 50-year-old female presents to the Emergency Department with a four-day history of right upper abdominal pain.

19.1.1.1 History of Presenting Complaint The pain has been constant but there are occasional episodes of more intense discomfort. She has also vomited twice over the last 24 hours but with no relief of the abdominal pain. Normally her appetite is good but it has decreased over the last week. She has also noticed her urine is darker than normal over the last couple of days.

    PMH: NAD
    SH:

- Has smoked all her life, now about 10 cigarettes per day.
- Drinks a half-bottle of wine per night.

    DH: NAD.

19.1.2 Examination

Clinical examination:

- Looks slightly jaundiced.
- Obese (BWI 31.0).
- Chest – clear.

- Heart sounds – normal.
- Tenderness and guarding on palpation of the right upper quadrant (RUQ).

Modified early warning signs (MEWS):

- Respiratory rate 18 rpm.
- SpO_2 94% on room air.
- Tympanic temp 37.3 °C.
- HR 76 bpm.
- BP 120/70 mmHg.
- Alert.

19.1.3 Blood Results

	Normal	Patient
Sodium	135–145 mmol/l	140 mmol/l
Potassium	3.5–5.0 mmol/l	4.0 mmol/l
Urea	2.5–6.7 mmol/l	6.0 mmol/l
Bilirubin	3–17 mmol/l	80.1 mmol/l
Alk. phosphatase	5–35 IU/l	810 IU/l
Gamma-glutamyl transpeptidase	11–51 IU/l	430 IU/l

19.1.4 Ultrasound

An ultrasound was arranged to assess the biliary tree (Figure 19.1).

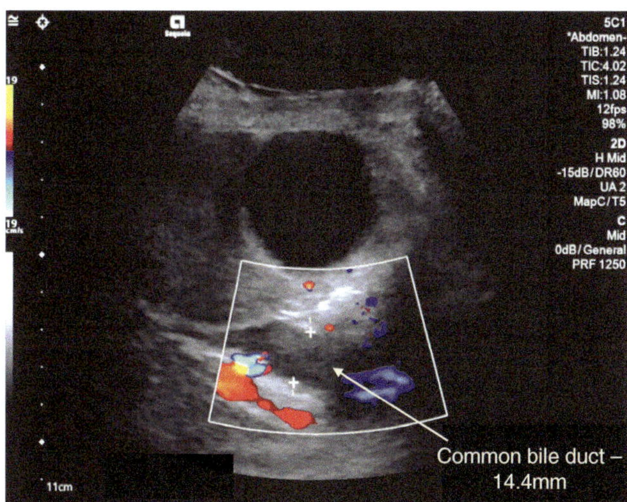

FIGURE 19.1 Patient A. Ultrasound of the RUQ, showing gallbladder and common bile duct.

19.1.5 Magnetic Resonance Cholangiopancreatography (MRCP)

Based on ultrasound findings an MRCP was arranged (Figure 19.2).

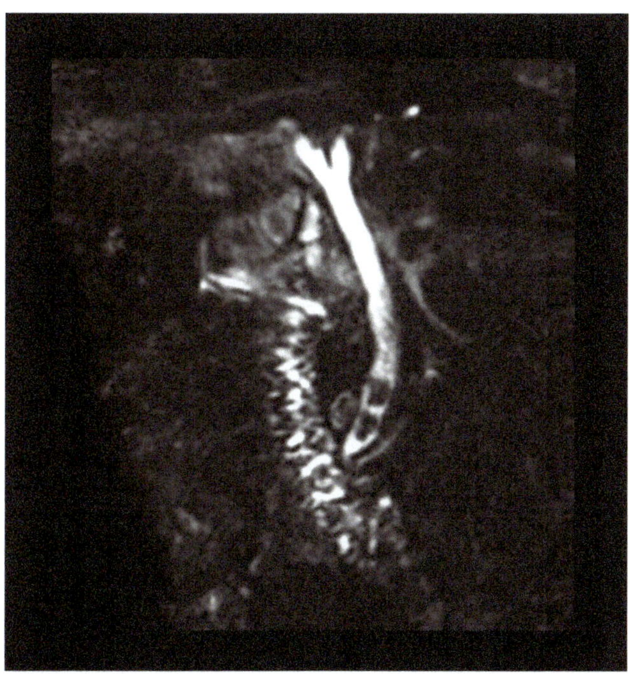

FIGURE 19.2 Patient A. MRCP, heavily T2-weighted coronal slice through the common bile duct.

> ## Clinical Case Questions
>
> - What is your differential diagnosis?
> - Why is ultrasound indicated?
> - Why is MRCP indicated?
> - What is your system for interpreting these images?
> - What is your final diagnosis?

19.2 Radiology Self-assessment

19.2.1 Technical

- When should ultrasound be performed in RUQ pain?
- What is magnetic resonance cholangiopancreatography (MRCP)?
- When should MRCP be arranged?

19.2.2 Correlating Gross Anatomy

- What do the gallbladder and biliary tree look like on ultrasound?
- What does the biliary tree look like on MRCP?

19.3 Key Radiology Review

19.3.1 Anatomy

An overview of the key anatomy is shown in Figure 19.3.

19.3.2 Technical

19.3.2.1 Ultrasound of the Biliary Tree This investigation is the first-line modality for assessing the liver and biliary tree. It has two big advantages over CT.

- It does not expose the patient to ionising radiation.
- It has a greater sensitivity for detecting gall stones (see Figures 19.7 and 19.8).

Ultrasound can also assess the common bile duct (CBD), so is an effective way to diagnose obstructive jaundice (Figure 19.4). However, the distal CBD is often obscured by bowel gas. Therefore, in the presence of obstructive jaundice, when ultrasound cannot find the cause, an MRCP or CT is often necessary.

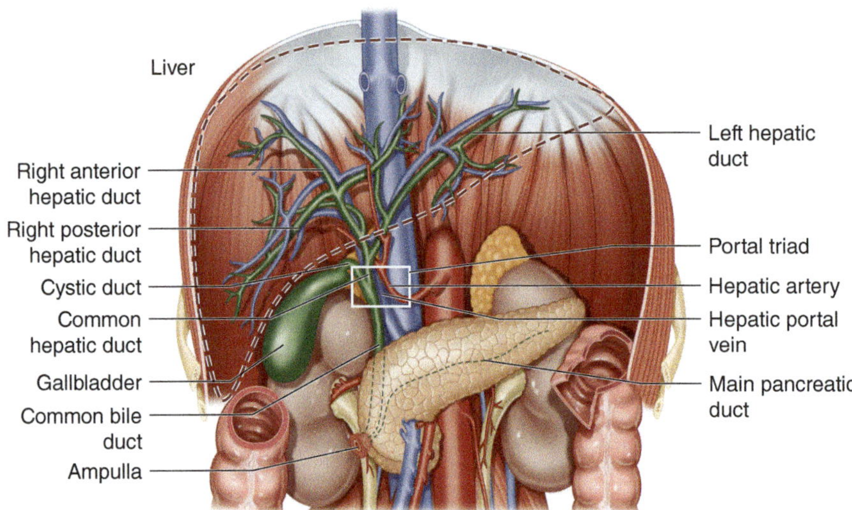

FIGURE 19.3 Diagram showing a coronal view of the biliary tree and surrounding organs. The liver has been removed to show the intrahepatic ducts. The common hepatic duct (CHD) becomes the CBD after the cystic duct confluence. The pancreatic duct can be identified, joining with the CBD at the ampulla. CHD, common hepatic duct; CBD, common bile duct; CD, cystic duct; GB, gallbladder. Box = porta hepatis.

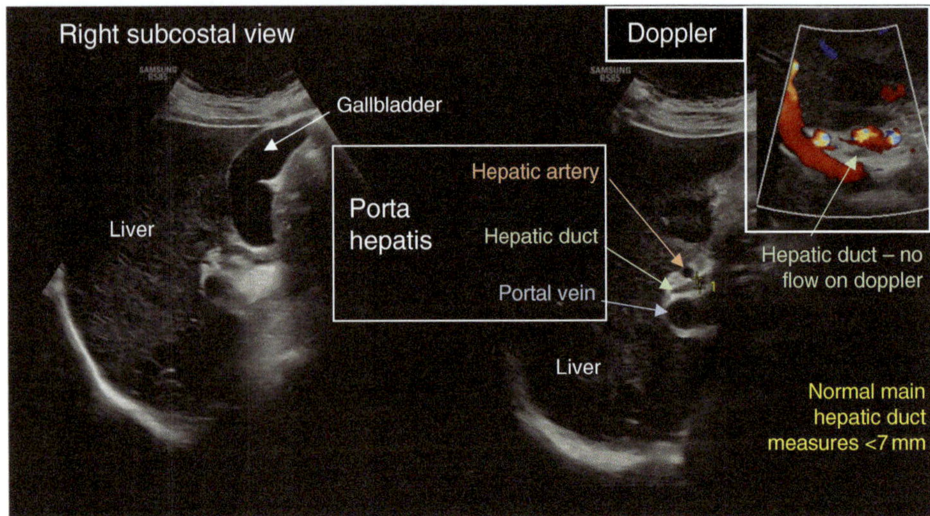

FIGURE 19.4 Normal right upper quadrant (RUQ) ultrasound, subcostal view showing gallbladder (left) and common hepatic duct (right). The gallbladder should be completely anechoic (black). The common hepatic duct can be identified at the porta hepatis, immediately anterior to the portal vein. The normal hepatic artery and duct are similar in calibre, but the hepatic artery tends to be more tortuous. Colour Doppler can be used to distinguish between the two as there will be no detectible flow in the biliary ducts (right upper image).

19.3.2.2 Magnetic Resonance Cholangiopancreatography (MRCP) This investigation uses a specialist MRI technique called a 'heavily T2-weighted sequence'. Fluid is bright on a standard T2 sequence. An MRCP takes this concept one step further with a sequence that *only* shows the fluid. All the other tissues become black and are invisible. The result is a scan showing *only* structures which contain fluid. This is very useful in the biliary tree as the surrounding pancreas and liver are removed, making the CBD more obvious.

Because the normal organs are invisible, it can be helpful to imagine where they are, in order to orientate the image (Figure 19.5).

19.4 Review of the Clinical Case

- What is your differential diagnosis?
- Why is US indicated?

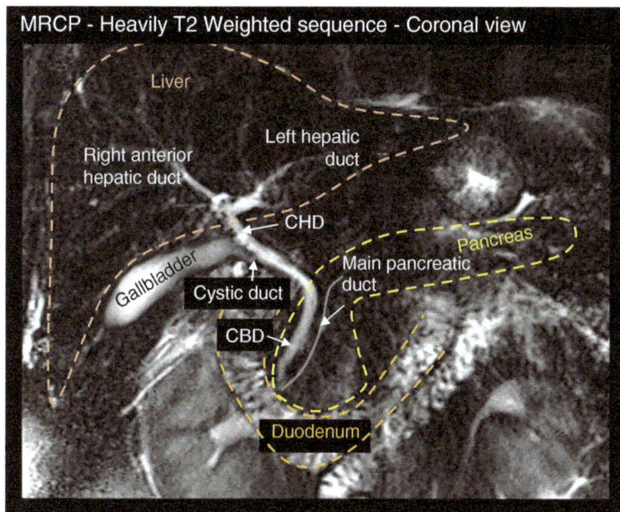

FIGURE 19.5 Normal MRCP, heavily T2-weighted coronal view. The positions of the liver, duodenum and pancreas have been superimposed (dotted lines). The main biliary duct should be less than 7 mm in diameter and hyperintense (bright). An internal blockage will appear as a filling defect (Figure 19.8).

- Why is MRCP indicated?
- What is your final diagnosis and immediate management?

19.4.1 Differential Diagnosis

Painful jaundice usually suggests gallstone disease with intraductal stones causing obstruction of the biliary drainage. Patients may also develop pancreatitis if the blockage involves the pancreatic duct.

- Mirizzi syndrome is when a gallstone in the gallbladder neck or cystic duct causes extrinsic compression of the common hepatic duct or CBD. These patients will present in a similar way to those with obstructed intraductal stones.
- Bouveret syndrome is when a gallstone fistulates into the stomach or duodenum, resulting in gastric outlet obstruction. These patients will present with vomiting as the primary symptom. This can be considered a proximal form of gallstone ileus.

Painless jaundice should raise suspicion of pancreatic cancer.

19.4.2 Ultrasound

The ultrasound shows CBD dilation (Figure 19.6)

19.4.3 MRCP

As only 20% of gallstones are dense on CT, it is a relatively insensitive test to pick up distal CBD stones (Figure 19.7). Consequently, MRCP is required (Figure 19.8)

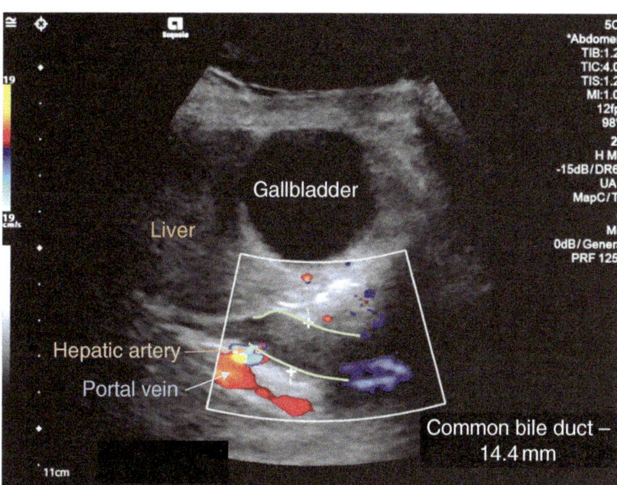

FIGURE 19.6 Patient A. Ultrasound of the RUQ, showing gallbladder and common bile duct (CBD). The CBD is dilated to 14.4 mm, suggesting obstructive jaundice. The gallbladder is also distended, which is often the case in obstructive jaundice. No gallstones are shown in this image. Doppler mode has been applied to the porta hepatis. Note the absence of flow in the CBD. Be aware that the colours on the Doppler relate to the direction of flow, *not* the oxygen content of the blood. As such, the portal vein here appears red and the hepatic artery blue.

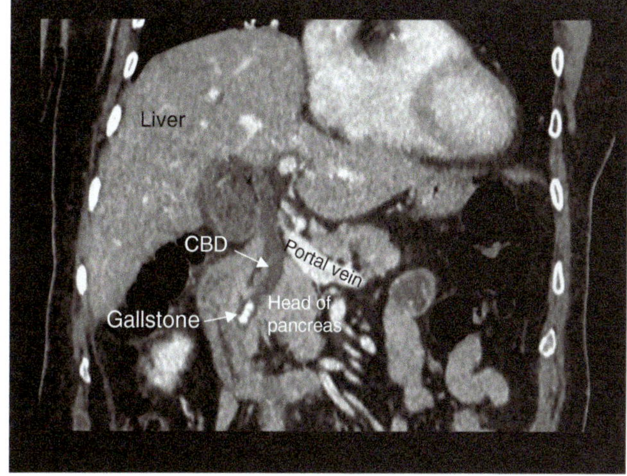

FIGURE 19.7 CT upper abdomen with contrast, coronal plane, soft tissue window. A calcified gallstone is seen impacted in the distal CBD. It is possible for CT to identify stones, but it lacks sensitivity as the majority of stones are not calcified.

19.4.4 Painless Jaundice

Painless obstructive jaundice usually represents pancreatic cancer rather than gallstone disease. If this is suspected, CT scans of the thorax, abdomen and pelvis are usually required.

MRCP can detect external compression of the biliary tree but is poor at delineating pancreatic malignancy. It is also unable to stage the nodal and metastatic cancer extent.

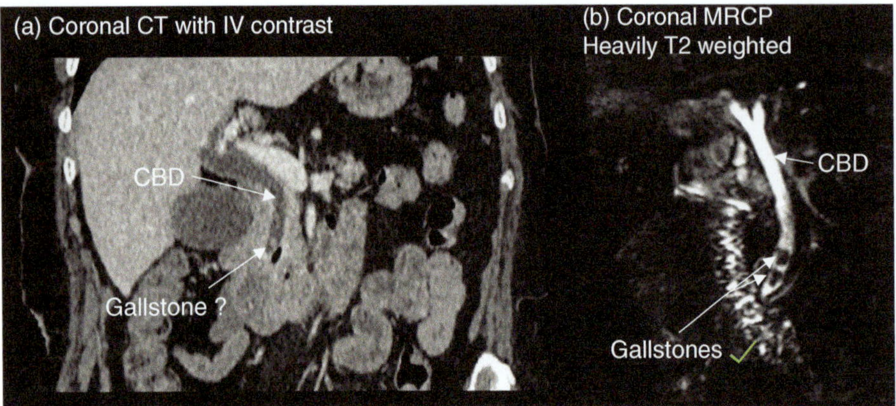

FIGURE 19.8 (a) CT upper abdomen with contrast, coronal plane, soft tissue window. (b) MRCP, coronal heavily T2-weighted sequence. This is a more typical case of distal CBD stone. The CT scan shows a dilated common bile duct but the stone is difficult to see as it is not calcified. It is much clearer on the MRCP which shows two filling defects in the distal CBD. These represent stones.

19.4.5 Final Diagnosis

Choledocholithiasis, causing obstructive jaundice. The patient went on to have an endoscopic retrograde cholangiopancreatography (ERCP).

19.5 Other Related Conditions

19.5.1 Gallstones and Cholecystitis on Ultrasound

Ultrasound is useful for diagnosing cholecystitis. The most sensitive sign is the presence of gallstones (Figure 19.9a) and sonographic Murphy's sign (pain during ultrasound probe pressure over the gallbladder). Gallbladder wall thickening and sludge are other features (Figure 19.9b).

19.5.2 Cholecystitis on CT

Although CT is not the preferred imaging modality for biliary pathology, it is sometimes performed when the history is atypical. In these circumstances an important clue is 'fat stranding' around the gallbladder due to adjacent inflammation. This is essentially oedema extending into the adjacent fat and appears as grey streaks through the otherwise hypodense (black) fat (Figure 19.10).

Recognising fat stranding is very useful as it provides a big clue for nearby pathology. It is seen in any inflammatory pathology (e.g. appendicitis and diverticular abscess).

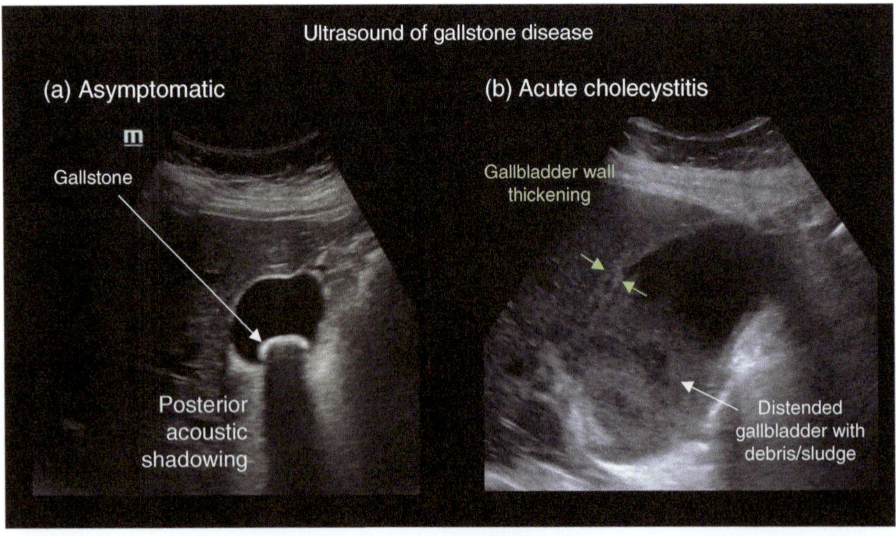

FIGURE 19.9 Ultrasound of RUQ showing two different patients with gallstones. (a) A simple gallstone in the gallbladder but no cholecystitis. Gallstones will appear as hyperechoic lesions inside the gallbladder. If calcified, they show posterior acoustic shadowing due to complete reflection of the ultrasound waves. (b) Acute cholecystitis. The gallbladder is distended with internal gallstones and sludge. There is thickening of the gallbladder wall and hyperechoic pericholecystic fat, representing inflammation. This patient was also tender over the gallbladder during the ultrasound examination (i.e. a sonographic Murphy's sign).

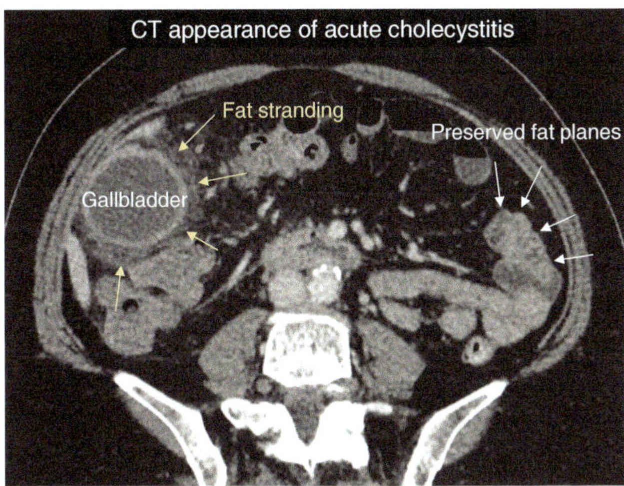

FIGURE 19.10 Axial CT of abdomen with IV contrast, soft tissue window. This patient has acute cholecystitis. Compare the fat around the gallbladder to the intact fat planes around the bowel in the left side of abdomen.

19.6 Take-home Message – Imaging in Gallstones

- Ultrasound is the first-line investigation for gallstones and has higher sensitivity than CT owing to the high proportion of non-calcified gallstones.
- MRCP is performed if the ultrasound shows biliary dilation which is suspected to be due to intraductal gallstones but not positively identified on ultrasound.
- CT is performed in suspected pancreatic malignancy.
- Endoscopic ultrasound of the biliary tree may be considered if these non-invasive modalities cannot provide a diagnosis.

Further Reading

National Institute for Health and Care Excellence. Gallstone disease: diagnosis and management. CG 188. www.nice.org.uk/guidance/cg188

CHAPTER 20

General Abdominal Pain

Joshua Lauder[1], Benjamin Layton[2], and Peter Driscoll[3]

[1] East Lancashire Hospitals NHS Trust, University of Central Lancashire and University of Manchester, UK
[2] Morecambe Bay Hospitals Trust, Lancaster, UK
[3] School of Medicine and Dentistry, University of Central Lancashire, Preston, UK

20.1 Primary Case

20.1.1 Presentation

A 60-year-old female presents to the Emergency Department with intermittent acute abdominal pain and vomiting.

20.1.1.1 History of Presenting Complaint The pain started 10 hours ago and is growing in severity. The vomit has been profuse and bile-stained but no blood was noted. She last opened her bowels 24 hours ago and that was normal.

SH:

- Previous cholecystectomy which was converted to an open procedure.

No other relevant past medical history or drug history.

20.1.2 Examination

- Looks in pain.
- Chest – clear.
- Heart sounds normal.
- Abdomen:
  - Midline laparotomy scar.
  - Distended.
  - Guarding and rebound tenderness noted in the supraumbilical region.

Modified early warning signs (MEWS):

- Respiratory rate 18 rpm.
- SpO_2 98% on room air.
- Tympanic temp. 37.1 °C.
- HR 90 bpm.
- BP 120/80 mmHg.
- Alert.

20.1.3 X-ray

A plain abdominal X-ray (AXR) was carried out (Figure 20.1).

20.1.4 CT

Subsequently an abdominal CT was arranged (Figure 20.2).

Clinical Case Questions

- What is your differential diagnosis?
- When should a plain AXR be requested?
- When should CT be requested?
- What is your final diagnosis?

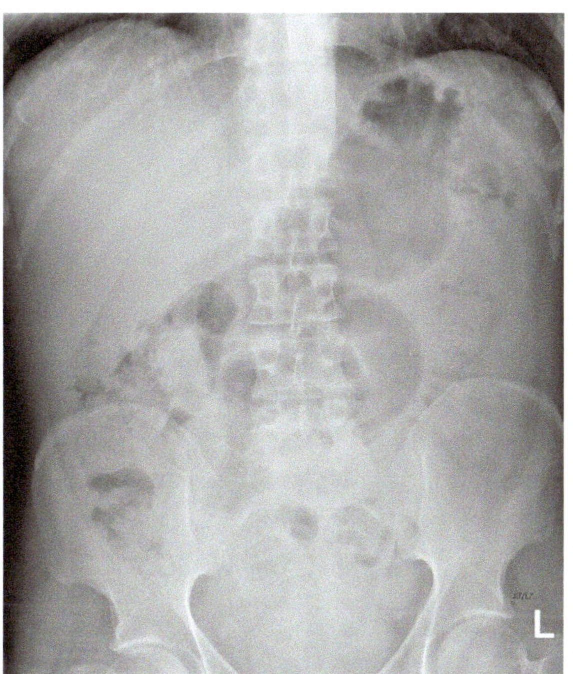

FIGURE 20.1 Patient A. Abdominal X-ray.

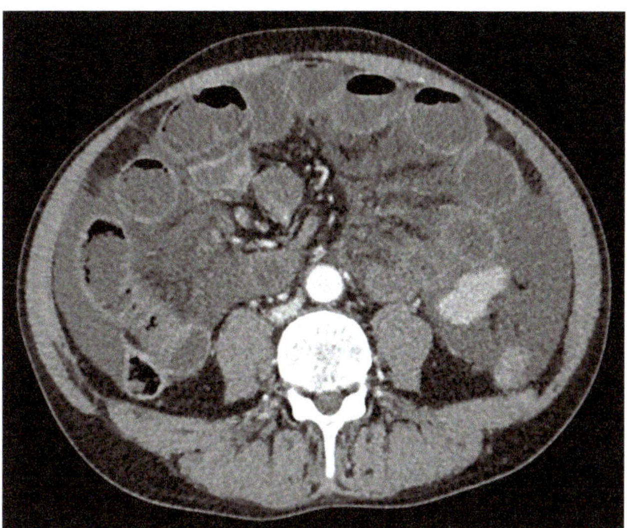

FIGURE 20.2 Patient A. Axial CT of the mid-abdomen with contrast.

20.2 Radiology Self-assessment

20.2.1 Technical

- What are the limitations of plain X-ray when looking at the gastrointestinal (GI) tract?

20.2.2 Correlation of Gross Anatomy

- What does the GI tract look like on CT?
- How can you trace the GI tract on CT?

20.3 Key Radiology Review

20.3.1 Technical Aspects and Anatomy X-ray

There is a tremendous variation in the appearance of the GI tract on X-rays. This is related to both the amount of bowel gas and the variable location of certain sections of the tract.

20.3.2 Gastrointestinal Tract on Plain Radiograph

Gas-filled bowel loops are visible on plain X-ray. As a result, occasionally most of the tract can be clearly seen (Figure 20.3a). However, if there is a lack of bowel gas, almost none of the GI tract will be visible (Figure 20.3b).

20.3.3 Gastrointestinal Tract on CT

As with plain radiographs, there is a huge variation in the appearance of the GI tract on CT, depending on the volume of gas/faeces in the lumen. The benefit of CT is that even when collapsed or fluid filled, the GI tract remains visible. This is thanks to visceral fat surrounding the abdominal organs (see previous chapter). As fat has a relatively low density on CT, it is easy to differentiate it from the lighter shaded adjacent organs, such as the bowel walls (Figure 20.4a,b).

20.3.4 Tracing the Bowel

Carrying this out on CT is notoriously difficult as it requires extensive scrolling up and down through the scan images while focusing on the same segment of bowel. A certain level of 3D spatial awareness is needed, along with knowledge of the anatomy of the GI tract. This is demonstrated in the accompanying online video (see Further Resources) but a summary of the key points is provided in Figure 20.5.

Awareness of the anatomically fixed parts of the bowel is very useful as they provide visual anchors for identifying certain sections of bowel. In particular, the third part of the duodenum, rectum, ascending and descending colon are reliable fixed sites visible on CT.

20.4 Review of the Clinical Case

- What is your differential diagnosis?
- When should a plain AXR be requested?
- When should CT be requested?
- What is your final diagnosis?

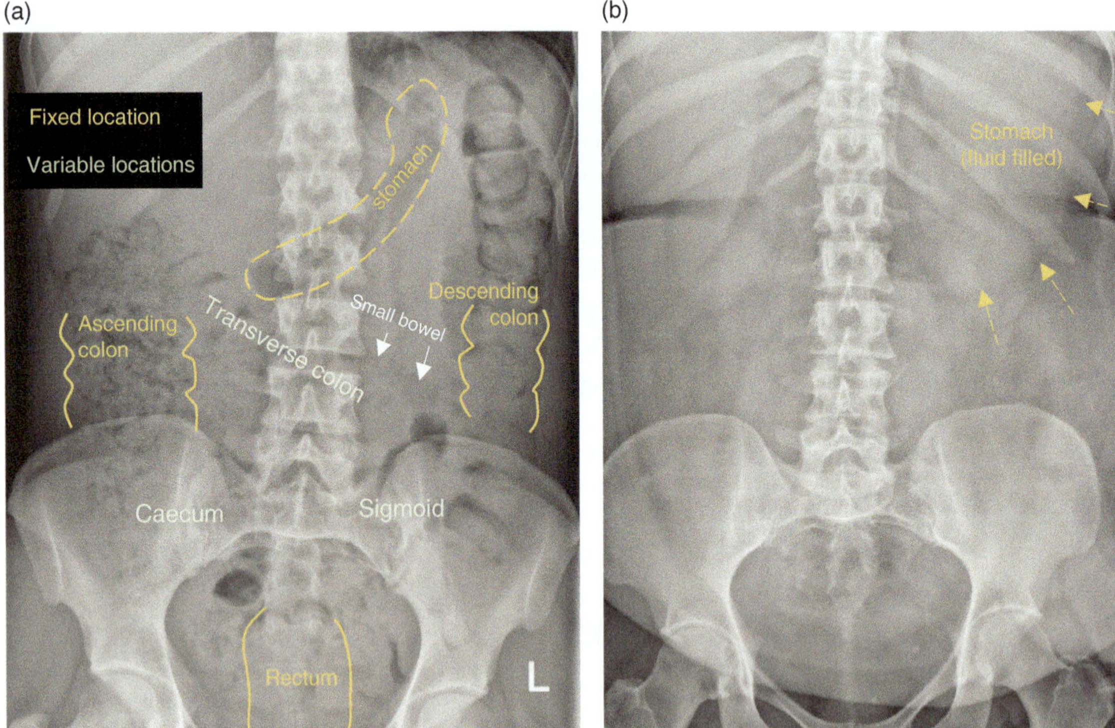

FIGURE 20.3 Examples of normal abdominal X-rays. (a) This patient has gas in the GI tract, making identification of the stomach, small and large bowel possible. The stomach, second and third parts of duodenum, ascending colon, descending colon and rectum are in anatomically fixed locations so will always be found at those sites. In contrast, the caecum, transverse colon and sigmoid have a variable location, depending on the length of bowel and accompanying mesocolon. For example, it is not uncommon for the transverse colon to be adjacent to the bladder and the sigmoid colon to be under the diaphragm. Although the small bowel loops are not fixed in position and can move to some extent, they will always be central in the abdomen (white arrows). Small bowel loops often extend into the pelvis to abut the urinary bladder. (b) This patient has a paucity of bowel gas so assessment of the GI tract is very limited. Occasionally, a very large fluid-filled stomach may be visible as a dense (white) object in the left upper quadrant (dashed orange arrows).

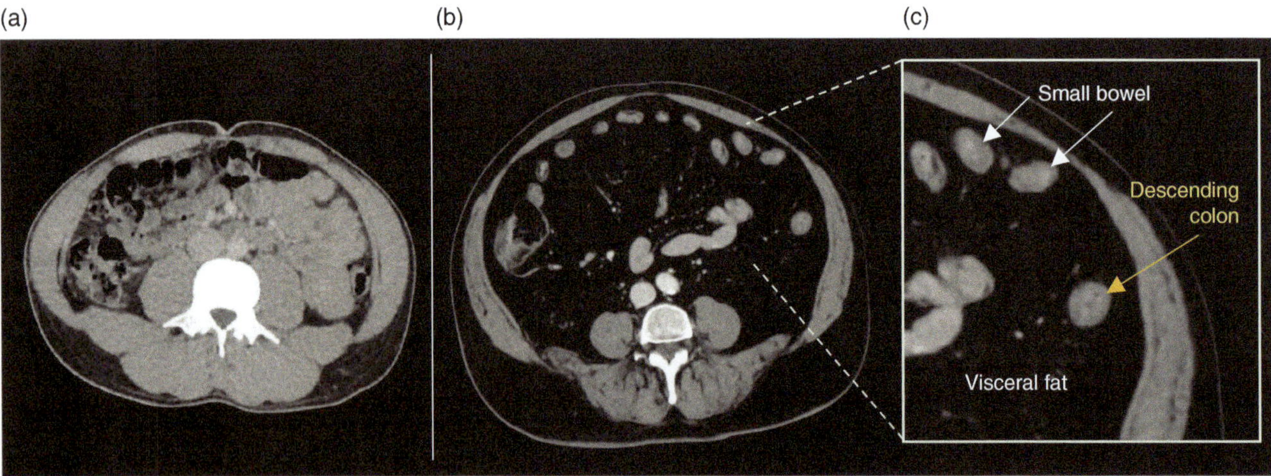

FIGURE 20.4 Axial CT through the mid-abdomen with contrast. (a) Minimal visceral fat – the bowel loops lie together, making it difficult to distinguish individual segments. (b) Significant visceral fat – the bowel loops are separated by fat (dark), making them easier to trace. (c) Contrary to traditional anatomy diagrams, the small and large bowel can look very similar when collapsed (compare descending colon to small bowel loops). The only reliable way to distinguish between them is by tracing the bowel. The haustra and valvulae conniventes are less obvious on CT in general and cannot be seen when the bowel is collapsed.

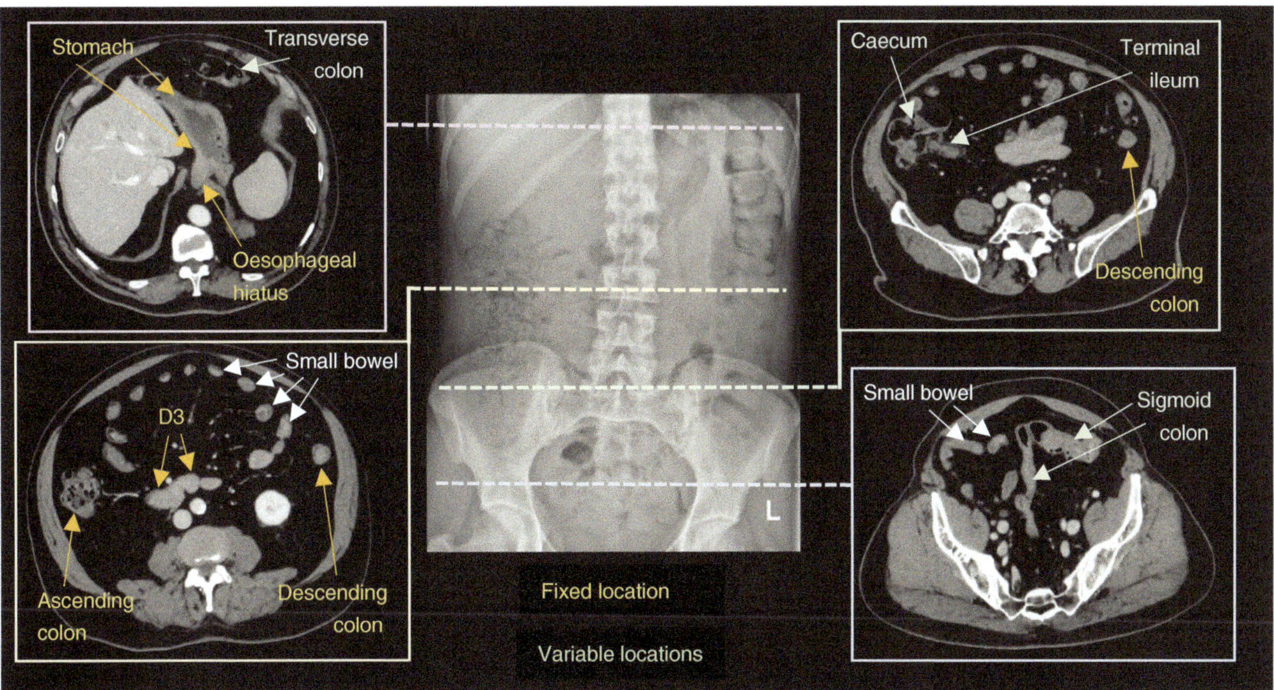

FIGURE 20.5 Selected axial CT slices of the abdomen, post contrast. AXR from Figure 20.3a is given to show corresponding level. Pink – oesophageal hiatus: find the oesophageal hiatus in the midline and the stomach on the left. By scrolling down you will see the stomach cross the midline with the pylorus on the right. The transverse colon often travels anterior to the stomach. Yellow – D3 (third part of duodenum): follow the duodenum as it crosses the midline back to the left. This is a fixed retroperitoneal location. If you follow the duodenum distally you will find the small bowel. This is the longest part of the bowel and can be followed from the jejunum (mostly in left upper quadrant) to the ileum (mostly in right iliac fossa [RIF]). On its journey it will twist and turn through the abdomen and pelvis but will remain inside the peritoneum. Green – ileocaecal valve: the caecum will usually lie in the RIF but this can be variable. Find the valve where the terminal ileum enters the caecum. From here, you can follow the colon through the fixed retroperitoneal ascending colon, back to intraperitoneal transverse colon. This has a variable location but will always cross the midline back to the left. Follow it to the fixed retroperitoneal descending colon. Blue – sigmoid colon: finally follow the intraperitoneal sigmoid colon which is the most variable segment of the GI tract. It can be very short and confined to the left iliac fossa but it may also have a long course, crossing over to the right side or even travelling up near the liver or spleen. Those patients with a long sigmoid mesocolon are more at risk of volvulus. Eventually the sigmoid will return to the midline posterior pelvis and continue to the extraperitoneal rectum.

20.4.1 Differential Diagnosis

The symptoms of acute-onset severe abdominal pain and vomiting are suggestive of GI tract obstruction. The most likely site is the small bowel as the pain is in the upper abdomen and vomiting is a prominent early feature. However, confirming the cause of small bowel obstruction can be difficult clinically but there are some clues. These are listed below in descending order of frequency but, for the purpose of memory recall, it can also be helpful to classify the causes in terms of location (i.e. inside lumen, inside the wall and outside the wall).

- Adhesions (outside the wall) – this is the most common cause of bowel obstruction. There must be a history of abdominal surgery or peritonitis. The risk of adhesions increases with handling of the bowel so is more common after open surgery as opposed to laparoscopic intervention.

- Hernia (outside the wall) – in the cohort of patients who have not had surgery, incarcerated external hernias are the next most common cause. Careful examination of the inguinal and femoral areas is required. Internal hernias (e.g. foremen of Winslow) are possible but much less common.
- Inflammatory (inside the wall) – patients with Crohn's disease can develop strictures, usually with a long history of frequent flare-ups prior to obstruction.
- Intussusception (inside the lumen) – this is a common cause of bowel obstruction in children but is rare in adults.
- Gallstone ileus (inside the lumen) – this is a very rare condition that can be difficult to distinguish from other causes of small bowel obstruction. There may be a clue in the history of intermittent abdominal pain, related to repeated bouts of cholecystitis prior to fistulation into the small bowel.
- Tumours (inside the wall) – small bowel tumours are also very rare but can cause small bowel obstruction.

20.4.2 Imaging in Small Bowel Obstruction

It is possible to have small bowel obstruction with a normal plain AXR. Furthermore, even when it is visible, it is unlikely that a radiograph will show you the cause. Therefore, if a patient has convincing symptoms of bowel obstruction, CT is the definitive investigation and plain radiographs are not usually required. The exceptions are when the obstruction occurs in patients with co-existing inguinal/femoral hernias. These can sometimes be picked up on plain X-ray with a pinched loop extending into the respective canal. Clinical examination is also helpful in these cases.

20.4.3 Review the X-ray (Figure 20.6)

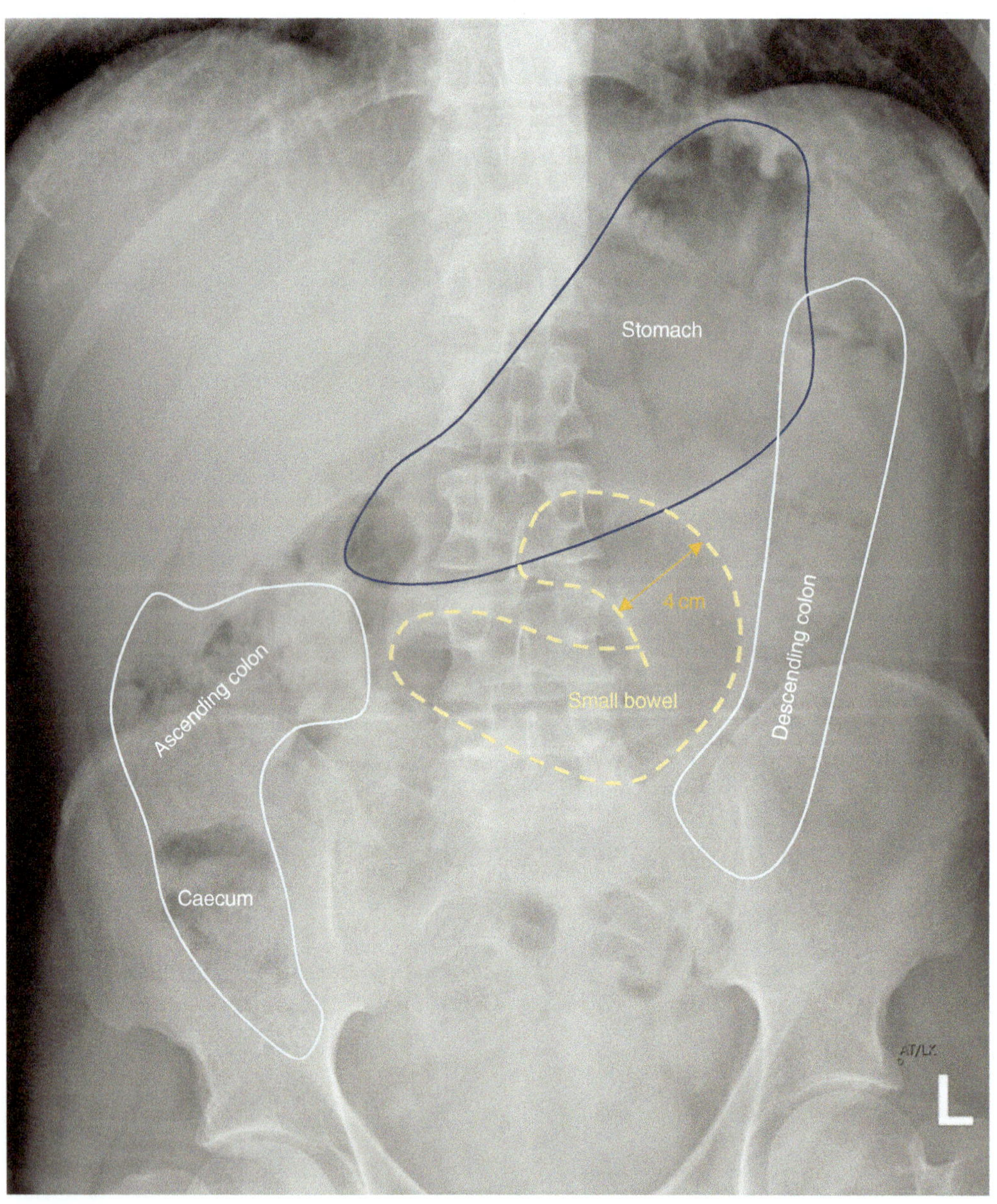

FIGURE 20.6 Patient A. Abdominal X-ray. There is a centrally dilated loop of small bowel, measuring 4 cm in diameter. A generally agreed cut-off for the maximum diameter of bowel is: small bowel <3 cm; large bowel <6 cm; caecum <9 cm; However, it is not uncommon to see bowel of this calibre in asymptomatic patients and so these measurements are not reliable, stand-alone, diagnostic criteria for bowel obstruction.

20.4.4 **Review the CT** (Figure 20.7)

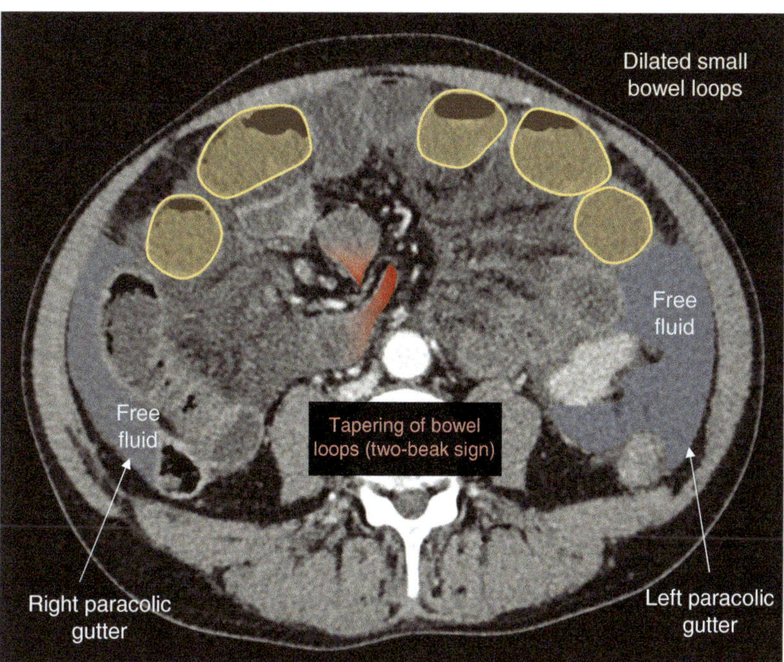

FIGURE 20.7 Patient A. Axial CT of the mid-abdomen with contrast. There is a mechanical small bowel obstruction secondary to an adhesional band in the central abdomen. On this CT slice, there are two transition points visible, which abruptly narrow in calibre. This is called the two-beak sign and suggests a closed loop obstruction (see Figure 20.8). There is also a large volume of free fluid in the peritoneum which can be a sign of early bowel ischaemia.

20.4.4.1 Closed Loop Obstruction (Figure 20.8)

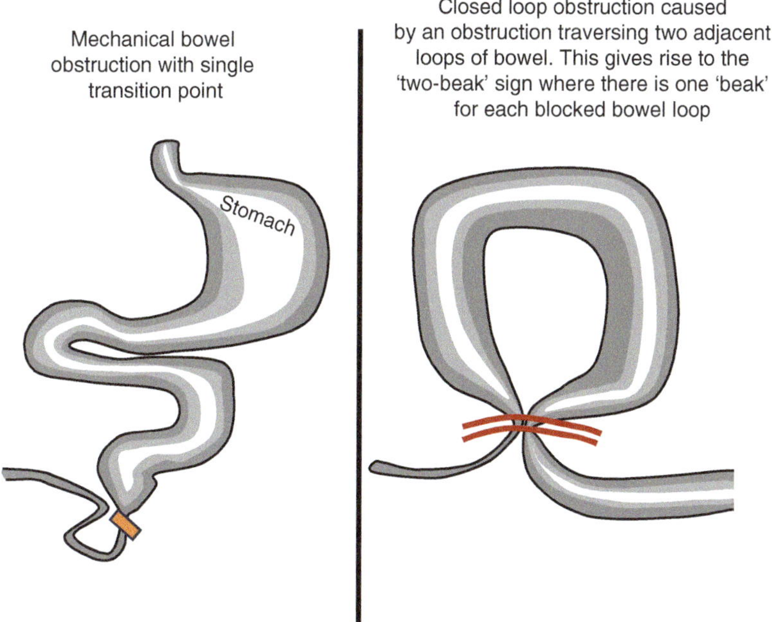

FIGURE 20.8 Types of bowel obstruction. It is important to distinguish between a single transition point (mechanical bowel obstruction) and closed loop obstruction. In single-point obstruction, the bowel can decompress upstream to the stomach and eventually through vomiting. This is why an NG tube is an important initial step in obstruction. These patients are often able to wait and be monitored, with IV fluids to maintain hydration. In contrast, with closed loop obstruction the bowel cannot decompress so the pressure builds up, resulting in vascular compromise. Bowel ischaemia is ultimately what causes the morbidity and mortality associated with closed loop obstruction. This is a surgical emergency and cannot be managed in the same way as single-point obstruction.

20.4.5 Final Diagnosis Closed loop small bowel obstruction secondary to an adhesional band.

20.5 Take-home Message – Imaging in Obstruction

- Plain AXRs have a place in assessing obstruction in patients who are not clinically unwell. Gas-filled dilated loops are easily picked up. However, fluid-filled loops will not be visible and a normal AXR does not exclude obstruction.
- For this reason, CT abdomen/pelvis with contrast is the definitive imaging modality in suspected obstruction. This can identify all segments of the GI tract, regardless of gas content, and will often show the underlying cause of obstruction.

Further Resources

Nelms, D.W. and Kann, B.R. (2021). Imaging modalities for evaluation of intestinal obstruction. *Clin Colon Rectal Surg* 34 (4): 205–218.

Video: https://shorturl.at/uvdKq

CHAPTER 21

Flank Pain

Joshua Lauder[1], Benjamin Layton[2], and Peter Driscoll[3]

[1] East Lancashire Hospitals NHS Trust, University of Central Lancashire and University of Manchester, UK
[2] Morecambe Bay Hospitals Trust, Lancaster, UK
[3] School of Medicine and Dentistry, University of Central Lancashire, Preston, UK

21.1 Primary Case

21.1.1 Presentation

A 38-year-old male presents to the Emergency Department with a 12-hour history of severe left loin pain, radiating his left groin area. He describes it as coming and going but it is making him nauseous. He has vomited twice but this made no difference to the pain.

21.1.1.1 History of Presenting Complaint His appetite is normally good and he had a normal bowel movement yesterday. There has been no dysuria or haematuria.

PMH: NAD.

SH:

- Non-smoker.
- Drinks around 7 units of alcohol per week.

DH: NAD.

21.1.2 Clinical Examination

- Looks in pain.
- Chest is clear on auscultation.
- Heart sounds are normal.
- Abdomen – tender left loin.

Modified early warning signs (MEWS)

- Respiratory rate 16 rpm.
- SpO_2 96% on room air.
- Tympanic temp. 37.2 °C.
- HR 98 bpm.
- BP 120/80 mmHg.
- Alert.

21.1.3 Blood Results

	Normal	Patient
Sodium	135–145 mmol/l	136 mmol/l
Potassium	3.5–5.0 mmol/l	4.7 mmol/l
Urea	2.5–6.7 mmol/l	7.2 mmol/l
Creatinine	3–17 mmol/l	15 mmol/l
Haemoglobin	115–157 g/l	143 g/l
White cell count	$3.5–11 \times 10^9$/l	9.6×10^9/l

Urinalysis: + protein; +++ blood

Diagnostic Imaging and Anatomy in Acute Care, First Edition. Edited by Joshua Lauder and Peter Driscoll.
© 2025 John Wiley & Sons Ltd. Published 2025 by John Wiley & Sons Ltd.
Companion website: www.wiley.com/go/DiagnosticImaginginAcuteCare

21.1.4 CT KUB (Kidney, Ureter, Bladder)

(Figure 21.1)

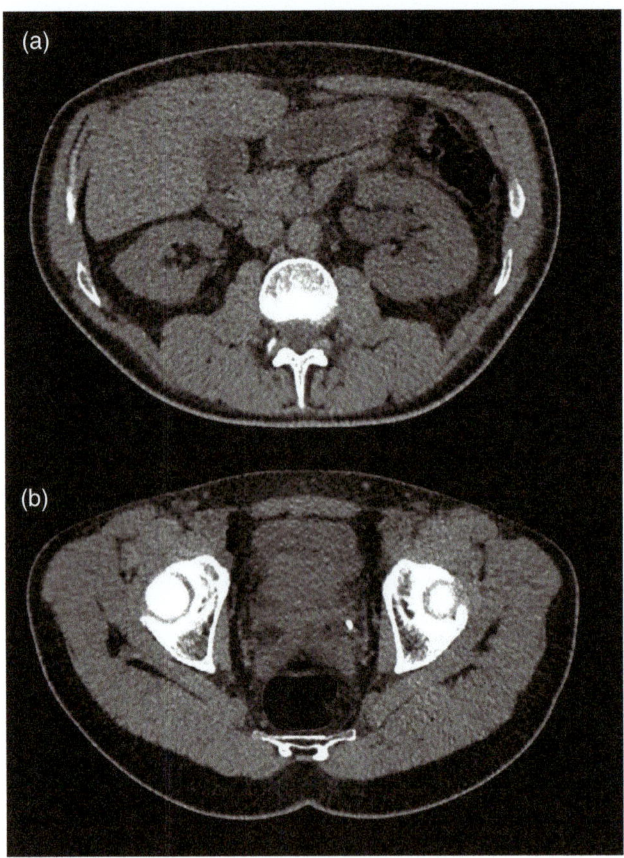

FIGURE 21.1 CT KUB of patient A. (a) Axial slice at level of the kidneys. (b) Axial slice at level of the distal ureter.

> ### Clinical Case Questions
> - What is your differential diagnosis?
> - When is CT indicated?
> - What is your system for interpreting these images?
> - What is your final diagnosis and immediate management?

21.2 Radiology Self-assessment

21.2.1 Technical

- How is a CT KUB performed?

21.2.2 Correlating Gross Anatomy

- What do the kidneys and urinary tract look like on CT?
- How does contrast affect the appearance of the urinary tract?

21.3 Key Radiology Review

21.3.1 Anatomy

An overview of the key anatomy is shown in Figure 21.2, along with sites of normal ureteric narrowing.

21.3.2 Technical Aspects

A CT KUB has two main differences compared to a standard CT of the abdomen. First, the scan is performed *without* contrast. This is because most kidney stones are calcified, so easily visualised on CT. Thanks to the fat in the renal pelvis, it is also possible to see hydronephrosis on CT, even without contrast (Figure 21.3).

The second difference is that the patient lies prone. This is to differentiate between loose stones in the bladder and stones stuck in the vesicoureteric junction (VUJ) (Figure 21.4).

21.4 Review of the Clinical Case

- What is your differential diagnosis?
- When is CT indicated?
- What is your system for interpreting these images?
- What is your final diagnosis

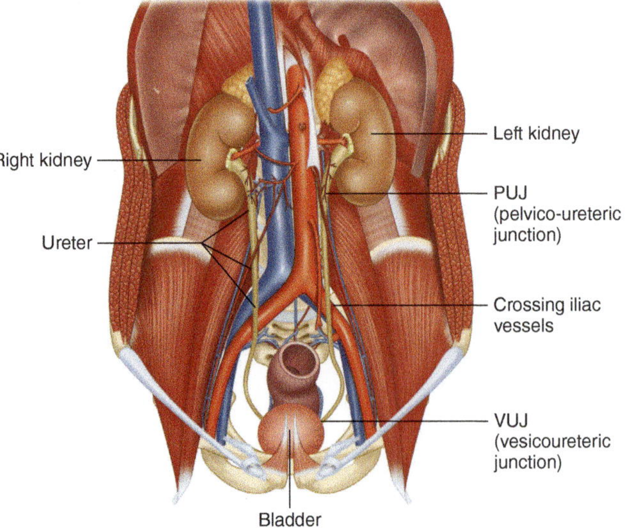

FIGURE 21.2 The urinary tract and the anatomical sites of ureteral narrowing.

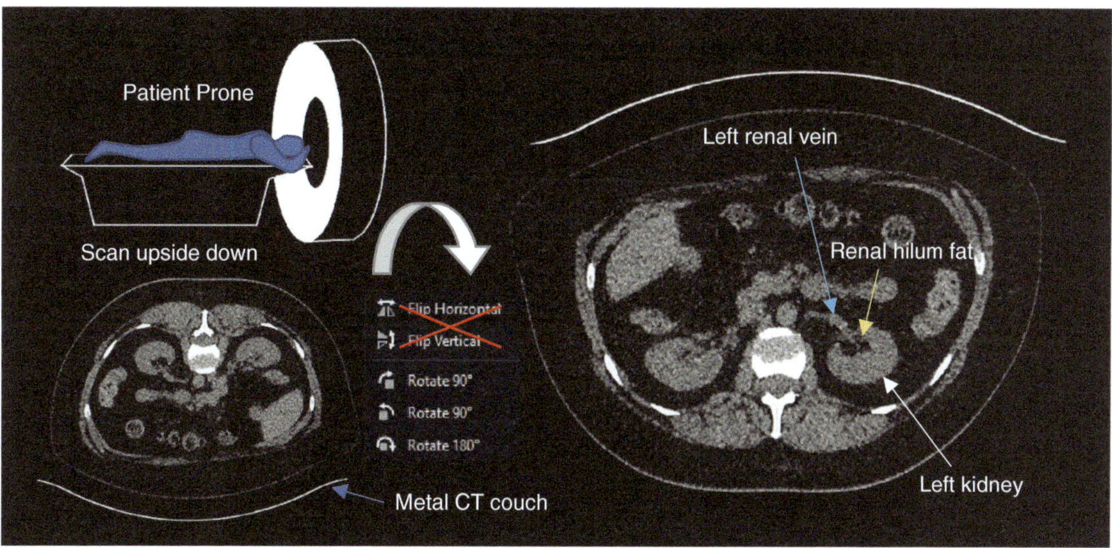

FIGURE 21.3 CT KUB technique. The scan is performed with the patient prone. This sometimes results in the image being upside down on the PACS viewer. In these situations, rotate the image through 180° to achieve the normal orientation. Never use the 'flip' function as this will result in the left and right sides being the wrong way round. The right image shows the normal renal hila containing low-density fat (so nearly black) interspersed with lighter coloured renal vessels. The normal renal collecting system is collapsed so is not clearly identified.

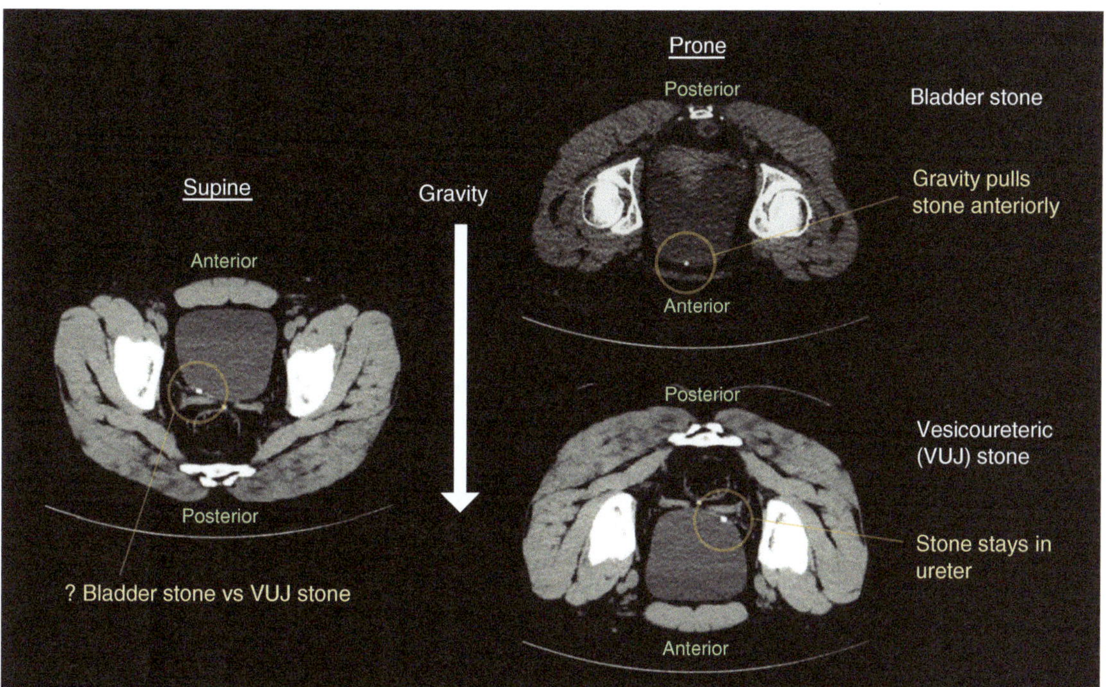

FIGURE 21.4 Rationale for prone CT KUB. On a supine CT, when a stone is seen in the region of the VUJ, it cannot be certain if this lies in the ureter or a dependent position in the posterior bladder. In the prone position, bladder stones are pulled anteriorly by gravity, whereas VUJ stones remain posterior.

21.4.1 Differential Diagnosis

- Renal tract calculi.
  - Loin to groin pain is a classic presentation of a ureteric calculus. The pain is usually described as severe and may be associated with nausea and vomiting. Urinalysis may contain blood.

- Pyelonephritis.
  - If there is a fever and/or elevated inflammatory markers, then this should be considered. It can occur as a complication of ureteric obstruction.

21.4.1.1 Modified Stone Score (Figure 21.5) This scoring system can aid in treatment planning, but local pathways vary.

Modified Stone Scoring System		
Categories		**Score**
Gender (Over 18's)		
	Female	0
	Male	2
Timing (duration of colicky pain to presentation)		
	>24 hours	0
	6–24 hours	1
	<6 hours	3
Nausea and vomiting		
	None	0
	Nausea alone	1
	Vomiting	2
Dipstick haematuria		
	Absent	0
	Present	3
Total		0–10

Probability	Total Score	Imaging Outcome
Low	0–4	No imaging
Moderate	5–7	Non-urgent CT KUB – within 72 hrs
High	8–10	Urgent CT KUB – within 24 hrs

FIGURE 21.5 Example of a modified stone score and investigation pathway. This applies to patients with classic history for kidney stones, who are clinically well (i.e. not septic) and when abdominal aortic aneurysm has been excluded if the patient is over 55 years old (see Chapter 22).

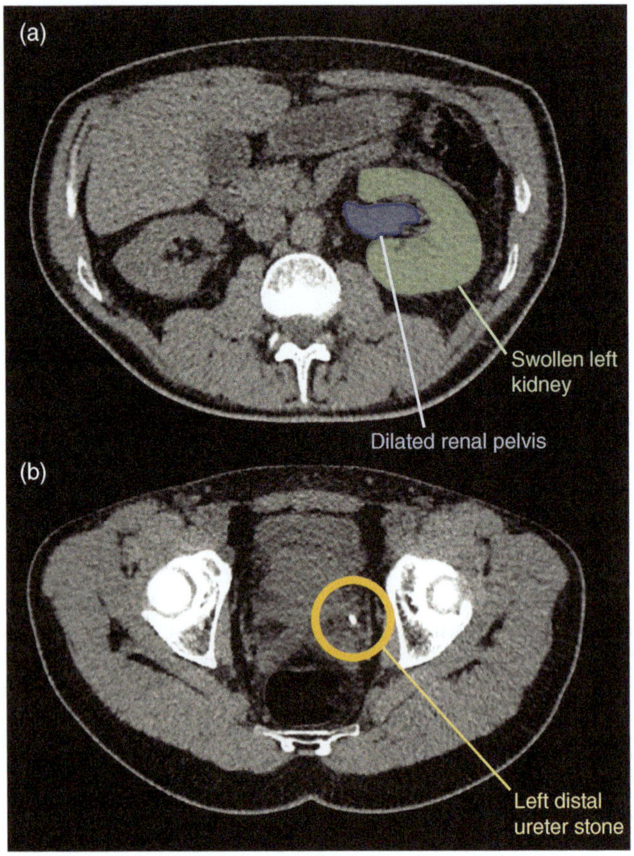

(a)

Swollen left kidney

Dilated renal pelvis

(b)

Left distal ureter stone

FIGURE 21.6 CT KUB of patient. (a) Axial slice at the level of the kidneys showing left hydronephrosis. The left renal pelvis and calyces are dilated. The left renal parenchyma is also swollen. (b) Once the ureter is identified, it should be followed along the retroperitoneum to the pelvic side wall and bladder. In this case a small impacted calculus lies in the left distal ureter. The size of the calculus should be described. Those less than 4 mm in length are likely to pass on their own within 31 days. Bigger stones are less likely to pass spontaneously and may require urological intervention.

21.4.2 Review the CT

21.4.2.1 Check the Urinary Tract Carry out a systematic inspection of the urinary tract starting with the kidneys. If there is hydronephrosis, the renal pelvis and calyces will be dilated, which replaces the dark fat in the renal hilum (Figure 21.6a). Compare the left and right kidneys for asymmetry. Look for any dense foci in the renal collecting system. If small, these may be non-obstructive renal calculi or Randall's plaques (see Figure 21.8).

Follow the ureter down from the renal pelvis looking for hydroureter. The distal ureter can be difficult to follow – it should curve along the pelvic side wall before joining to the bladder base. Look for calculi in the distal ureter but beware of phleboliths in the pelvis (see Figure 21.7).

21.4.2.2 Distinguishing Stones from Phleboliths Phleboliths are benign vascular calcifications which very commonly occur in the pelvis. These can easily be mistaken for ureteric stones as they lie in a similar position to the distal ureters (Figure 21.7). Useful discriminating features which favour phleboliths are central lucency and a round contour. Renal tract calculi tend to be more oval shaped and uniformly calcified.

21.4.2.3 Non-obstructive Renal Calculi Renal stones are formed at the renal papilla. They begin as a Randall's plaque which are less than 2 mm in size. These can then act as a focus for deposition of calcium oxalate and progress to renal calculi which detach and fall into the calyx (Figure 21.8).

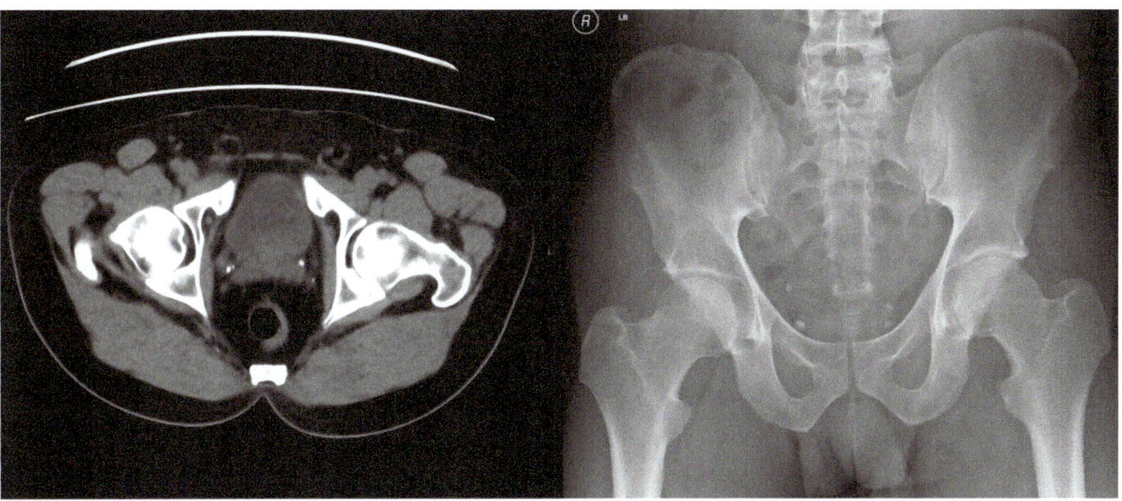

FIGURE 21.7 (Left) Axial CT KUB at the level of the bladder. (Right) AP pelvis X-ray of the same patient. There are multiple calcified phleboliths in the pelvis. This patient has no hydronephrosis so these are unlikely to represent calculi.

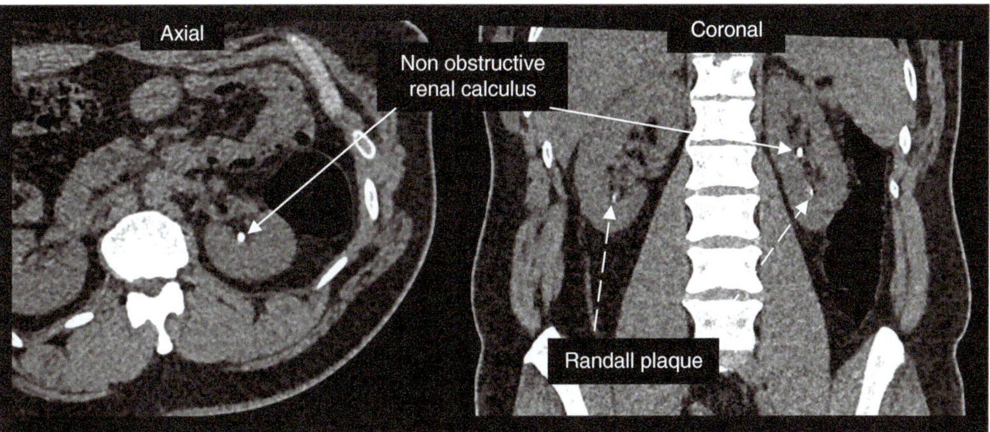

FIGURE 21.8 Axial and coronal CT KUB of the kidneys. There are Randall's plaques in the lower poles of both kidneys (dashed arrows). A non-obstructive renal calculus is present in the mid-pole of the left kidney (white arrows). Note the preserved renal hilar fat, with no dilation of renal pelvis or calyces.

21.4.3 Role of Ultrasound

Ultrasound is a useful test to exclude hydronephrosis (Figure 21.9).

Therefore, if expertise is available, point-of-care ultrasound can help to triage patients with suspected obstructive uropathy (Figure 21.10). However, it has poor sensitivity for renal tract calculi and the ureters cannot be seen. Consequently, a small ureteric calculus with no hydronephrosis will be missed.

21.4.4 Final Diagnosis

Left distal ureteric calculus causing hydronephrosis. There are no features of secondary pyelonephritis.

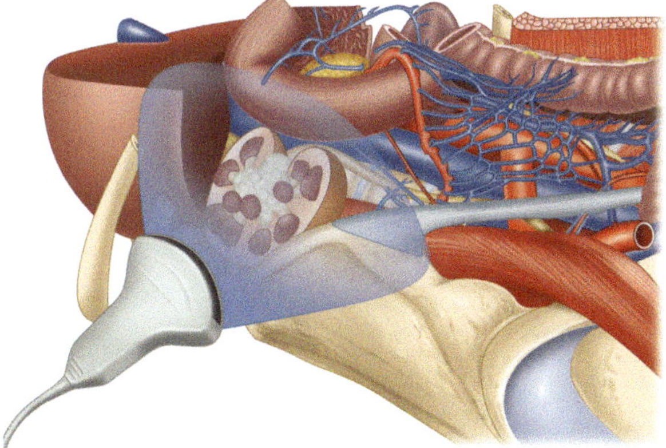

FIGURE 21.9 Ultrasound technique. The kidneys are relatively posterior in location so are often best seen from the flank. In this way, the gas in the anterior lying bowel does not obstruct the view. It is also helpful to get the patient to lift their ipsilateral arm above their head as this spreads the ribs.

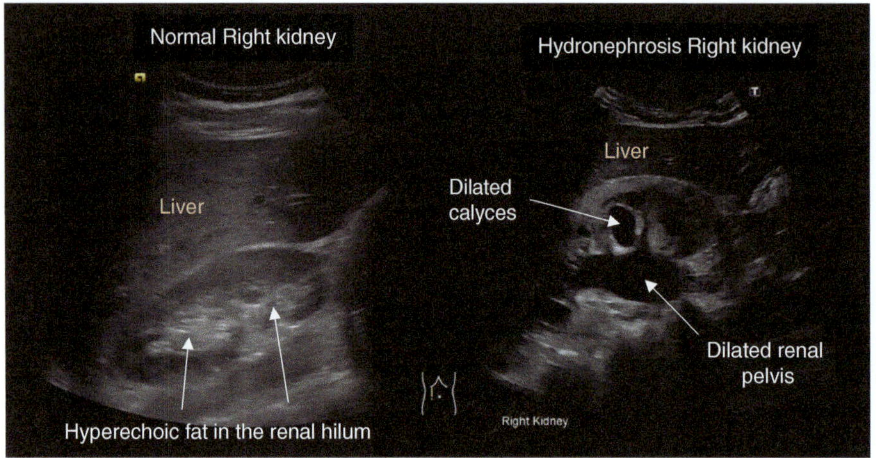

FIGURE 21.10 Long axis ultrasound of the right kidney. Normal (left image), hydronephrosis (right image). The normal kidney will have hyperechoic fat in the hilum, with the renal pelvis barely visible. In hydronephrosis there is dilation of both the renal pelvis and calyces.

21.5 Take-home Message – Imaging in Kidney Stones

- Ultrasound is a useful screening test for obstructive uropathy but cannot identify the ureters so will not always show the cause of obstruction.

- CT KUB is the gold standard for diagnosing kidney stones. The urgency of investigation will depend on the presenting symptoms.

Further Resources

Arac, M., Celik, H., Oner, A.Y. et al. (2005). Distinguishing pelvic phleboliths from distal ureteral calculi: thin-slice CT findings. *Eur Radiol* 15 (1): 65–70.

Malik, A., Mohkummudin, S., Yousaf, S. et al. (2020). Validity of STONE score in clinical prediction of ureteral stone disease. *Pak J Med Sci* 36: 1693–1697.

Jendeberg, J., Geijer, H., Alshamari, M. et al. (2017). Size matters: the width and location of a ureteral stone accurately predict the chance of spontaneous passage. *Eur Radiol* 27 (11): 4775–4785.

CHAPTER 22

Back Pain

Joshua Lauder[1], Shofiq Al-Islam[2], Benjamin Layton[3], and Peter Driscoll[4]

[1]*East Lancashire Hospitals NHS Trust, University of Central Lancashire and University of Manchester, UK*
[2]*East Lancashire Hospitals NHS Trust, Blackburn, UK*
[3]*Morecambe Bay Hospitals Trust, Lancaster, UK*
[4]*School of Medicine and Dentistry, University of Central Lancashire, Preston, UK*

22.1 Primary Case

22.1.1 Presentation

A 72-year-old male presents to the Emergency Department with sudden-onset severe abdominal pain radiating to his back.

22.1.1.1 History of Presenting Complaint The symptoms started two hours ago and he felt faint. The latter has eased since lying flat, but the pain has not settled.

PMH:

- Known cardiovascular disease with a previous myocardial infarction and a history of hypertension, taking amlodipine 5 mg and ramipril 10 mg.
- Smoker (40 pack-years).

22.1.2 Examination

- Obese (BWI 30.2).
- Chest clear on auscultation.
- Heart sounds normal.
- Tenderness in the epigastric and umbilical area.

Modified early warning signs (MEWS):

- Respiratory rate 16 rpm.
- SaO_2 95% on room air.
- Tympanic temp 36.5 °C.
- HR 70 bpm.
- BP 110/70 mmHg.
- Alert.

22.1.3 Blood Results

	Normal	Patient
Sodium	135–145 mmol/l	140 mmol/l
Potassium	3.5–5.0 mmol/l	4.7 mmol/l
Urea	2.5–6.7 mmol/l	6.0 mmol/l
Haemoglobin	115–157 g/l	143 g/l
White cell count	$3.5–11 \times 10^9/l$	$7.11 \times 10^9/l$

22.1.4 CT Angiogram

In view of his presenting signs and symptoms a CT angiogram was arranged (Figure 22.1).

Clinical Case Questions

- What is your differential diagnosis?
- When is CT indicated?
- What is your system for interpreting these images?
- What is your final diagnosis and immediate management?

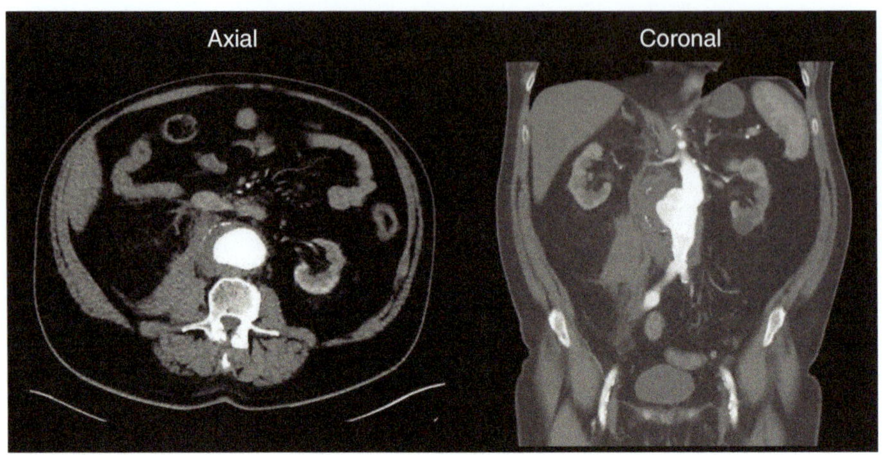

FIGURE 22.1 Patient A. CT angiogram. (Left) Axial slice at the level of the renal hilum. (Right) Abdominal coronal view.

22.2 Radiology Self-assessment

22.2.1 Technical

- What imaging is used to assess the aorta?
- How is an aortic angiogram performed?

22.2.2 Correlation of Gross Anatomy

- What is the normal calibre for the aorta?
- What does the aorta look like on CT?

22.3 Key Radiology Review

22.3.1 Technical Aspects and Anatomy

22.3.1.1 CT Angiogram CT angiogram is the most comprehensive way to assess the aorta (Figure 22.2). This requires intravenous contrast, with the scan usually performed at around 20–30 seconds after injection.

22.3.2 Imaging of Abdominal Aortic Aneurysm

22.3.2.1 Ultrasound of Aorta Ultrasound is used in the screening and monitoring of abdominal aortic aneurysms (AAA). This is a quick and cheap option, without the need for IV contrast and radiation.

When measuring aortic diameter, the AP measurement is typically used and should be measured in the transverse plane (Figure 22.3). Anything above 3 cm is considered aneurysmal, but the risk of rupture increases with increasing size. The chance is exceedingly low if the AP diameter is less than 4 cm. However, this increases to over a 30% risk of rupture per year when the sac is over 8 cm. Another risk factor for rupture is an expansion rate of over 0.5 cm in six months, hence patients with known aneurysms have serial scans to assess for growth. NICE recommends referral to vascular surgeon when the AP diameter is greater than 5.5 cm.

In England, AAA screening is offered to men when they turn 65 years old.

Ultrasound has limitations; bowel gas often obscures the aortic bifurcation and common iliac arteries, so aneurysms here can be missed (Figure 22.4). It is also insensitive to retroperitoneal haemorrhage so cannot reliably exclude an aneurysm rupture.

22.4 Review of the Clinical Case

- What is your differential diagnosis?
- When should CT aorta be arranged?
- What is your final diagnosis and immediate management?

22.4.1 Differential Diagnosis

- Ruptured AAA.
  - If an elderly patient presents with abdominal pain radiating to the back, with clinical features of hypovolaemic shock, then a ruptured AAA should be excluded.
  - If there is a large retroperitoneal haemorrhage involving the psoas muscle, there may be reduced hip flexion which can be a useful sign. If expertise is available then a bedside ultrasound can be used to assess for a AAA. If the aorta is normal in calibre, then rupture can be excluded.

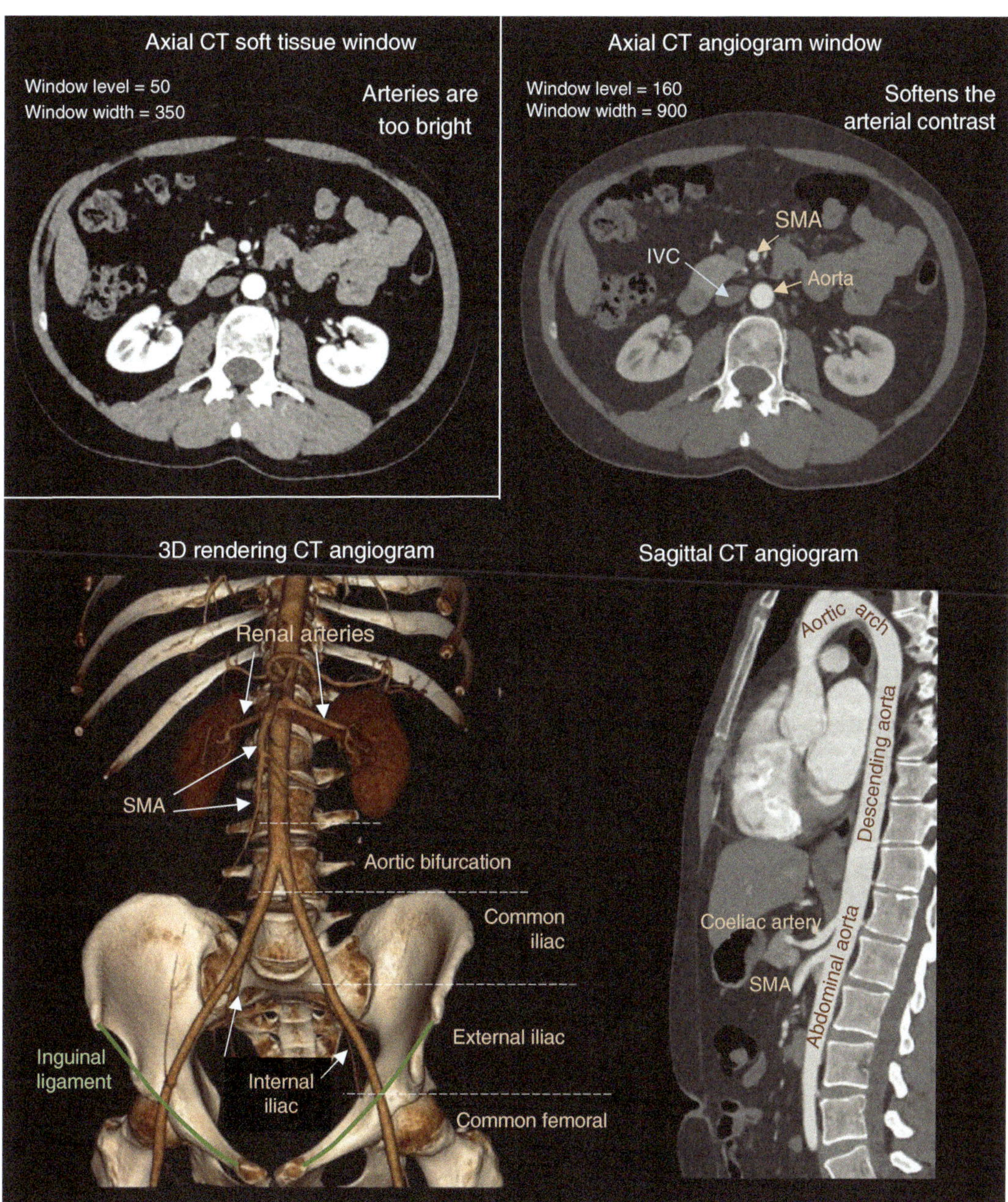

FIGURE 22.2 Normal CT angiogram aorta. The top two images are axial slices through the infrarenal abdominal aorta. On the soft tissue window (top left), the contrast in the arteries is too white, blanching out the vessel lumen. Therefore, an angiogram window should be used (top right) as this softens the vessel, allowing better assessment of the lumen. This is particularly important for spotting dissection flaps. (Bottom left) 3D CT angiogram reformat frontal view. The entire abdominal aorta can be traced to the bifurcation and onwards to the femoral arteries. (Bottom right) Sagittal CT angiogram on angiogram window.

If the aorta is aneurysmal or cannot be positively identified on ultrasound, then urgent CT angiogram is indicated.

- Aortic dissection.
  - This may present in a similar manner to a ruptured abdominal aneurysm but is more likely to have pain higher up in the chest and thoracic spine region. Furthermore, the amount of blood loss is less. Therefore, the patient may have unequal blood pressure in the upper limbs but should not have hypovolemic signs.
- Renal pathology.
  - Both hydronephrosis and pyelonephritis can present with back pain (see Chapter 21).
- Musculoskeletal back pain is very common and can occasionally mimic aortic pain.

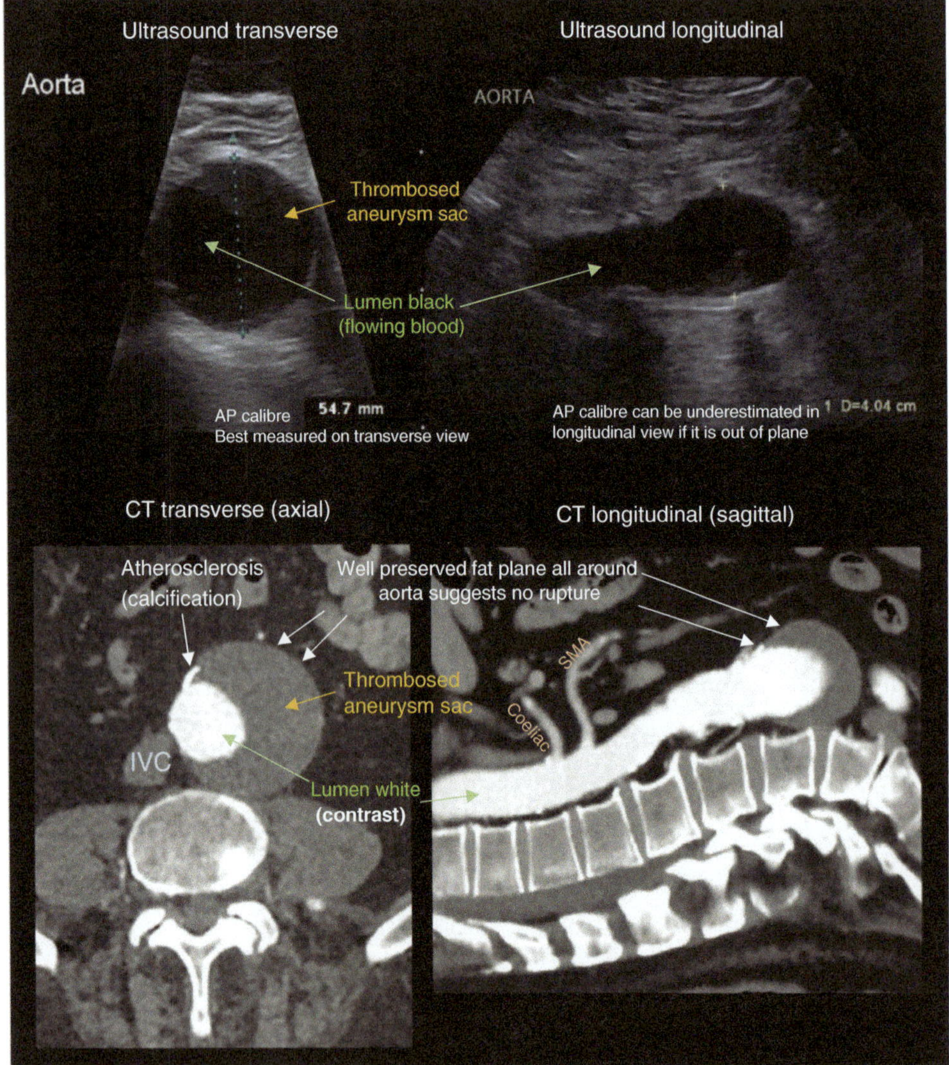

FIGURE 22.3 Ultrasound and CT images of an infrarenal abdominal aortic aneurysm. (Top images – US) The lumen of the aorta appears black on ultrasound as it is filled with flowing blood: this can be confirmed with Doppler (not shown). A thrombus is visible in the aneurysm sac. This appears as a peripheral hypoechoic crescent. (Bottom images – CT angiogram) Same patient. The extent of the thrombosis is more easily seen than on US. The clear demarcation between the vessel wall (grey) and the surrounding fat (black) indicates there is no rupture or inflammation.

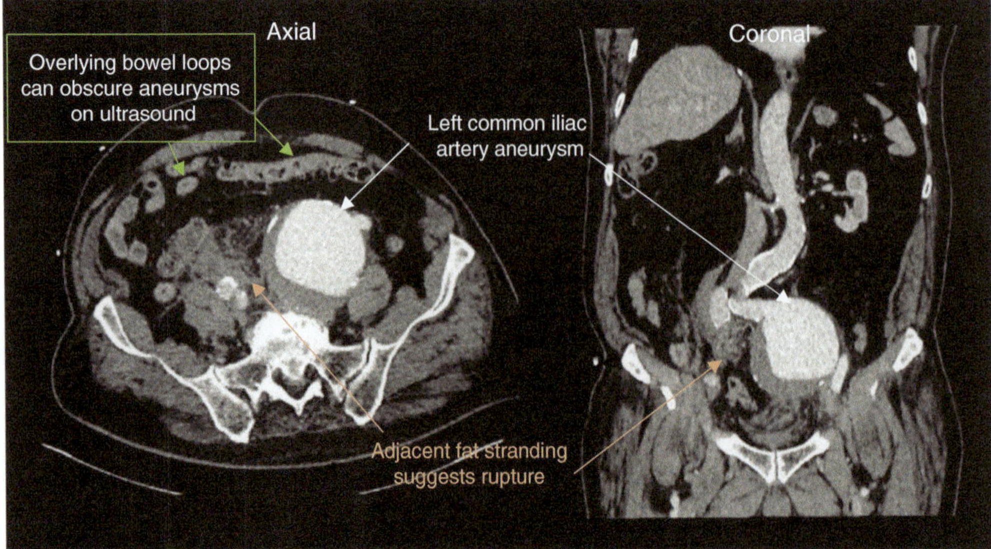

FIGURE 22.4 Axial and coronal CT angiogram aorta, showing a left common iliac artery aneurysm. There is fat stranding around the right side of the aneurysm, representing recent haemorrhage, which was managed conservatively in this case. Distal aortic and common iliac artery aneurysms can be missed on ultrasound due to overlying bowel gas.

22.4.2 Review the CT

The CT shows a relatively small abdominal aortic aneurysm measuring 5 cm in AP dimension. However, there is a focal bulge on the right side representing a penetrating ulcer, giving a transverse dimension of 6.6 cm (Figure 22.5). Therefore, the morphology of the aneurysm can be important, and it is not always appropriate to rely solely on the AP dimension.

There is fat stranding in the right retroperitoneum representing haemorrhage.

This aneurysm is infrarenal. This distinction is important when it comes to treatment, as the renal arteries must maintain patency.

22.4.3 Final Diagnosis

Ruptured abdominal aortic aneurysm.

22.4.4 Management

Ruptured AAA can be managed with open or endovascular repair (Figure 22.6).

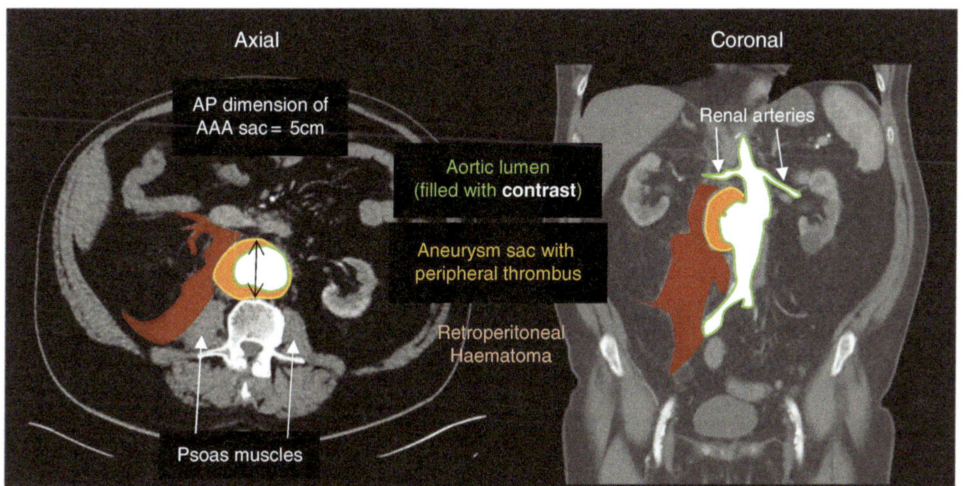

FIGURE 22.5 Patient A, CT angiogram aorta. There is an infrarenal abdominal aortic aneurysm (AAA). This has a focal bulge on the right side, best appreciated on coronal plane. The contrast fills the lumen of the aorta, with thrombosis peripherally inside the aneurysm sac. The fat plane around the aorta is lost with fat stranding, representing blood. The haematoma is extending into the right side of the retroperitoneum and tracking down along the psoas muscle. There is no extravasation of contrast in this example. Extravasation of contrast may be seen in AAA rupture, but its absence does not exclude active bleeding.

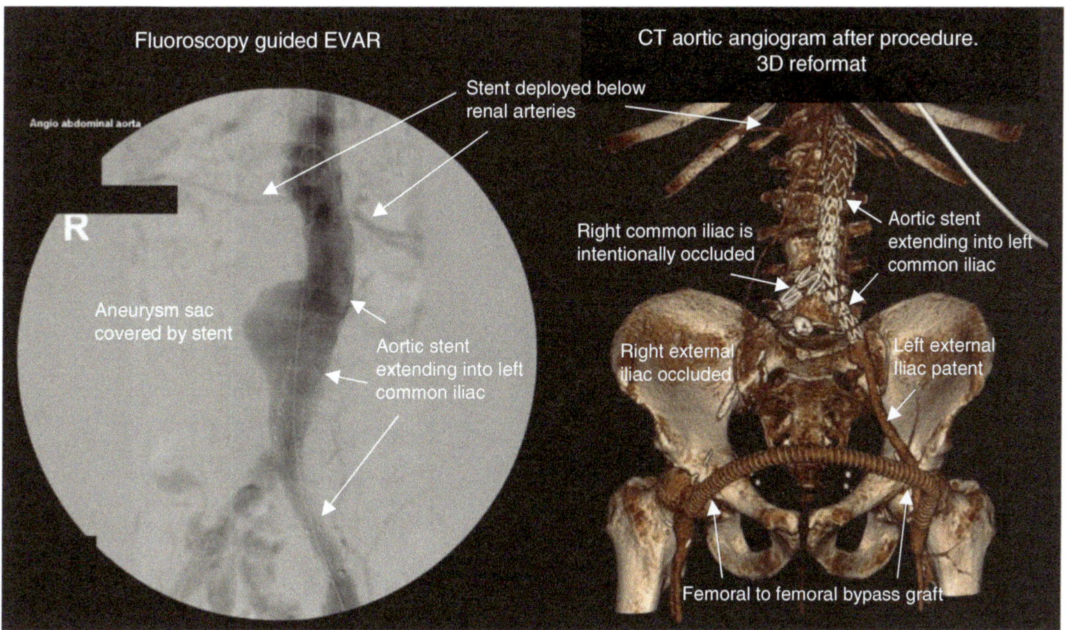

FIGURE 22.6 Patient A underwent emergency endovascular aneurysm repair (EVAR). To save time in planning the procedure, only the left iliac artery is stented from the aorta, with intentional occlusion of the right external iliac. A femoral-to-femoral bypass is then performed to maintain circulation to the right lower limb.

22.5 Take-home Message – Imaging in Abdominal Aortic Aneurysm

- Ultrasound is used for AAA screening and can accurately measure the size of the aneurysm sac.

- CT aorta is used in suspected AAA rupture as it shows the retroperitoneum better than ultrasound and can identify active bleeding if contrast is used.

Further Resources

Aggarwal, S., Qamar, A., Sharma, V., and Sharma, A. (2011). Abdominal aortic aneurysm: a comprehensive review. *Exp Clin Cardiol* 16 (1): 11–15.

AAA screening: standard operating procedures: www.gov.uk/government/publications/aaa-screening-standard-operating-procedures

Spine Section

CHAPTER 23

Acute Back Pain

Joshua Lauder[1], Eoghan Donnelly[2], and Peter Driscoll[3]

[1] *East Lancashire Hospitals NHS Trust, University of Central Lancashire and University of Manchester, UK*
[2] *NHS Greater Glasgow and Clyde, Glasgow, UK*
[3] *School of Medicine and Dentistry, University of Central Lancashire, Preston, UK*

23.1 Primary Case

23.1.1 Presentation

A 78-year-old woman presents to the Emergency Department following acute onset of lower back pain.

23.1.1.1 History of Presenting Complaint She describes bending over to pick something up from the kitchen floor two days previously when there was a sudden pain in her back. She was subsequently able to walk to the living room but has not really been mobile since due to pain. Her daughter has brought her into hospital as she was concerned the pain wasn't settling with simple analgesia.

PMH: hypertension; chronic obstructive pulmonary disease; previous bilateral wrist fractures (two and four years ago), managed conservatively; right hemiarthroplasty for hip fracture; gastro-oesophageal reflux disease; renal cell carcinoma treated with surgery two years ago.

SH: ex-smoker 20/day stopped 30 years ago. She mobilises in the house with one stick and outside with a frame.

DH: calcium supplementation, steroid and salbutamol inhalers, an ACE inhibitor, omeprazole.

23.1.2 Examination

Bony tenderness over the thoracic spine. Restricted movements of the spine due to pain. No neurological deficit.

Modified early warning signs (MEWS): 0

23.1.3 Blood Results

- Chronic microcytic anaemia.
- Normal inflammatory markers and renal function.
- Alkaline phosphatase is mildly raised.

23.1.4 Imaging

In view of the signs and symptoms, plain radiographs of the thoracolumbar region was requested (Figure 23.1).

> **Clinical Case Questions**
> - What is your differential diagnosis?
> - When is CT indicated?
> - What is your system for interpreting these images?
> - What is your final diagnosis and immediate management?

23.2 Radiology Self-assessment

23.2.1 Technical

- What are the standard plain radiology projections of the spine?

Diagnostic Imaging and Anatomy in Acute Care, First Edition. Edited by Joshua Lauder and Peter Driscoll.
© 2025 John Wiley & Sons Ltd. Published 2025 by John Wiley & Sons Ltd.
Companion website: www.wiley.com/go/DiagnosticImaginginAcuteCare

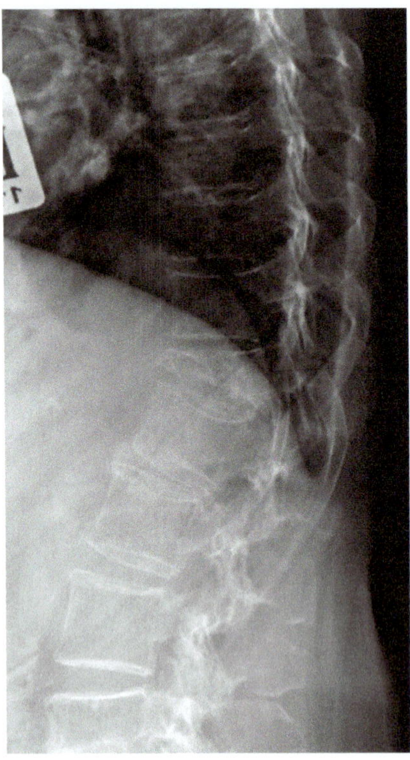

FIGURE 23.1 Patient A. Lateral thoracolumbar spine X-ray.

23.2.2 Correlation with Gross Anatomy

- What is the normal alignment of the spine?

23.3 Key Radiology Review

23.3.1 Technical Aspects and Anatomy

A lumbar spine X-ray has a relatively high radiation dose compared to chest and extremity X-rays. This is worth taking into consideration when requesting because most patients with mechanical back pain require no imaging. However, imaging is indicated following trauma when vertebral bony tenderness is found during examination.

The main anatomical features of the thoracolumbar spine can be identified on the standard AP and lateral projections (Figure 23.2a,b). Clinically, the lateral view is by far the most useful when looking for fractures and malalignment (Figures 23.2b and 23.3).

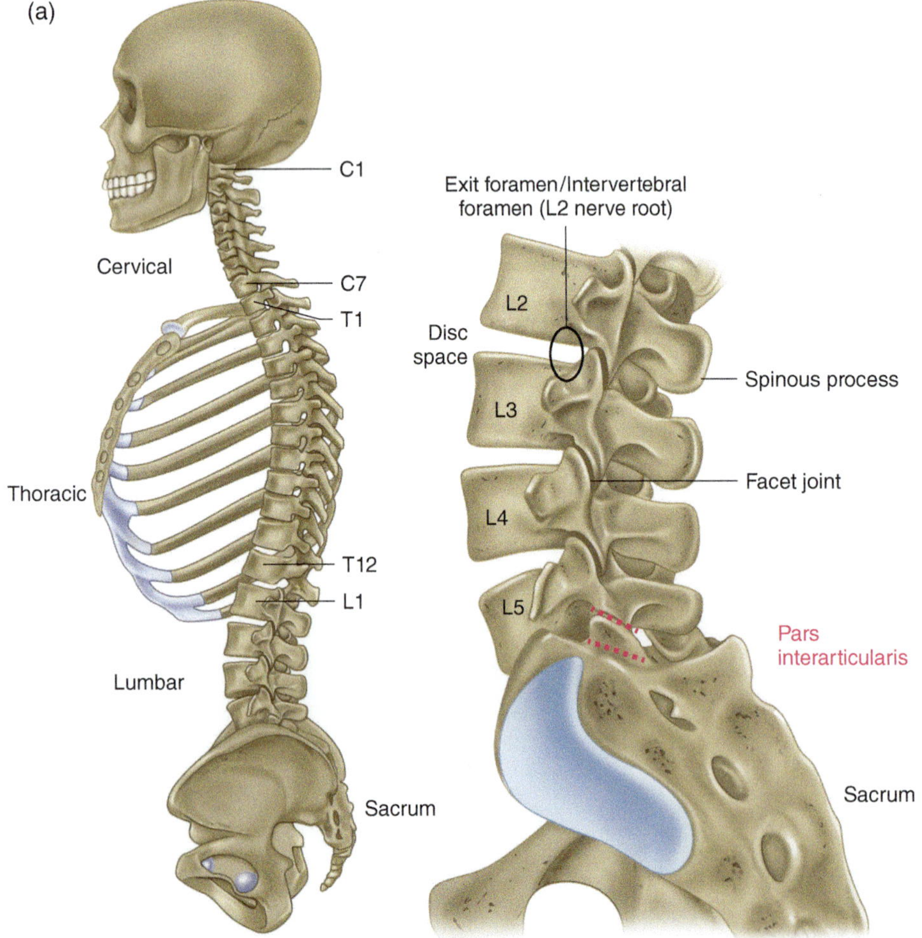

FIGURE 23.2 (a) Lateral anatomical view of the vertebral column. The right image shows a focus on the lumbar spine. (b) Normal lumbar spine X-ray: AP (left image) and lateral (right) projections.

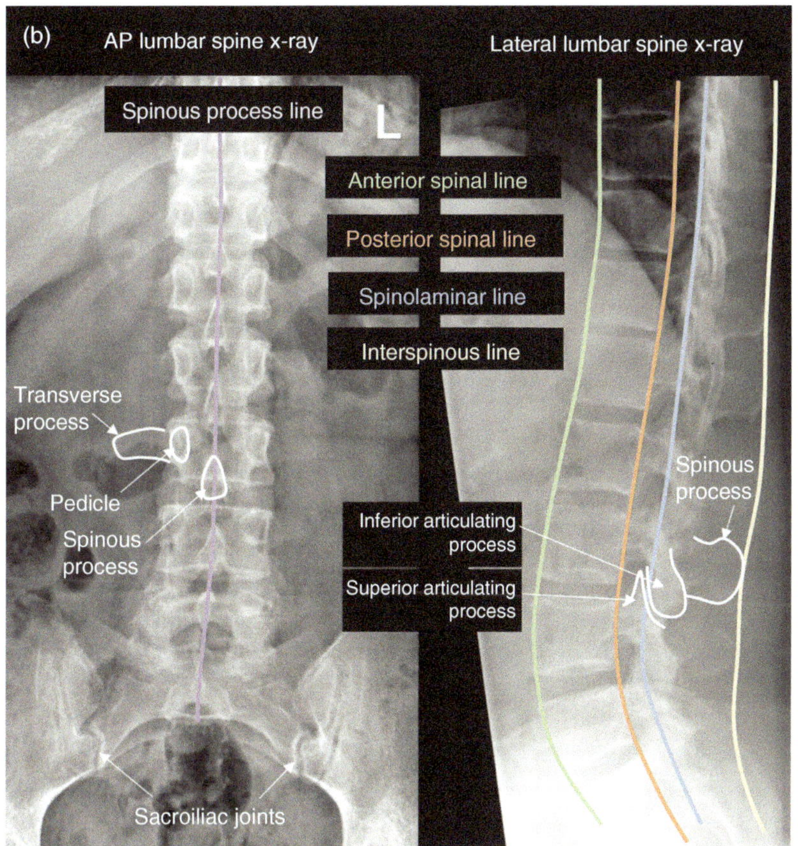

FIGURE 23.2 (Continued)

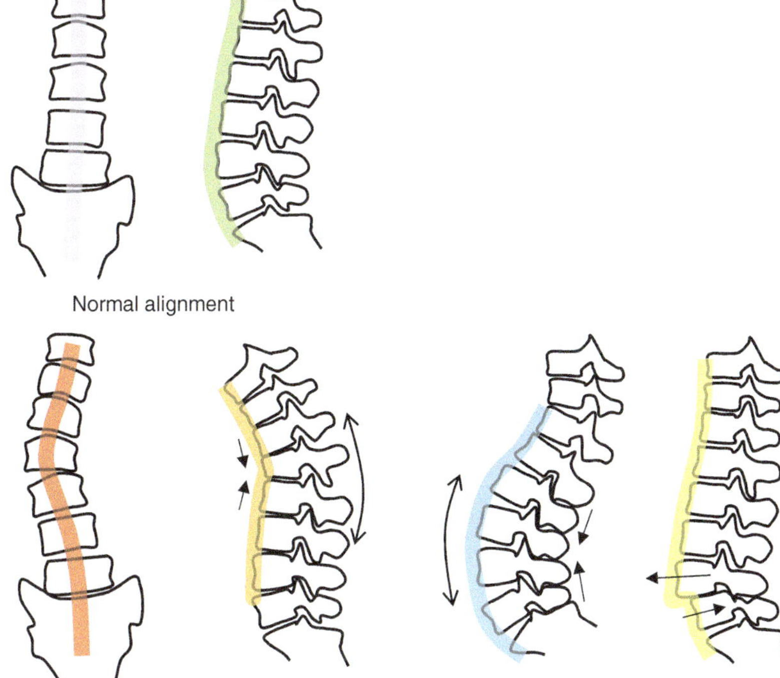

FIGURE 23.3 Spinal alignment in the thoracolumbar region. Most malalignments occur in the anterior–posterior plane, so are best shown on a lateral projection. Kyphosis is exaggerated flexion deformity, commonly related to wedge fractures of the vertebral bodies. Lordosis is exaggerated extension deformity. When this is extreme enough to allow the lumbar spinous processes to contact each other, it is termed Baastrup's syndrome. Listhesis is a slipping between adjacent vertebral segments. This suggests compromise of the disc and facet joint complex. A common non-traumatic cause is a pars defect (see Figure 23.9).

23.4 Review of the Clinical Case

- What is your differential diagnosis?
- When is plain radiology indicated?
- When is a DEXA scan indicated?
- When is CT/MRI indicated?
- What is your final diagnosis and immediate management?

23.4.1 Differential Diagnosis

The clinical index of suspicion for spinal fracture depends on the mechanism of injury and density of bone. If there are risk factors for osteoporosis then vertebral fragility fracture should be investigated. This may require X-rays of the spine for innocuous trauma as in this case (Figure 23.4).

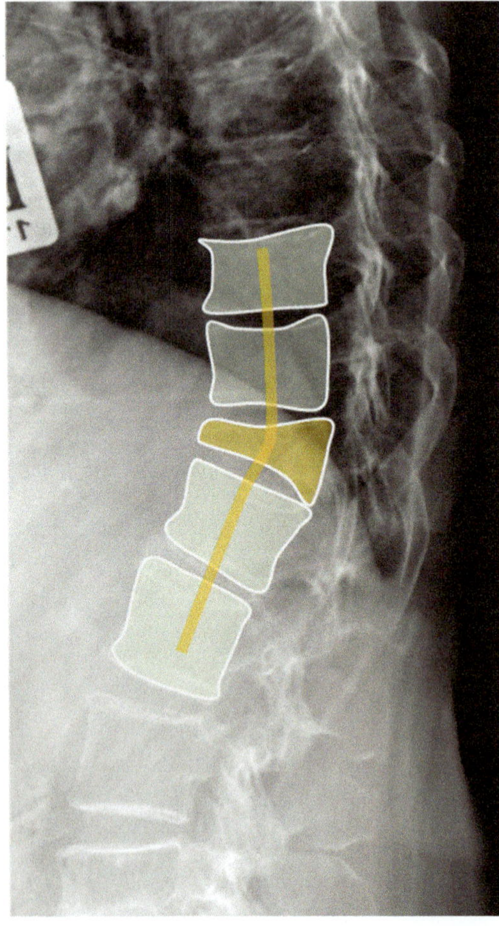

FIGURE 23.4 Patient A. Lateral thoracolumbar spine X-ray. There is a wedge fracture of T12 with resultant kyphotic deformity. There is no spondylolisthesis. The interspinous line remains intact with no evidence of posterior ligamentous complex injury (see Spine Chapter 24).

23.4.2 Review the X-ray

The X-ray shows the typical features of a vertebral fragility fracture at T12 (Figure 23.4).

23.4.3 Dual Energy X-ray Absorptiometry (DEXA)

If a patient suffers a fracture after minimal trauma, a DEXA scan should be arranged to identify underlying osteoporosis (Figure 23.5). This is a special type of X-ray which measures bone density. Various osteoporotic fracture risk algorithms exist (e.g. QFracture and FRAX), and these can help to guide use of DEXA scanning.

23.4.4 CT and MRI

Cross-sectional imaging of the spine is often not required if the history and X-ray are convincing for a vertebral fragility fracture (see Figure 23.4).

In patients who have sustained significant energy transfer, the clinical suspicion is higher and it may be appropriate to go straight to CT. If this is the case then a whole-body major trauma CT should be considered, as there may be multiple injuries in different anatomical regions.

MRI spine has several indications following trauma.

- Neurological deficit (e.g. cord/cauda equina syndrome or new radicular symptoms).
- If the X-ray or CT raises suspicion of ligamentous injury (e.g. widening of spinous processes or spondylolisthesis). This is because visualisation of the soft tissue ligamentous complexes will be crucial in determining the need for surgical intervention. Several classifications exist to aid in surgical decision making, one example being the Thoracolumbar Injury Classification and Severity score (TLICS) (Figure 23.6).
- Suspected pathological fracture secondary to malignancy.

Given patient A has a history of renal cell carcinoma, CT and MRI were performed to assess for underlying malignancy (Figure 23.7).

23.4.5 Final Diagnosis

T12 acute vertebral fragility fracture.

TLICS = 1 suggesting non-surgical management.

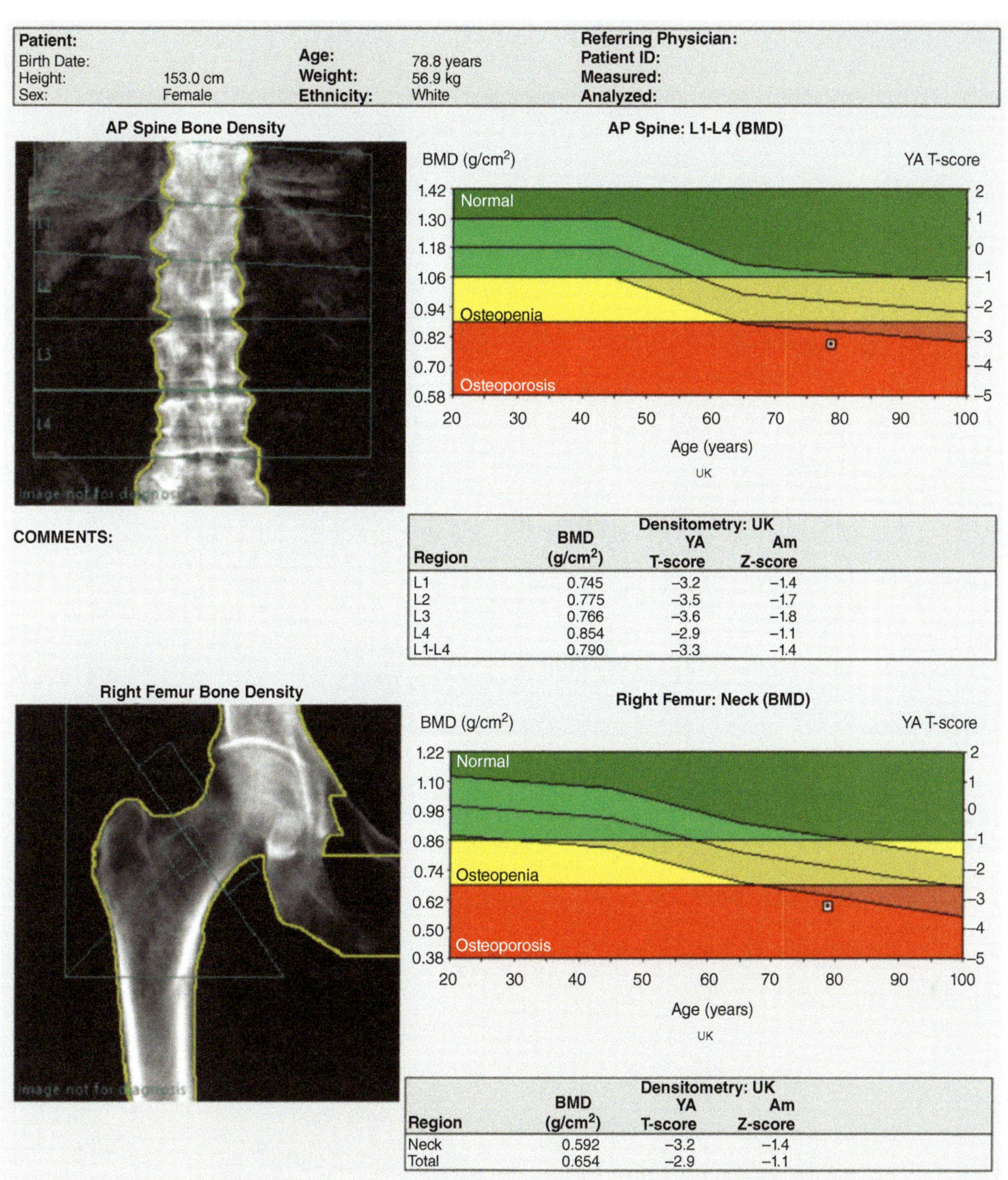

FIGURE 23.5 DEXA scan showing osteoporosis. The process consists of firstly imaging the lumbar spine and femoral neck using low-resolution X-ray. The bone mineral density is then calculated using computer software with the value plotted on a graph. This allows the patient's gender and age to be considered when deriving a T score so that a quantitative diagnosis of osteoporosis can be made.

TLICS	3 independent predictors		
1	**Morphology** immediate stability	- Compression - Burst - Translation/rotation - Distraction	1 2 3 4	- Radiographs - CT
2	**Integrity of PLC** longterm stability	- Intact - Suspected - Injured	0 2 3	- MRI
3	**Neurological status**	- Intact - Nerve root - Complete cord - Incomplete cord - Cauda equina	0 2 2 3 3	- Physical examination
Predicts	- **Need for surgery**		0 – 3 4 > 4	- nonsurgical - surgeon's choice - surgical

FIGURE 23.6 Thoracolumbar Injury Classification and Severity score (TLICS), Posterior ligamentous complex (PLC), composed of facet joint capsule, ligamentum flavum, interspinous ligament and supraspinous ligament. Combining these three features can help determine if surgery is required. For most vertebral fragility fractures, no surgery is required. For more information on how to use the system, see https://radiology assistant.nl/neuroradiology/spine/tlics-classification.

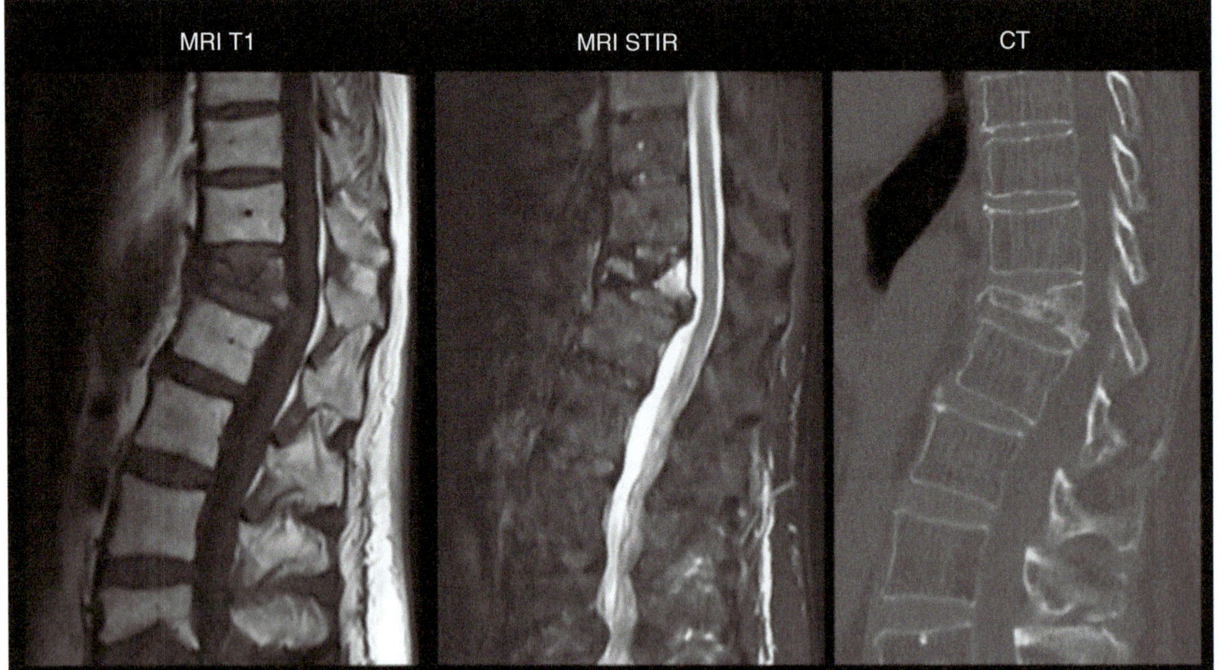

FIGURE 23.7 Patient A. Sagittal MRI and CT of lumbar spine. Acute vertebral fragility fracture of T12. The CT shows severe loss of vertebral body height anteriorly, resulting in a wedge shape. There is slight retropulsion of the posterior vertebral body into the spinal canal. T1 shows loss of the bright fat marrow signal in T12 vertebra, with corresponding high T2 signal on STIR. This represents bone marrow oedema secondary to an acute fracture. The bone is not expanded, suggesting no underlying malignancy. It is important to be aware that bone marrow oedema can persist for several months after a fracture so its exact age cannot be determined on MRI. There is no oedema in the posterior ligaments or spinous process, suggesting a stable injury. TLICS = 1; morphology compression 1; intact posterior ligamentous complex 0; neurological status intact 0.

23.4.6 Pars Defect

This tends to occur in patients with normal bone density, with increased incidence amongst athletes and children. It is hypothesised to result from exaggerated lumbar lordosis, which puts strain on the pars interarticularis (Figure 23.8). In these cases, the pars can fracture, allowing the lumbar vertebra to slide anterior to the sacrum. This is known as spondylolisthesis (Figure 23.9). A similar situation can arise in some people who are born with a defect in the pars interarticularis.

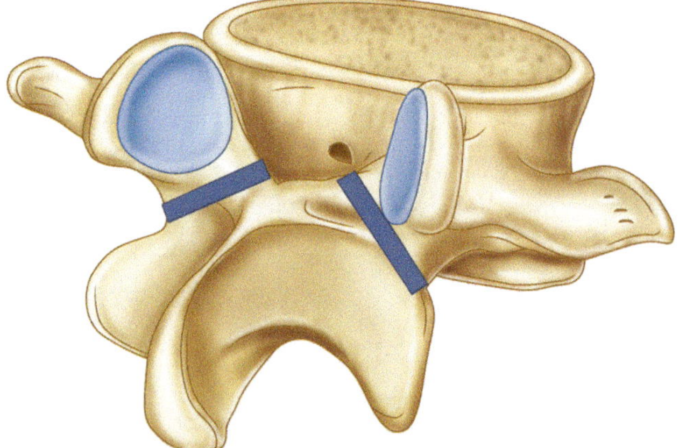

FIGURE 23.8 Posterior view of the fourth lumbar vertebra showing the right and left pars interarticularis. This is so named because it lies between the superior and inferior facet joints.

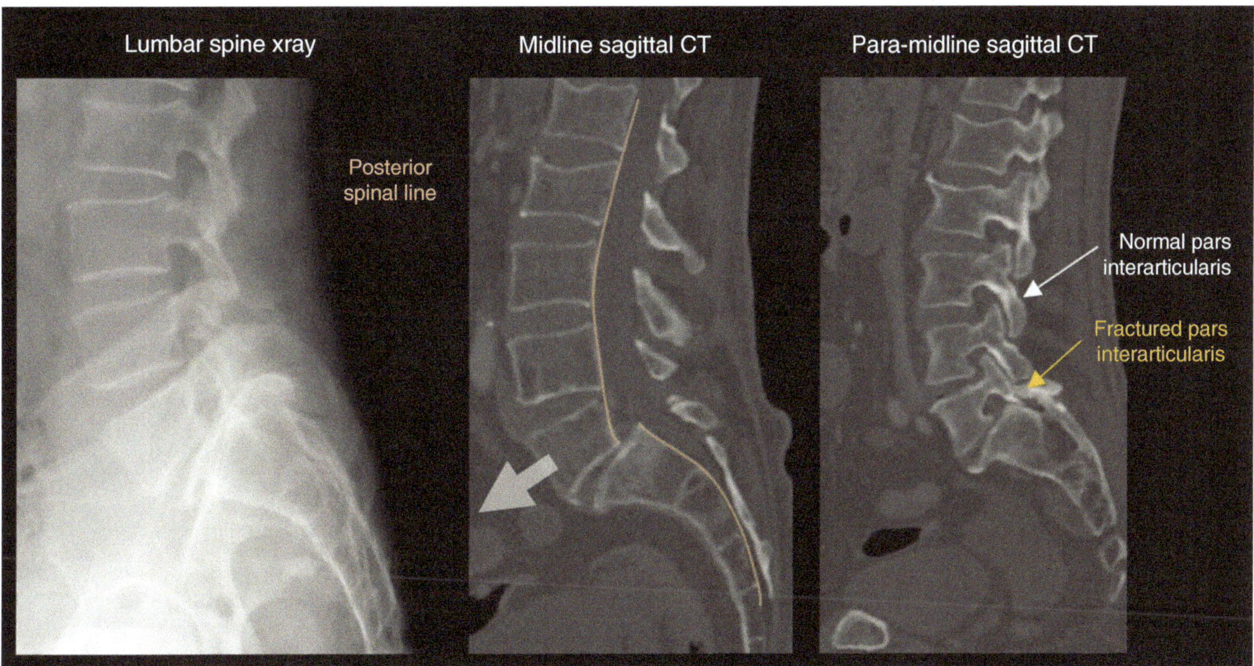

FIGURE 23.9 Lateral X-ray and sagittal CT scan showing a pars defect. There is a chronic fracture through the inferior articulating process of L5, shown on the para-midline sagittal plane. Due to loss of the stabilising facet joints, there is an anterior listhesis of L5 on S1.

23.5 Take-home Message – Imaging in Back Pain

- Chronic back pain is very common and can be managed without imaging, provided there are no associated radicular symptoms. If that is the case then the patient requires an MRI (see Chapter 24).

- Suspected vertebral fragility fractures may occur with innocuous trauma and can be investigated with X-ray.
- If there is a suspicious mechanism of injury (e.g. high energy transfer, compression, rotation), then spinal CT is indicated. MRI is also required if there is neurology or suspected ligamentous injury on X-ray/CT.

Further Resources

Tawfik, S., Phan, K., Mobbs, R.J., and Rao, P.J. (2020). The incidence of pars interarticularis defects in athletes. *Global Spine J* 10 (1): 89–101.

CHAPTER 24

Back Pain and Leg Weakness

Joshua Lauder[1], Eoghan Donnelly[2], and Peter Driscoll[3]

[1]*East Lancashire Hospitals NHS Trust, University of Central Lancashire and University of Manchester, UK*
[2]*NHS Greater Glasgow and Clyde, Glasgow, UK*
[3]*School of Medicine and Dentistry, University of Central Lancashire, Preston, UK*

24.1 Primary Case

24.1.1 Presentation

A 34-year-old male presents to the outpatient orthopaedics spine clinic with a six week history of back pain radiating down his right lower limb.

24.1.1.1 History of Presenting Complaint On further questioning, he related that the pain initially started in the lower back and came on suddenly whilst he was on the toilet. After 24–48 hours it slowly shifted to the right and began to radiate down his lower limb. He describes a shooting and burning pain down the back of the leg to the lateral aspect of the ankle and occasionally into the sole of his foot. This has been constant and not helped by simple medications. His general practitioner has recently started him on amitriptyline but this has not really helped.

Over the last two weeks he has noticed some numbness in his lower leg but on questioning denies any saddle anaesthesia, change in micturition, incontinence or signs of sexual dysfunction.

PMH: nil
SH: nil.
DH: paracetamol and ibuprofen.

24.1.2 Examination

On clinical examination, he has a straightened lumbar spine with no obvious evidence of kyphoscoliosis. His spinal movements are restricted in all directions due to pain and he is tender to palpate in the right paraspinal region.

Straight leg raising at 10° elevation reproduces the pain symptoms in his leg.

Neurological examination of the lower limbs demonstrates normal power, tone and reflexes in the left side. On the right side he describes numbness in the posterior part of the calf and lateral border of the foot, with four out of five MRC graded power on plantarflexion of the right ankle.

His right ankle reflex is absent.

Perianal examination is normal. His postvoid bladder scan carried out in clinic shows 22 ml residual.

His upper limb neurological examination is normal and there are no features of an upper motor neurone lesion in the lower limbs; he denies any issues with balance.

Modified early warning signs (MEWS): 0

24.1.3 MRI Lumbar Spine

In view of the signs and symptoms an MRI scan was requested (Figure 24.1).

Clinical Case Questions

- What is your differential diagnosis?
- When is MRI indicated in cases of back pain?
- What is your system for interpreting these images?
- What is your final diagnosis and immediate management?

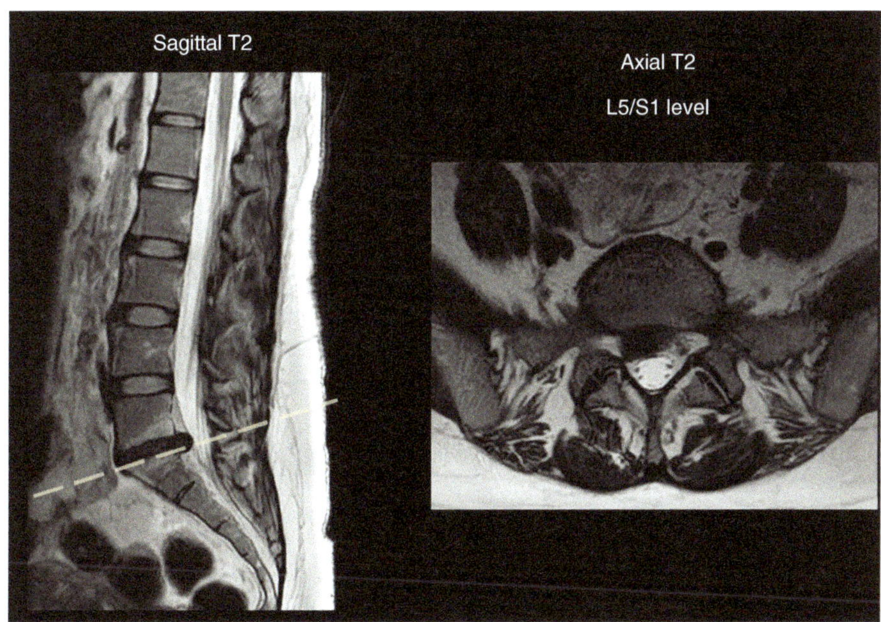

FIGURE 24.1 Patient A, MRI lumbar spine. The axial slice is at the level indicated by the dotted line on the sagittal view.

24.2 Radiology Self-assessment

24.2.1 Technical

- What are the standard MRI sequences for viewing the spine?

24.2.2 Correlation of Gross Anatomy

- What is the MRI anatomy of the spine cord, cauda equina and nerve roots?

24.3 Key Radiology Review

24.3.1 Technical Aspects and Anatomy

The standard MRI sequences for viewing the spine are sagittal T1 and T2, plus selected axial T2 through the discs of interest. As described in Chapter 1, these views allow different types of tissues to be identified (Figure 24.2).

- Fat is bright on both T1 and T2 sequences, best identified in the subcutaneous tissue and fatty bone marrow.
- Fluid is bright on T2 but dark on T1.
- Nerve tissue (spinal cord and spinal nerves) appear dark – especially on T2 views where they contrast with the surrounding CSF which is white.
- Fibrous tissue like ligaments and the annulus fibrosus will be dark on both sequences, as will cortical bone.

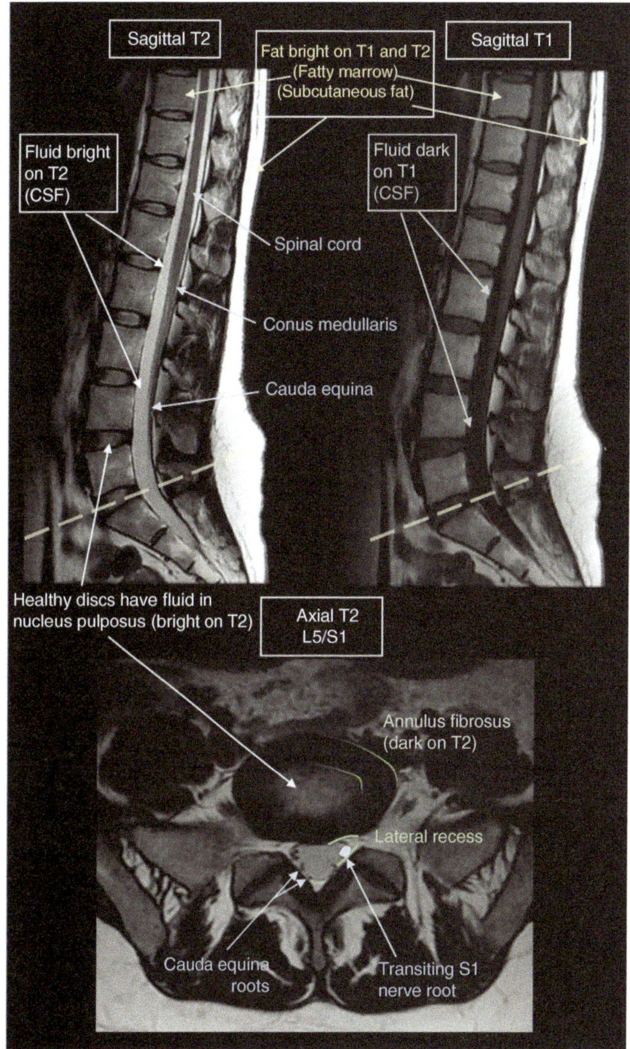

FIGURE 24.2 Sagittal T2 and T1 of the normal lumbar spine, axial T2 through L5/S1 disc. The spinal cord usually ends between T12 and L2 at the conus medullaris. The cauda equina nerve roots then continue in the spinal canal (Figure 24.3).

24.3.2 **Nerve Roots**

The nerve roots leave the spinal cord and travel in the CSF for a variable distance, depending on the number of the nerve root (Figure 24.4). Spinal nerve roots are named after the vertebral level from which they arise. However, remember there are eight cervical spinal nerves even though there are only seven cervical vertebrae (Figure 24.4). This is because the top seven exit the vertebral column *above* their corresponding vertebral level (i.e. the C2 nerve root lies above the C2 vertebral pedicle). In contrast, all the spinal nerves from C8 downwards leave the spinal canal *below* their corresponding vertebral level (i.e. the L2 nerve root lies below the L2 vertebral pedicle).

The cauda equina is a collection of the lumbar nerve roots inside the dura (Figure 24.3). When the nerve roots are nearing their exiting level, they become lateralised inside the lateral recess of the spinal canal and are termed the transiting nerve roots (Figures 24.2 and 24.5). This anatomical narrowing is the most common site of compression from disc bulges.

The nerve roots leave the spinal canal through the exit foramen. This is another common site of compression (Figure 24.6).

24.4 Review of the Clinical Case

- What is your differential diagnosis?
- When is MRI indicated?
- What is your final diagnosis and immediate management?

24.4.1 **Differential Diagnosis**

When there is back pain with radicular symptoms (nerve root compression symptoms), an MRI is indicated. The specific symptoms will depend on the level of the involved nerve root. L5 is the most common and usually manifests as pain radiating down the lateral leg into the foot. Examination may reveal weakness in hallux extension, foot eversion, inversion and foot dorsiflexion.

The urgency of investigation will depend on the severity of neurology. Motor weakness is more concerning than isolated pain in a dermatome. Equally, if the symptoms are rapidly progressive then urgent investigation is required.

Although radicular symptoms (i.e. spinal nerve root irritation) are often the result of disc herniation or degenerative changes in the spine, differentials including cancer and spinal infection should also be considered.

24.4.2 **MRI**

MRI of the spine is not always helpful, due to the large number of abnormal findings in the asymptomatic population. For example, it is not unusual to find disc disease and facet joint disease in completely asymptomatic patients. Therefore, it is vital that the clinical symptoms correlate with the imaging findings before further intervention can be considered (Figure 24.7).

24.4.3 **Disc Pathology Terminology**

The language used to describe disc pathology is relatively standardised to aid communication between healthcare professionals (Figure 24.8).

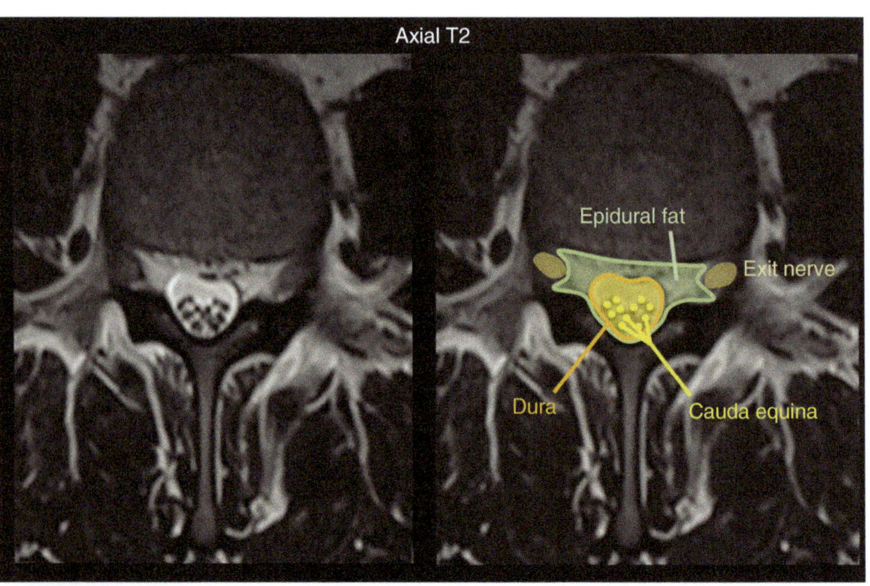

FIGURE 24.3 Axial T2 MRI through the spinal canal at L4. Note the dark spinal roots of the cauda equina compared to the surrounding CSF which appears white on a T2-weighted image.

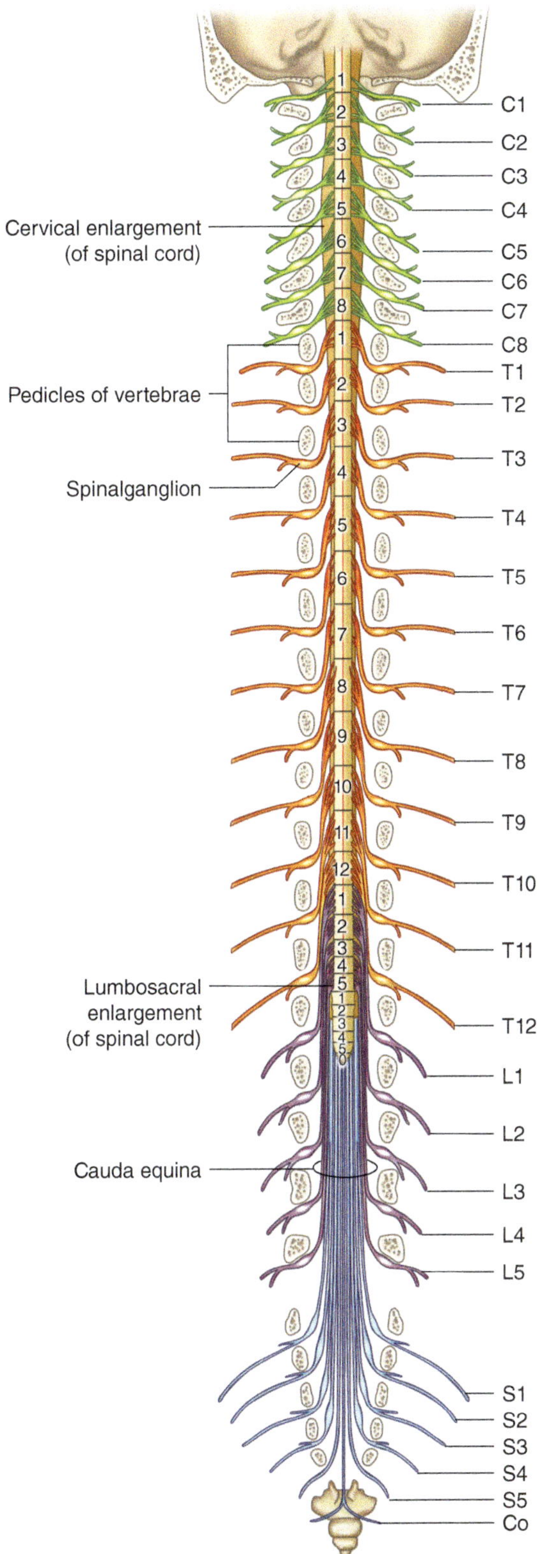

FIGURE 24.4 Distribution of the spinal nerves. Note there are eight cervical spinal nerves even though there are only seven cervical vertebrae.

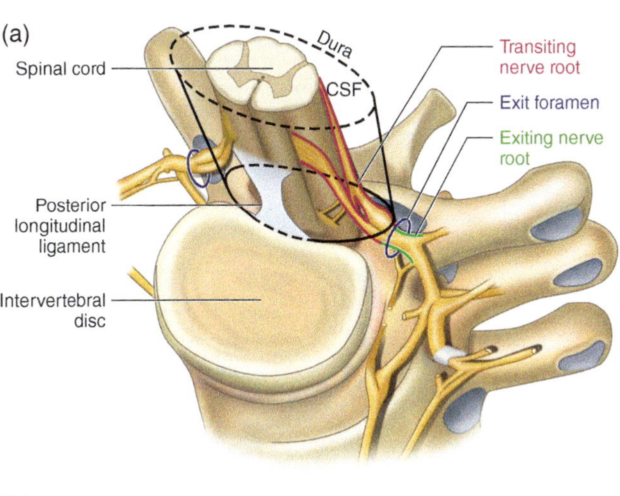

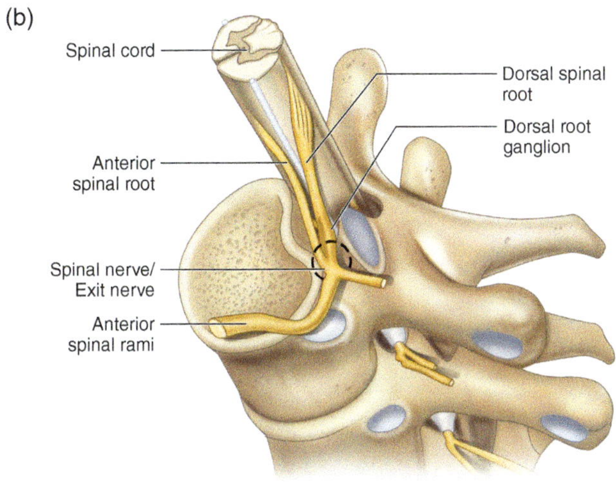

FIGURE 24.5 Relationship between spinal cord, nerve roots and spinal canal in the thoracic spine. The arrangement is similar in the lumbar spine, except the cord will no longer be present and instead the cauda equina roots lie centrally in the spinal canal. (a) Note that the posterior longitudinal ligament only lies in the midline. Disc bulges are most common posterolateral to this ligament (see Figure 24.8: disc bulge terminology). (b) The spinal nerve/exit nerve is formed by the merging of the anterior and posterior spinal roots as they run through the intervertebral foramen (dotted circle).

24.4.4 Final Diagnosis

L5/S1 right paracentral disc bulge extending into the right lateral recess and compressing transiting S1 nerve root.

Treatment options include conservative medicinal therapy, nerve root injections and surgical laminectomy and discectomy.

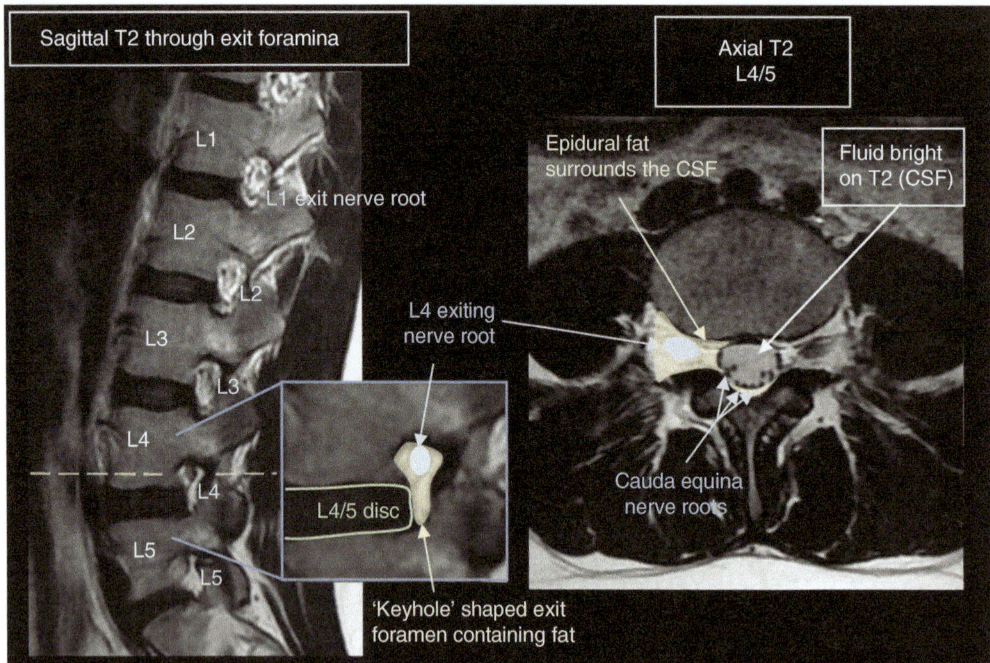

FIGURE 24.6 Sagittal T2 through the exit foramina. Axial T2 through L4/5 exit foramen. The L4 exiting nerve leaves in the exit foramen *below the L4 vertebral pedicle*. The exit foramen is a keyhole shape in the sagittal plane, with the nerve lying superiorly and the L4/5 disc making the anteroinferior wall.

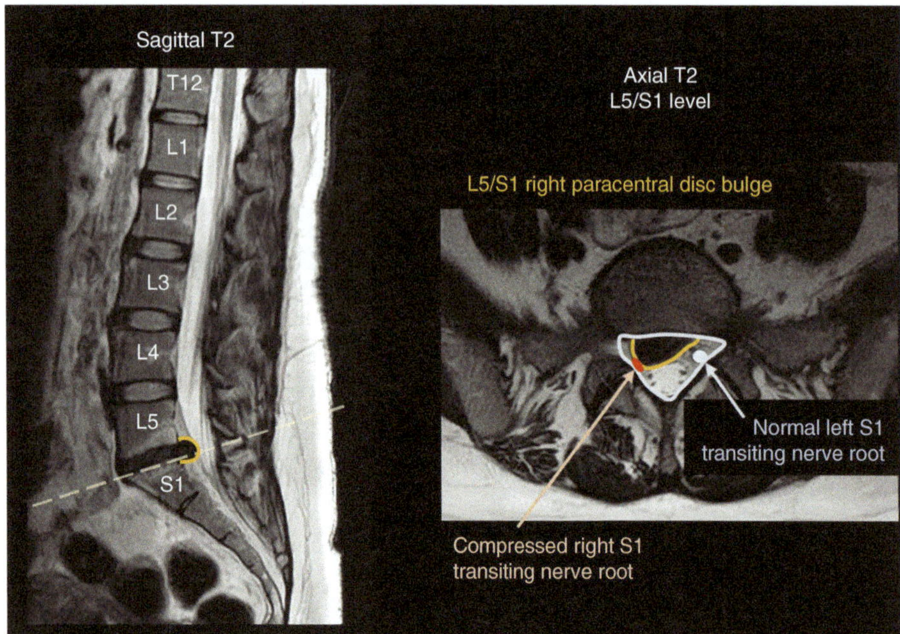

FIGURE 24.7 MRI lumbar spine annotated. There is low T2 signal in the L5/S1 disc indicating dehydration. There is a large disc bulge in the right paracentral region which extends into the right lateral recess, compressing the right S1 transiting nerve root.

24.5 Take-home Message – Imaging in Back Pain

- Chronic back pain is very common and can be managed without imaging, provided there are no associated radicular symptoms. Chronic back pain with radicular symptoms should be investigated with MRI.

- Suspected vertebral fragility fractures can be investigated with plain X-ray (see Chapter 23).
- If there is a suspicious mechanism of injury (e.g. high energy transfer), then CT spine is indicated. MRI is also required if there is neurology or suspected ligamentous injury on X-ray/CT. The latter would indicate a spinal cord at risk because of a potentially unstable vertebral column.

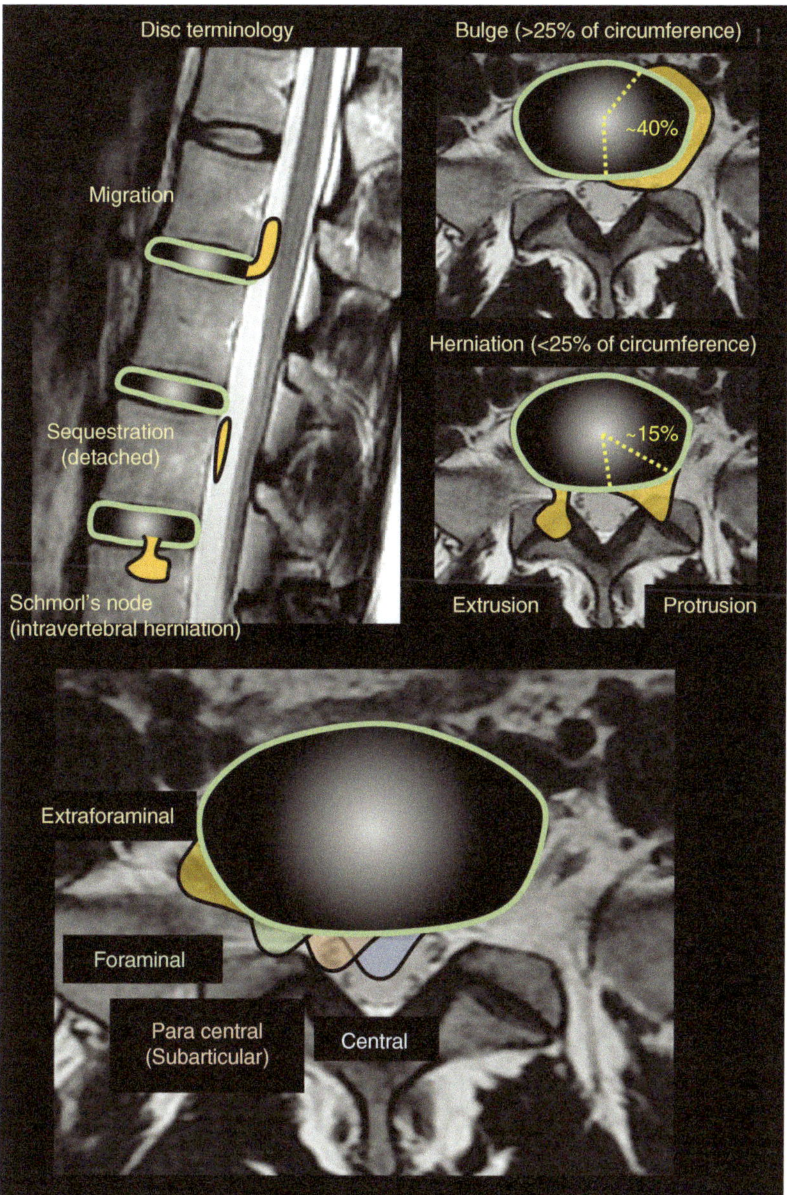

FIGURE 24.8 Disc pathology terminology.

When over 25% of the disc extends outwards, this is termed a 'bulge'. These may be completely circumferential.

If less than 25% of the disc perimeter extends outwards, this is termed a 'herniation'. These are subdivided into protrusion (where the width of the hernia is less than the width of the base) and extrusion (where the width of the hernia is larger than the width of the base).

The location of posterior herniations is described anatomically.

- Central are in the midline, directly under the posterior longitudinal ligament which is relatively protective of herniations.
- Paracentral are at the facet joint so are also termed subarticular. These lie immediately lateral to the posterior longitudinal ligament and are the most common form of disc bulge. They invariably extend into the lateral recess.
- Foraminal extend into the exit foramen, usually below the level of the nerve root (see Figure 24.6).
- Extraforaminal occur outside the exit foramen.

Migration is when a disc extrusion travels far from the site of herniation but remains attached. Sequestration is when the disc material detaches and lies distant from the site of herniation. Schmorl's nodes are intraventricular disc herniation through the vertebral endplate. These are more common with osteoporosis but also occur commonly in the general population. They are often an incidental finding but can cause back pain.

Further Resources

Brinjikji, W., Luetmer, P.H., Comstock, B. et al. (2015). Systematic literature review of imaging features of spinal degeneration in asymptomatic populations. *Am J Neuroradiol* 36: 811–816.

Fardon, D.F., Williams, A.L., Dohring, E.J. et al. (2014). Lumbar disc nomenclature: version 2.0: recommendations of the combined task forces of the North American Spine Society, the American Society of Spine Radiology and the American Society of Neuroradiology. *Spine J* 14 (11): 2525–2545.

Macnab, I. (1971). Negative disc exploration: an analysis of the causes of nerve-root involvement in sixty-eight patients. *J Bone Joint Surg Am* 53: 891–903.

Orita, S., Inage, K., Eguchi, Y. et al. (2016). Lumbar foraminal stenosis, the hidden stenosis including at L5/S1. *Eur J Orthop Surg Traumatol* 26: 685–693.

Othman, M. and Menon, V.K. (2022). The prevalence of Schmorl's nodes in osteoporotic vs normal patients: a middle eastern population study. *Osteoporos Int* 33 (7): 1493–1499.

CHAPTER 25

Trauma with Limb Weakness

Joshua Lauder[1], Eoghan Donnelly[2], and Peter Driscoll[3]

[1] *East Lancashire Hospitals NHS Trust, University of Central Lancashire and University of Manchester, UK*
[2] *NHS Greater Glasgow and Clyde, Glasgow, UK*
[3] *School of Medicine and Dentistry, University of Central Lancashire, Preston, UK*

25.1 Primary Case

25.1.1 Presentation

A 67-year-old female presents to the Emergency Department following an unwitnessed fall at home.

25.1.1.1 History of Presenting Complaint She was found by her husband at the bottom of a flight of stairs and doesn't remember the incident. Paramedics attended and fully immobilised her on a spinal board prior to transfer. They also noted she was alert and orientated but complaining of severe neck pain and an inability to move her lower limbs since the fall.

PMH: hypertension, atrial fibrillation, chronic kidney disease.

SH: lives with husband, normally mobilises outside with one stick.

DH: apixaban, amlodipine.

25.1.2 Examination

Clinical examination:

- Mild bruising to the face and a laceration to the posterior occiput which has been bandaged by the ambulance crew.
- A neurological examination demonstrates:
  - flaccid paralysis of both lower limbs with no sensation or reflexes present
  - altered sensation on the ulnar border of both arms and hands with loss of finger flexion, elbow and wrist extension bilaterally
  - full power wrist and elbow flexion as well as shoulder abduction.

Modified early warning signs (MEWS):

- Respiratory rate 16 rpm.
- SpO_2 99% on room air.
- Tympanic temperature 37.2 °C.
- Pulse rate 90/min.
- BP 93/65.

25.1.3 CT Cervical Spine

An urgent CT cervical spine was arranged as part of a major trauma CT (Figure 25.1).

25.1.4 MRI Cervical Spine

An urgent MRI of the cervical spine was also arranged (Figure 25.2).

Clinical Case Questions

- What is your differential diagnosis?
- When is MRI indicated?
- What is your system for interpreting these images?
- What is your final diagnosis and immediate management?

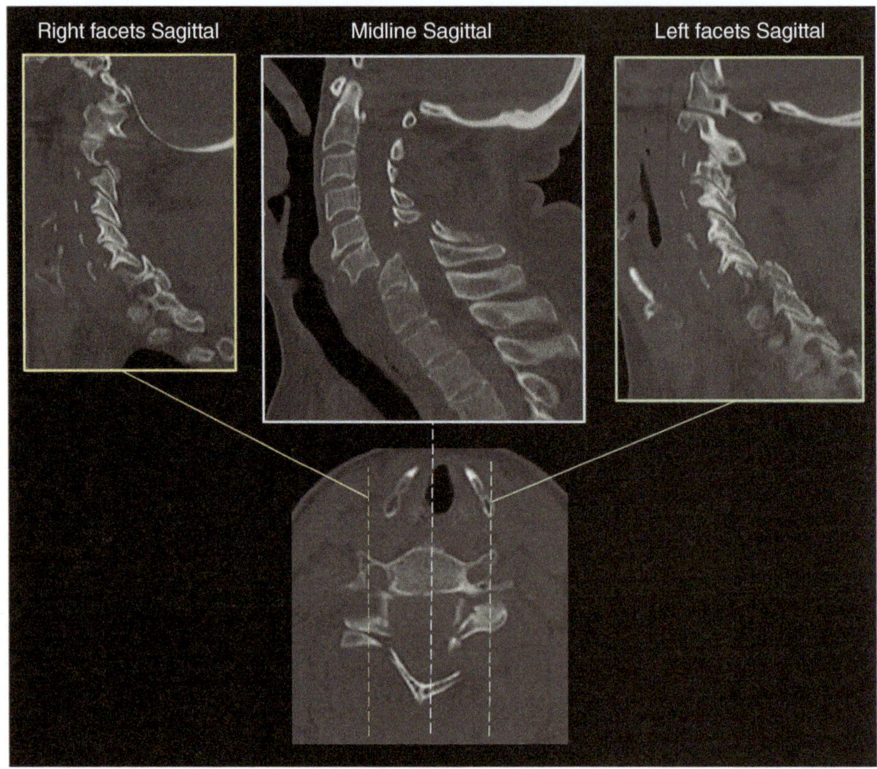

FIGURE 25.1 Patient A. CT cervical spine, showing a midline sagittal view and left and right facet joint sagittal views.

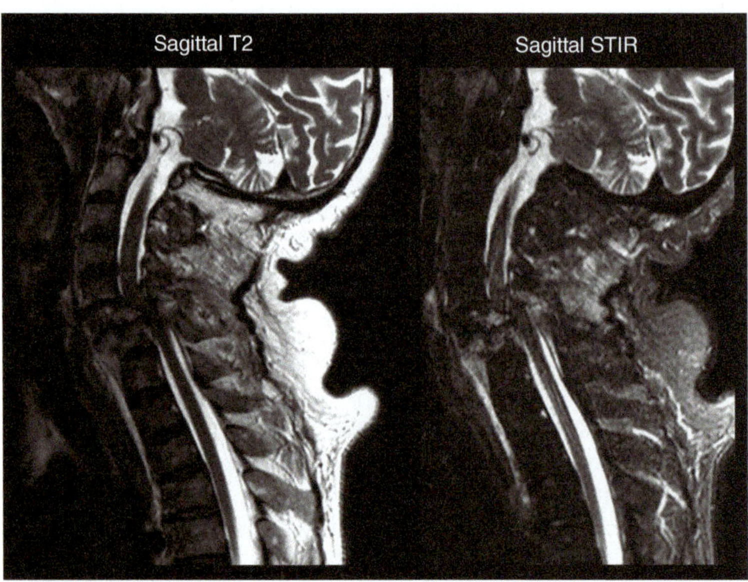

FIGURE 25.2 Patient A. MRI cervical spine, showing sagittal T2 and sagittal STIR (short tau inversion recovery) sequences.

25.2 Radiology Self-assessment

25.2.1 Technical

- What is a STIR sequence and when is it used?

25.2.2 Correlation of Gross and Radiological Anatomy

- How does the cervical spine differ from the lumbar spine?
- What does the cervical spine look like on plain radiographs and CT?

- What fracture patterns can occur in the cervical spine?

25.3 Key Radiology Review

25.3.1 Technical Aspects and Anatomy

When reviewing the cervical spine it is useful to have a system. To that end, we present the ABCS approach. This can be applied to both the lateral X-ray view and the sagittal CT view.

- *A Alignment*: observe the overall alignment by using the four spinal lines (Figure 25.3). Look for the malalignments described in Chapter 23 (Figure 23.3). Spondylolisthesis is particularly concerning as it indicates underlying fractures and ligamentous disruption (see Figure 25.6).
- *B Bones*: look at the shape and outline of each bone, checking for fracture lines and deformities (for example, wedging of vertebral bodies) (see Spine Chapter 23 – Figures 23.1 and 23.4).
- *C Cartilage*: look at the disc spaces and facet joints. Loss of joint space is most often related to degenerative joint disease but can also occur with ligamentous disruption in trauma. Widening of a joint space is highly suggestive of ligamentous injury.

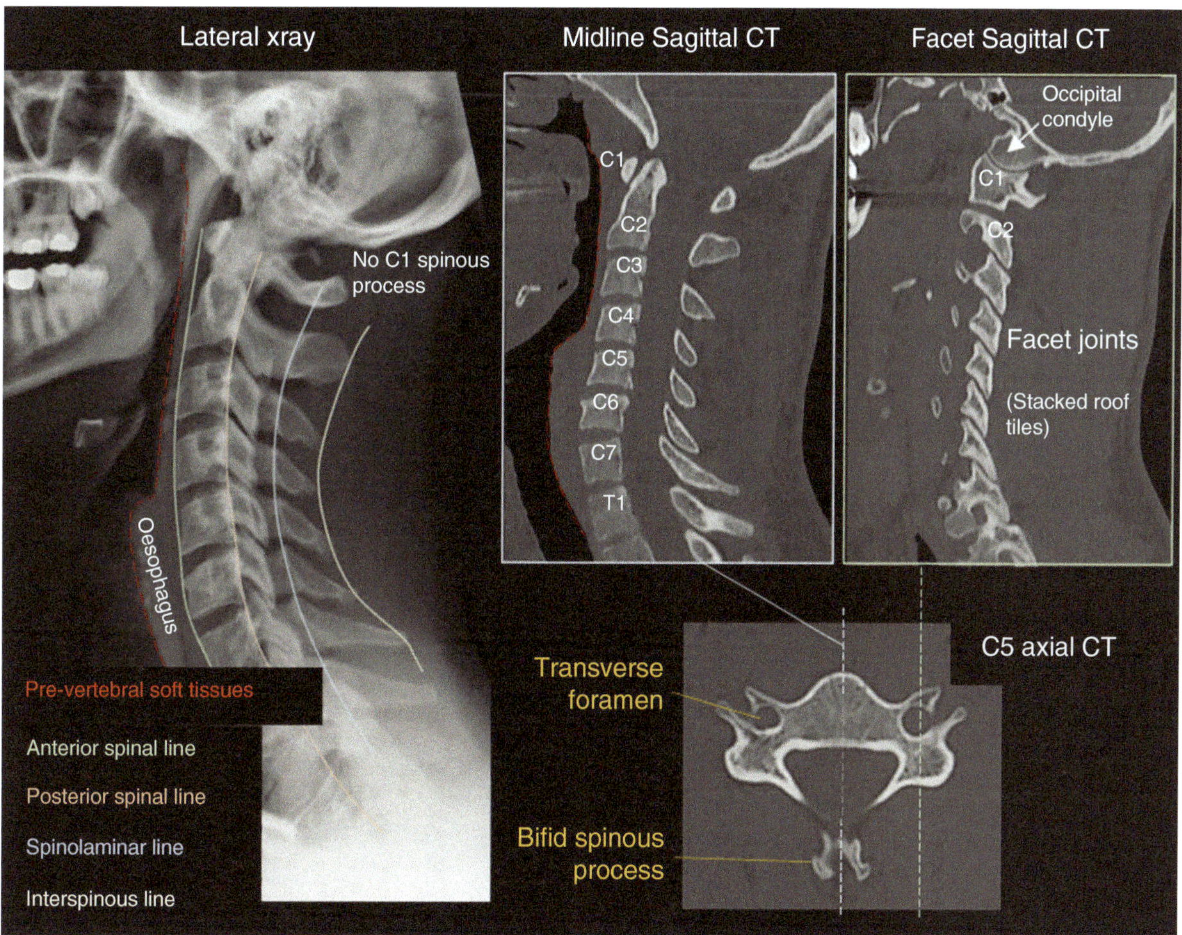

FIGURE 25.3 Normal cervical spine anatomy as seen on plain radiology and CT, bone window.
As in the thoracic and lumbar spine, the four longitudinal lines can be drawn onto the lateral X-ray or midline sagittal CT of the cervical spine. However, be aware that the interspinous line does not align with C1, owing to the absence of a spinous process at this level.

It is important to also appreciate the alignments of both the vertebral bodies and facet joints. On CT, this requires you to scroll to the paramidline sagittal view so the stacked facet joints can be seen (Figure 25.4).

Due to the unique anatomy of the atlantoaxial joint, the occipital condyle/C1/C2 articulations do not conform to the rest of the stacked facet joints and are better viewed in the coronal plate (see Figure 25.9, Jefferson's fracture).

The prevertebral soft tissues are an important review area.

- From C1 to C4, the prevertebral soft tissue space is less than one-third of the vertebral body AP thickness (<7 mm).
- From C5 and below, the oesophagus fills this space so its size increases but should remain less than one vertebral body AP thickness (<21 mm).
- In the context of trauma, prevertebral soft tissue thickening could represent a haematoma and is suggestive of a spinal fracture or ligamentous injury. Even on its own, this is an indication for an MRI scan.

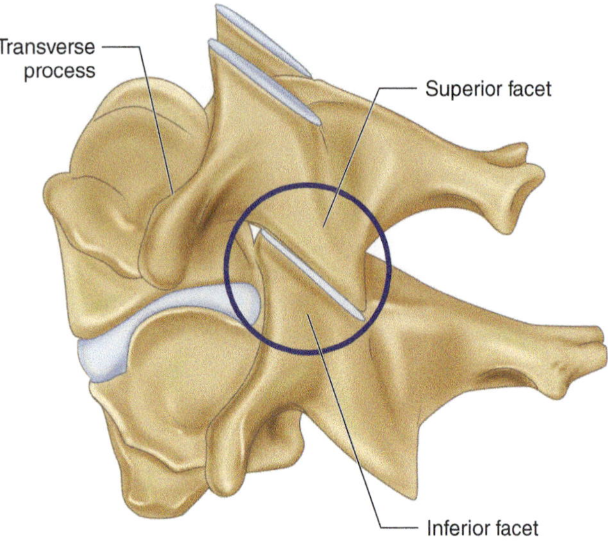

FIGURE 25.4 Anatomical diagram showing the facet joint (yellow ring). These are stacked on top of one another – similar to roof tiles. This arrangement helps resist listhesis (i.e. forward slippage) and rotation of one vertebra on another.

- *S Soft tissue*: look at the paraspinal soft tissues, particularly in the prevertebral region (see Figure 25.7). Widening here in the context of trauma suggests a paravertebral haematoma, heralding an underlying fracture or significant ligamentous injury.

25.3.2 MRI

Short tau inversion recovery (STIR) sequence is a T2 sequence with fat suppression. Fluid remains bright but the fat signal is dampened so it becomes dark on the image (Figure 25.5). This results in a very sensitive sequence for oedema in the soft tissues and bone marrow. For this reason, all spine MRI scans in trauma should include a STIR sequence, in addition to the standard images discussed previously.

25.4 Review of the Clinical Case

- What is your differential diagnosis?
- When is CT indicated?
- When is MRI indicated?
- What is your final diagnosis and immediate management?

25.4.1 Differential Diagnosis

Various decision pathways exist for assessing cervical spine injury, including NEXUS and Canadian C-spine rules (NICE 2016). It is generally accepted that CT is the most appropriate initial investigation if a cervical spine fracture is suspected. Therefore, when a plain X-ray shows

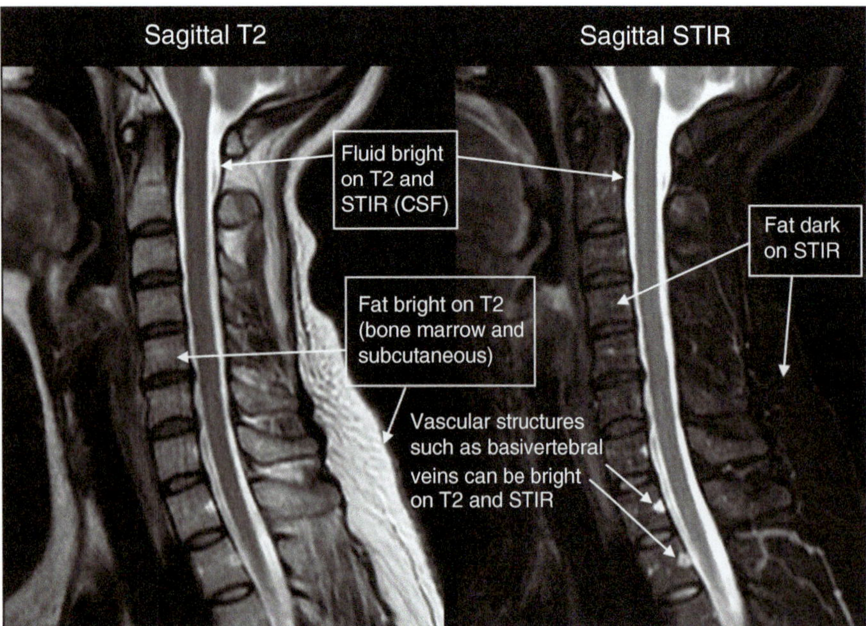

FIGURE 25.5 Normal MRI of the cervical spine, sagittal T2 and sagittal STIR sequences.

malalignment (Figure 25.6) or prevertebral soft tissue swelling (Figure 25.7) then a CT is indicated. If the patient has focal neurology then an MRI of the cervical spine is also indicated (Figure 25.8).

25.4.2 Review the CT

See Figure 25.6.

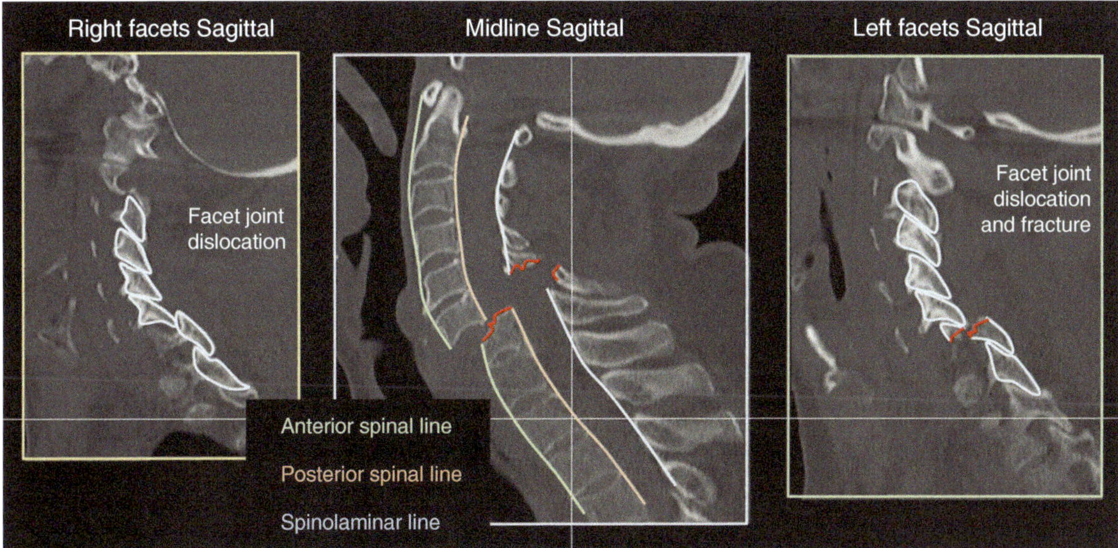

FIGURE 25.6 Patient A. CT cervical spine, showing a midline sagittal view and left and right facet joint sagittal views. There is a fracture at the C6/7 level involving disc space and lamina. There are bilateral facet joint dislocations, associated with a fracture of the superior articulating process on the left.

25.4.3 MRI (Figure 25.7)

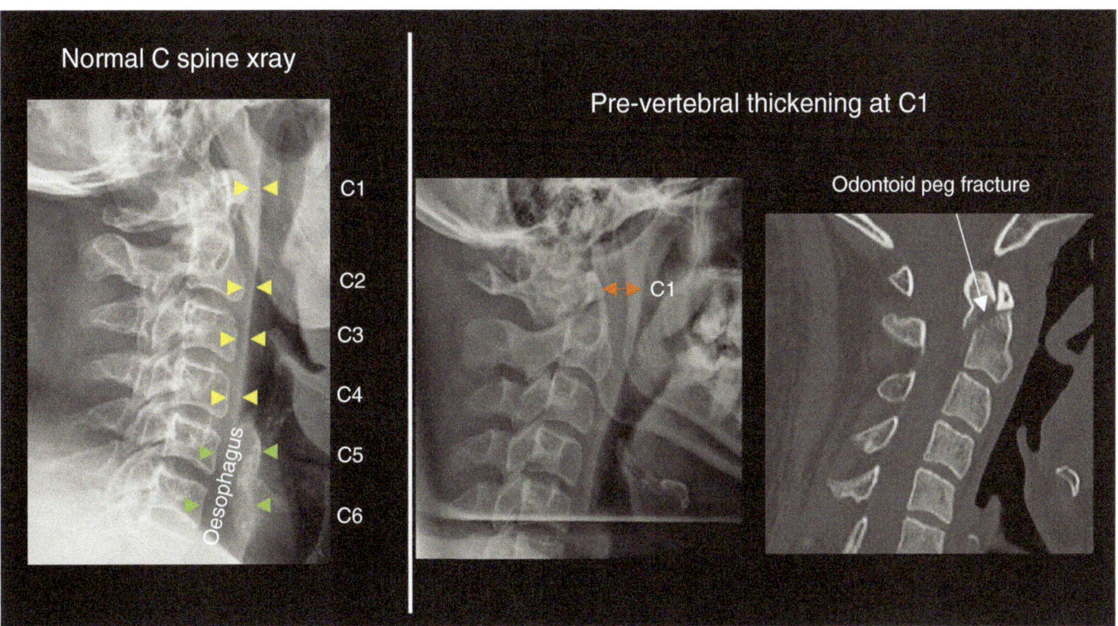

FIGURE 25.7 Prevertebral soft tissue swelling. Normal lateral C spine X-ray (left). Abnormal lateral C spine X-ray and CT (right). The prevertebral soft tissues can be easily identified on X-rays, due to the air column in the pharynx and trachea. Behind the pharynx from C1 to C4, the prevertebral soft tissues should be thin, i.e. less than one-third the AP thickness of a vertebral body. From C5 and inferiorly, the oesophagus forms resulting in natural thickening of the prevertebral soft tissues. Nevertheless, this should remain less than the AP thickness of a vertebral body. The X-ray and CT on the right show an odontoid peg fracture. The plain X-ray shows thickening of the soft tissues anterior to C1, prompting further investigation with CT.

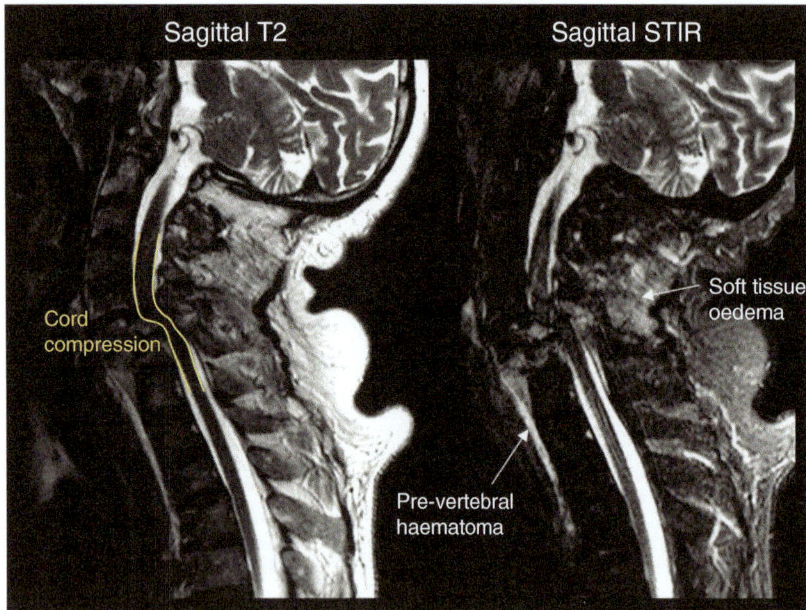

FIGURE 25.8 Patient A. MRI cervical spine, showing sagittal T2 and sagittal STIR sequences. The MRI confirms cord compression (compressive myelopathy). There may be associated high T2 signal inside the cord indicative of a central lesion (not shown here).

25.4.4 Other Cervical Fractures

See Figure 25.9.

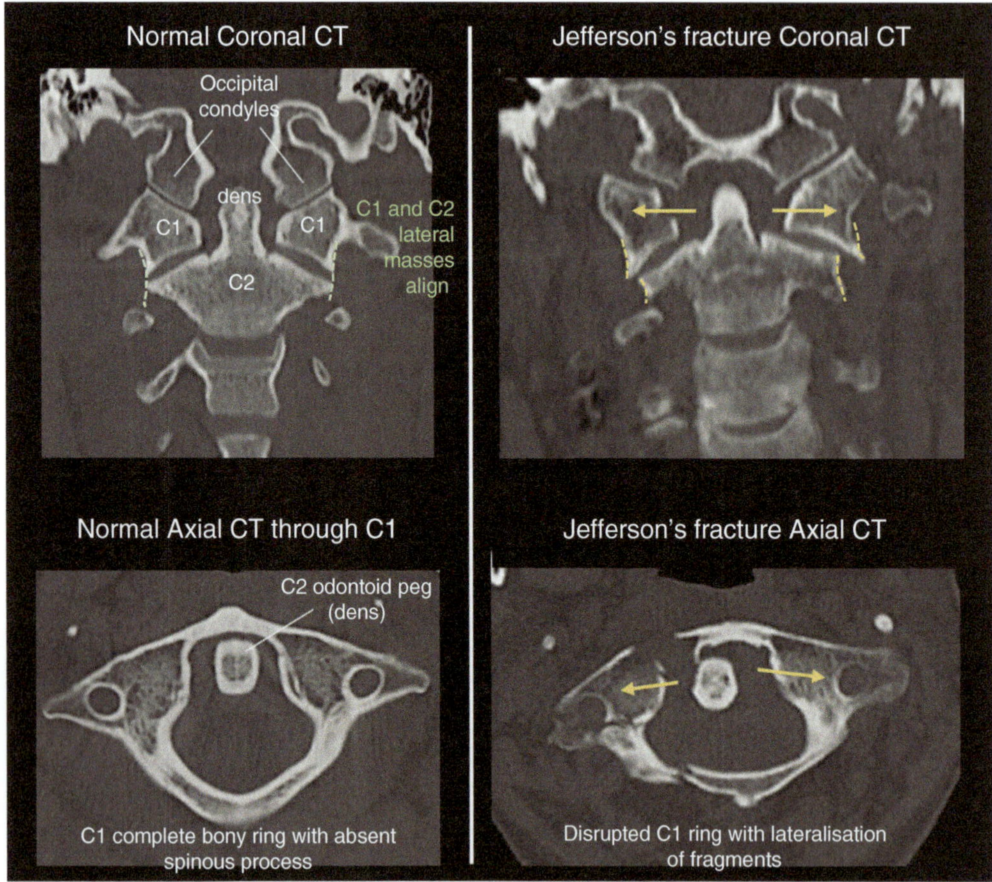

FIGURE 25.9 Anatomical relationship between occipital/C1/C2 articulation. Normal comparison and Jefferson's fracture. C1 assessment requires inspection of both the axial and coronal planes. The C1/C2 lateral masses should align at the lateral margins on the coronal view. This same alignment can be appreciated on an open mouth AP peg view (not shown). With a Jefferson's fracture, the C1 bony ring is fractured in more than one place, resulting in lateral shift of the lateral masses.

25.4.5 **Final Diagnosis**

C6/7 fracture with bilateral facet joint dislocation, resulting in compressive myelopathy. Urgent referral to neurosurgery is required for surgical fixation.

25.5 Take-home Message – Imaging in Traumatic Spine Injury

- When there is a low trauma mechanism with low clinical suspicion, a plain radiograph may be appropriate. Refer to your local guidelines which are often based around NEXUS and Canadian C-spine rules (NICE 2016).
- If there is a significant mechanism of injury (e.g. high energy transfer, compression or rotation), then CT spine is indicated. This may be as part of a major trauma CT.
- MRI is also required if there is neurology or suspected ligamentous injury on X-ray/CT.

Further Resources

Matar, L.D. and Doyle, A.J. (1997). Prevertebral soft-tissue measurements in cervical spine injury. *Australas Radiol* 41 (3): 229–237.

National Institute for Health and Care Excellence. (2016) *Spinal injury assessment: assessment and imaging for spinal injury. Methods, evidence and recommendations.* NG41. www.nice.org.uk/guidance/ng41/evidence/full-guideline-2358425776

Rojas, C.A., Vermess, D., Bertozzi, J.C. et al. (2009). Normal thickness and appearance of the prevertebral soft tissues on multidetector CT. *Am J Neuroradiol* 30 (1): 136–141.

Saragiotto, B.T., Maher, C.G., Lin, C.W.C. et al. (2018). Canadian C-spine rule and the National Emergency X-Radiography Utilization Study (NEXUS) for detecting clinically important cervical spine injury following blunt trauma. *Cochrane Database Syst Rev* 2018 (4): CD012989.

CHAPTER 26

Back Pain and Fever

Joshua Lauder[1], Eoghan Donnelly[2], and Peter Driscoll[3]

[1]East Lancashire Hospitals NHS Trust, University of Central Lancashire and University of Manchester, UK
[2]NHS Greater Glasgow and Clyde, Glasgow, UK
[3]School of Medicine and Dentistry, University of Central Lancashire, Preston, UK

26.1 Primary Case

26.1.1 Presentation

A 62-year-old woman presents to the Emergency Department with severe lower back pain and fever.

26.1.1.1 History of Presenting Complaint The pain started several days ago and is gradually getting worse. She describes feeling feverish and generally unwell but is unable to say how long for and further history is difficult to obtain.

She was found by her care support worker when she visited this morning. It was she who called for an emergency ambulance.

PMH: asthma, intravenous drug use.
SH: lives alone. Normally mobilises independently.
DH: methadone, paracetamol, dihydrocodeine.

26.1.2 Examination

Clinical examination: difficult and restricted due to pain. However, midline lumbar spinal tenderness is noted. Examination of the lower limbs is limited as it clearly provokes pain.

Her right hip is held in slight flexion and any attempt to extend it is met with protest.

Modified early warning signs (MEWS):

- Respiratory rate 25 rpm.
- Oxygen saturation 98% on 5 l O_2/min.
- Temperature 39.8 °C.
- Heart rate 123 bpm.
- Blood pressure 74/53 mmHg.

Bloods: WCC 18.4 10^9/l, CRP 278 mg/l, creatinine 244 µmol/l, eGFR 45.

26.1.3 MRI Spine

An urgent MRI spine with contrast is arranged (Figure 26.1).

Clinical Case Questions

- What is your differential diagnosis?
- When is MRI indicated?
- What is your system for interpreting these images?
- What is your final diagnosis and immediate management?

26.2 Radiology Self-assessment

26.2.1 Technical

- When is contrast indicated with spine MRI?

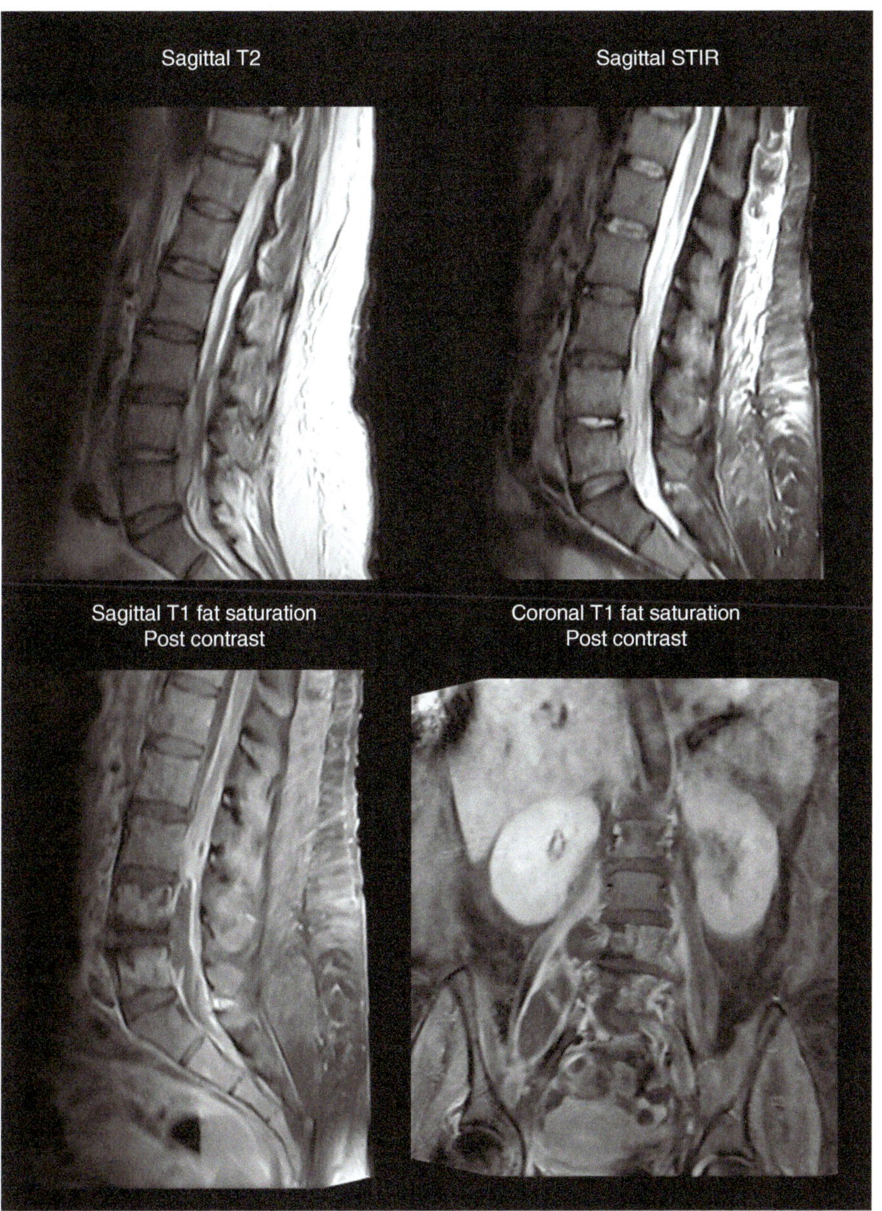

FIGURE 26.1 MRI lumbar spine with contrast.

26.2.2 Correlation of Gross and Radiological Anatomy

- What normal tissues can enhance in the spine after contrast?
- What is the appearance of the epidural space on MRI?
- What does the psoas muscle look like on MRI?

To help your understanding of the epidural space, you may it helpful to review the anatomy notes in Chapter 25 (Figure 25.3).

26.3 Key Radiology Review

26.3.1 Technical Aspects and Anatomy

Contrast is useful in spine MRI in several situations including discitis, osteomyelitis, postsurgical infection and characterisation of tumours. It can provide more information about the composition of tissue, compared to conventional T1, T2 and STIR sequences.

Postcontrast scans should always be performed with fat saturation as it makes pathological sites more

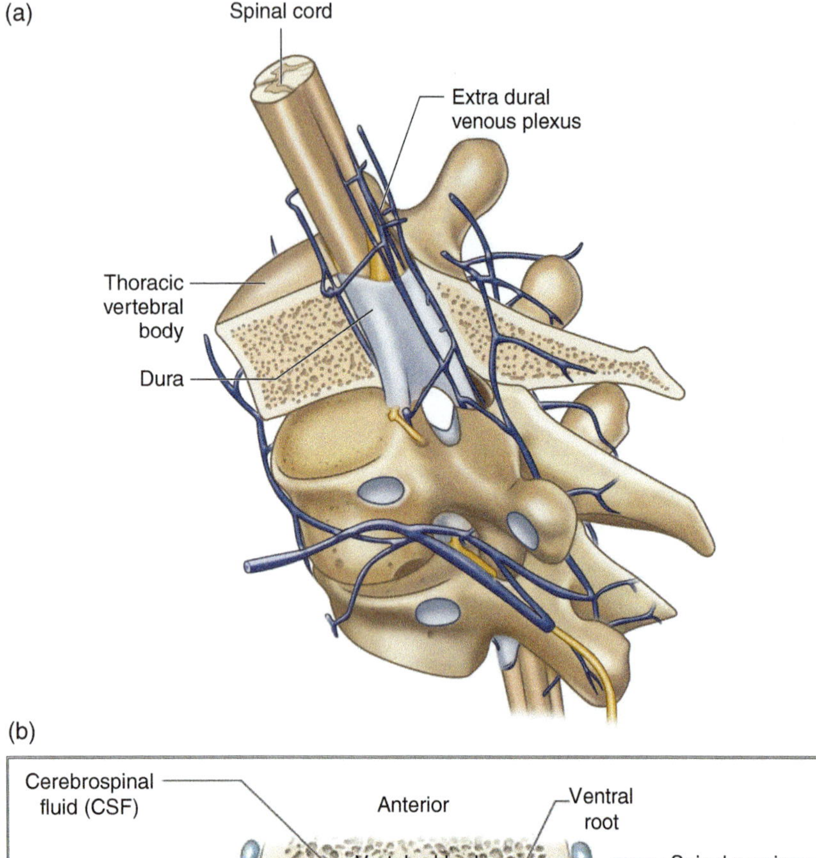

FIGURE 26.2 Cut-away diagrams of the thoracic spinal canal showing the epidural space lying between the dura and the boundary of the spinal canal. (a) Sagittal view showing the venous plexus lying in the epidural space. (b) Axial view showing fat lying in the epidural space.

noticeable. Various MRI techniques can be employed to suppress the signal from the fat. The underlying MRI mechanics is beyond the scope of this book but the end result of fat saturation is the same: the fatty tissues generate *less* signal and therefore appear *darker* (Figure 26.3).

This makes it easier to spot enhancing tissue which is abutting or inside fat. An epidural abscess provides a good example. The spinal epidural space lies between the dural membrane and the boundary of the spinal canal (Figure 26.2). As it normally only contains fat and a venous plexus, MRI scans using fat saturation significantly improves detection of pathology in this region.

26.4 Review of the Clinical Case

- What is your differential diagnosis?
- When is MRI indicated?
- What is your final diagnosis and immediate management?

26.4.1 Differential Diagnosis

Discitis will often present with severe pain, localised to a particular vertebral level, with associated bony tenderness on palpation. Fever is an inconsistent finding, as is a leucocytosis. However, most patients with discitis will have elevated inflammatory markers (e.g. CRP and ESR). If discitis is suspected, blood cultures should be taken. *Staphylococcus aureus* is the pathogen most often implicated.

Careful neurological examination is required. When there are focal signs or features of cauda equina, an epidural abscess should be suspected. These patients require an urgent MRI scan (Figure 26.3).

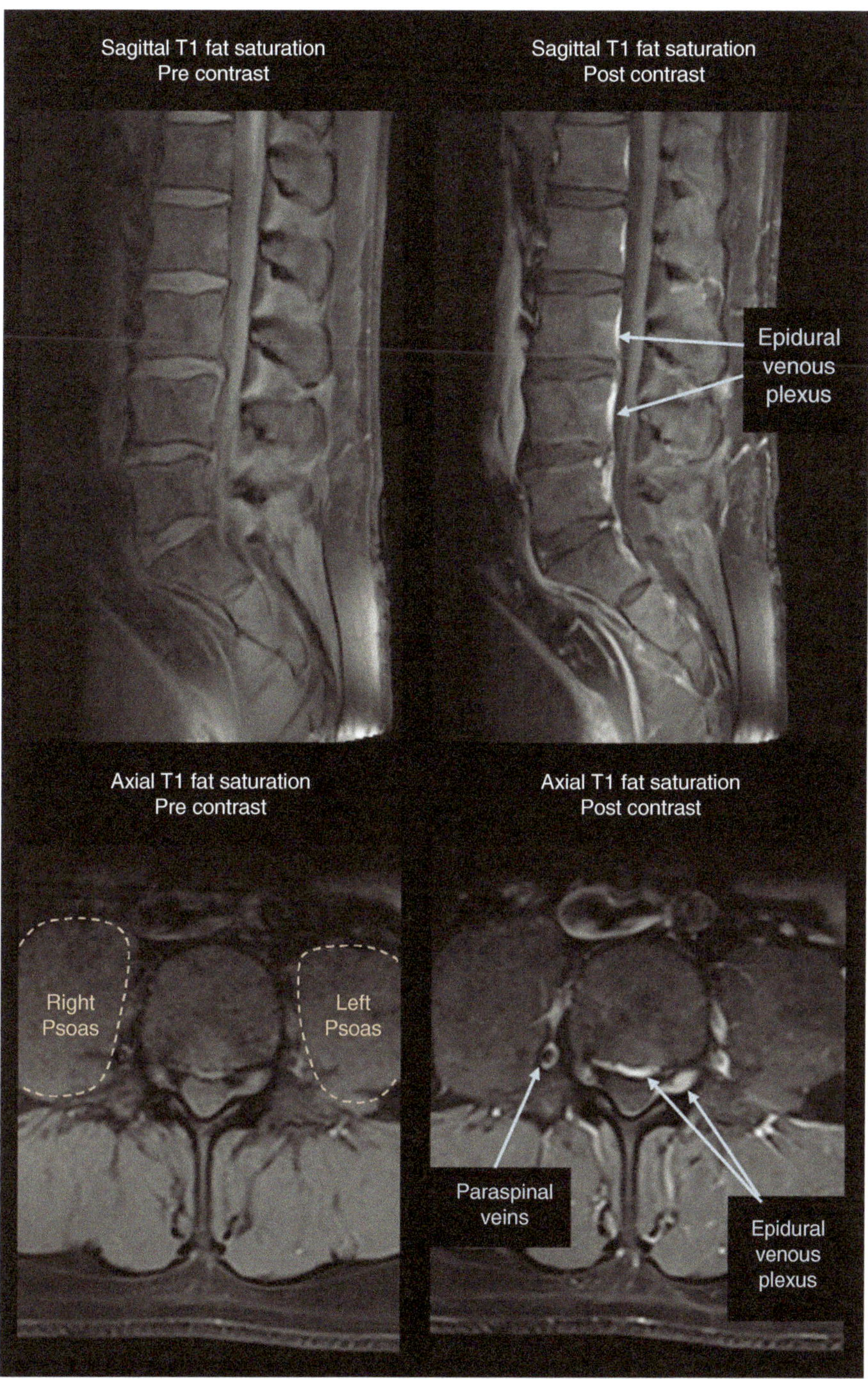

FIGURE 26.3 Pre- and postcontrast T1 fat saturation sequences (T1FS), sagittal and axial planes. Normal appearance. True enhancing tissue should be dark on the precontrast T1FS and bright on the postcontrast T1FS. It is therefore good practice to compare the pre- and post-contrast scans side by side. This is because something with an intrinsically high signal on T1 can be mistaken for enhancement if only the postcontrast images are viewed. Beware, normal vascular structures may variably enhance after contrast, depending on the timing of the scan after injection.

26.4.2 **MRI** (Figure 26.4)

Once an abscess is identified, adjacent areas need to be checked for signs of local spread (Figure 26.5).

26.4.3 **Discitis on CT**

Discitis may be first identified on CT, but the findings can be more subtle. If there is destruction of two adjacent vertebral endplates, then discitis should be considered (Figure 26.6).

26.4.4 **Final Diagnosis**

L4/5 discitis with an epidural abscess and right psoas abscess. *Staphylococcus aureus* is the pathogen most often implicated.

Urgent neurosurgical referral is required, to consider surgical decompression.

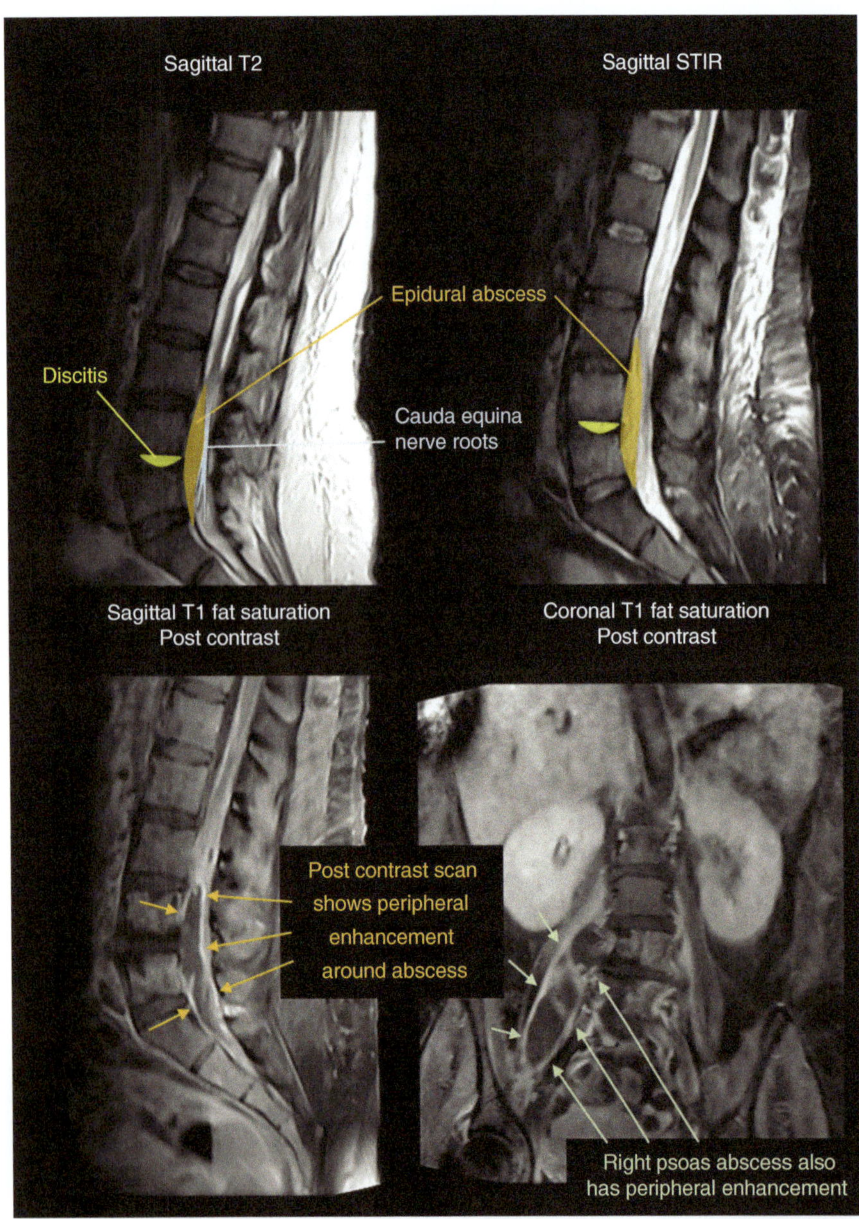

FIGURE 26.4 Patient A. MRI lumbar spine with contrast. The T2 and STIR sequences show a fluid signal in the L4 disc space. There may be adjacent bone marrow oedema in the vertebral endplates (not shown in this case). An epidural abscess is visible on the plain MRI as a space-occupying shape in the spinal canal which does not follow the signal intensity of fat or CSF. The abscess will generate a low signal on T1 (i.e. be darker), with variable intensity on T2 (due to inflammatory changes). Postcontrast MRI spine can help to delineate the size and extent of the abscess. An inflammatory phlegmon will centrally enhance, whereas abscesses peripherally enhance.

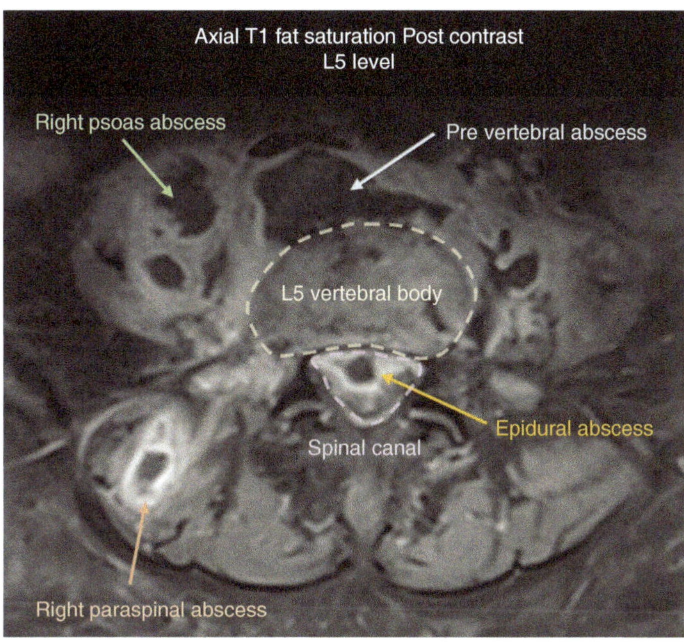

FIGURE 26.5 Patient A. Additional axial postcontrast T1FS through L5. This shows the epidural abscess and adjacent psoas, paraspinal and prevertebral abscesses.

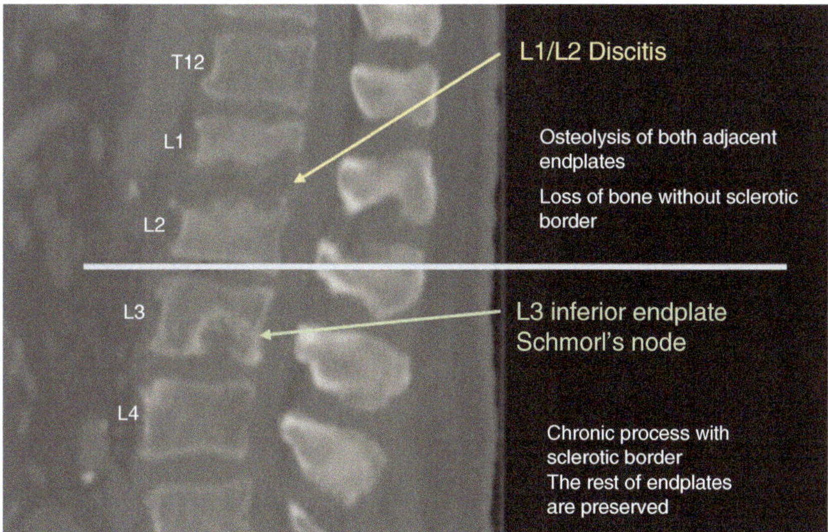

FIGURE 26.6 Sagittal CT of lumbar spine on bone windows comparing discitis and chronic Schmorl's node. Discitis will have changes on both sides of the disc space and there will be bone erosion (osteolysis). In the acute phase there will not be a sclerotic border. Schmorl's nodes are an intraosseous herniation of the disc (see Spine Chapter 25 – Figure 25.8). These will tend to be only on one side of the disc space. In the acute situation they may have an osteolytic appearance with bone marrow oedema on MRI. However, when chronic, they tend to develop a sclerotic border.

26.5 Take-home Message – Imaging in Suspected Discitis

- MRI is the most sensitive modality to diagnose discitis. Contrast should be used to improve sensitivity for paraspinal abscess.
- CT will spot later features such as erosion of the bony endplates and psoas abscess.

Further Resources

Dhodapkar, M.M., Patel, T., and Rubio, D.R. (2023). Imaging in spinal infections: current status and future directions. *N Am Spine Soc J* 16: 100275.

Head Section

CHAPTER 27

Sudden Severe Headache

Joshua Lauder[1], Aleksandr Valkov[2], and Peter Driscoll[3]

[1] *East Lancashire Hospitals NHS Trust, University of Central Lancashire and University of Manchester, UK*
[2] *Salford Royal Hospital and University of Central Lancashire, Salford, UK*
[3] *School of Medicine and Dentistry, University of Central Lancashire, Preston, UK*

27.1 Primary Case

27.1.1 Presentation

A 47-year-old female is brought to the Emergency Department by ambulance. She is complaining of a severe headache which started suddenly, about an hour ago.

27.1.1.1 History of Presenting Complaint Shortly afterwards she became unconscious for a couple of minutes before spontaneously recovering. She has been 'drowsy' ever since. Her husband called for an ambulance. While waiting for its arrival, his wife mentioned feeling sick and vomited twice.

27.1.2 PMH (from Husband)

- Two episodes of headache over the last month. Each had a sudden onset and were localised to the right orbital region and right side of forehead.
- These were associated with nausea and blurred vision but both settled over a period of hours. She had wondered if they were 'migraine' and had planned to see her GP. On enquiring, her husband said she had no history of headaches.
- This episode appeared to be more severe and was not resolving. She is also now confused which has not happened previously.

27.1.3 Examination

- Chest – no abnormality detected.

- Normal heart sounds on auscultation.
- Glasgow Coma Scale: Eye opening 3; Verbal response 4; Motor response 6.
- The motor response is equal on both sides.
- Eyes:
  - Left ptosis.
  - Pupils: left 5 mm diameter and less responsive than right (3 mm diameter).
  - Left eye abducted and inferior compared to the right.
  - Photophobic.
- Pain score 7/10 (0 = no pain and 10 = worse pain imaginable).
- Neck stiffness. Movement increases the neck pain.

Modified early warning signs (MEWS):

- Respiratory rate 22 rpm.
- SpO_2 98% on room air.
- Tympanic temperature 37.0 °C.
- HR 80 bt/min.
- BP 160/80 mmHg.
- Alert.

27.1.4 CT Head

In view of her presentation signs and symptoms, a CT head was performed (Figure 27.1).

27.1.5 CTA

Due to the findings on this non-contrast scan, a CT angiogram (CTA) was arranged (Figure 27.2).

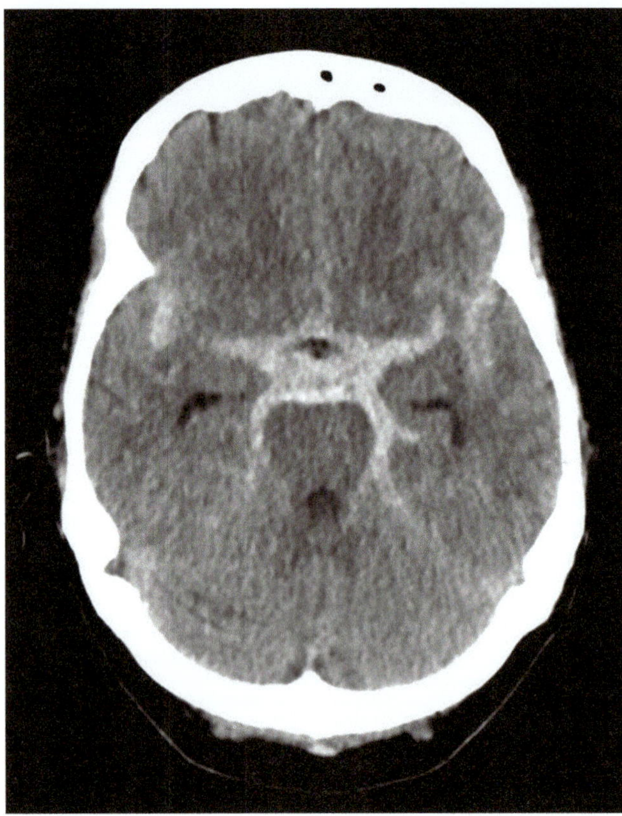

FIGURE 27.1 Patient A. Axial CT head on brain windows – non-contrast.

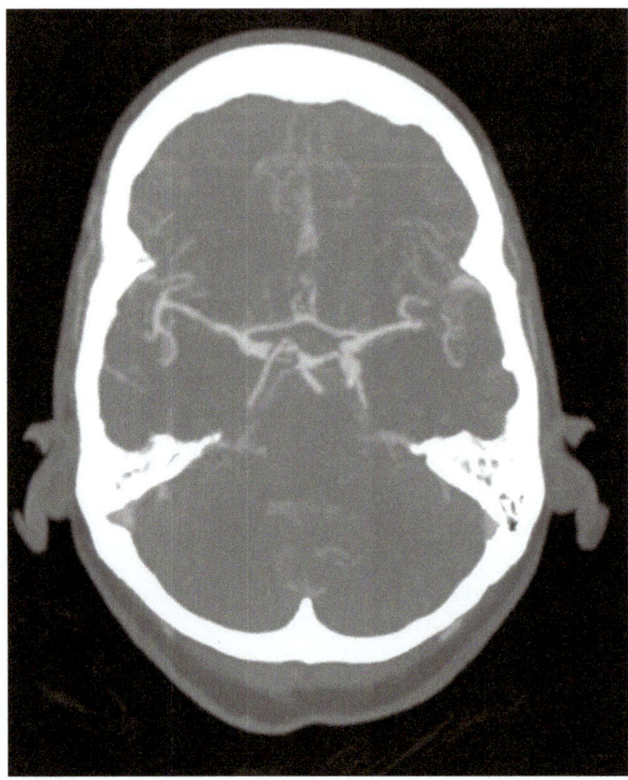

FIGURE 27.2 Patient A. Axial CT head angiogram maximum intensity projection (MIP) image.

Clinical Case Questions

- What is your differential diagnosis? Why?
- What is the location of the original lesion? Why?
- Why were these types of CT scans requested?
- What is your system for interpreting these images?
- What is your final diagnosis?

27.2 Radiology Self-assessment

27.2.1 Technical

27.2.1.1 Orientation

- In what anatomical plane is a CT head commonly viewed?
- How do you orientate the left and right sides of the image?

27.2.1.2 Density and Windowing

- What are the relative densities of tissues in the head?
- What CT windows are used to look at a head scan?

27.2.1.3 Blood on CT

- What do normal blood vessels look like on an unenhanced CT?
- What does clotted blood look like on CT?

27.2.1.4 CT Angiogram (CTA)

- How does a CTA differ from a standard CT head scan?

27.2.2 Correlating Anatomy to CT

27.2.2.1 Skull

- Where are the carotid canals?
- Where is the foramen magnum?

27.2.2.2 Ventricles and Cisterns

- What does cerebrospinal fluid (CSF) look like on CT?
- Where are the four ventricles on a CT scan? Which of these are visible on the midsagittal plane?
- On CT, how do you locate the following basal cisterns?
  - Suprasellar cistern.
  - Prepontine cistern.
  - Cerebellopontine angle cistern.
  - Ambient cistern.
  - Quadrigeminal cistern.
  - Cisterna magna.

27.2.2.3 Vessels

- What does the circle of Willis look like on a CTA?
- What does the basilar artery look like on a CTA?
- Can you identify the three paired cerebral arteries on a CTA?
- In which basal cisterns do the above vessels travel?

27.2.2.4 Meninges

- What do the dural venous sinuses look like on a CTA compared to a standard CT?
- How can you identify the following dural venous sinuses on CT?
  - Superior sagittal sinus.
  - Transverse sinus.
  - Sigmoid sinus.
  - Cavernous sinus.

27.2.3 The Ageing Brain

- What happens to the CSF spaces as the brain ages?
- Which structures normally calcify with ageing?

27.3 Key Radiology Review

27.3.1 Technical Aspects

A summary of the relevant terminology has been provided in Introduction Chapter 1; this includes a review of orientation, the sagittal plane, density of tissues and blood on CT.

27.3.2 Modified Axial Plane

A CT head is usually acquired in a modified axial plane to avoid irradiating the lenses of the eyes (Figure 27.3).

Modern PACS software allows the plane to be corrected if required.

27.3.3 CT Angiogram

Figure 27.4 provides an anatomical overview of the main cerebral arteries and their relationship to the underlying brain. Obtaining optimal views of these vessels on CT requires the administration of intravenous contrast (Figure 27.5). For a more comprehensive review of contrast protocols see the Introduction Chapter 1 (contrast protocols).

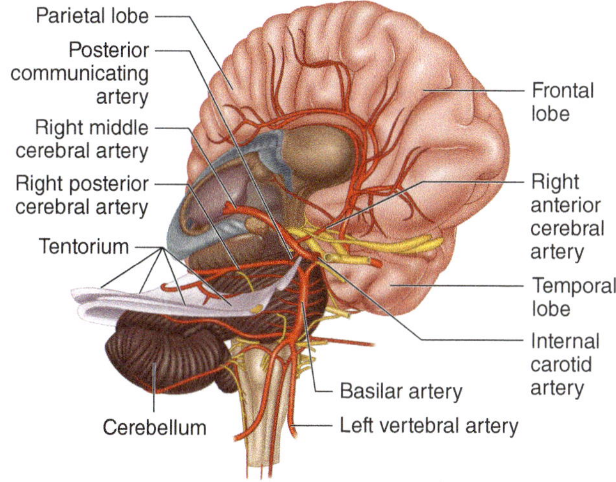

FIGURE 27.4 Right anterior view showing the main cerebral arteries and their relation to the underlying brain. The right tentorium cerebelli is included to demarcate the roof of the posterior cranial fossa. ACA, anterior cerebral artery; MCA, middle cerebral artery; PCA, posterior cerebral artery.

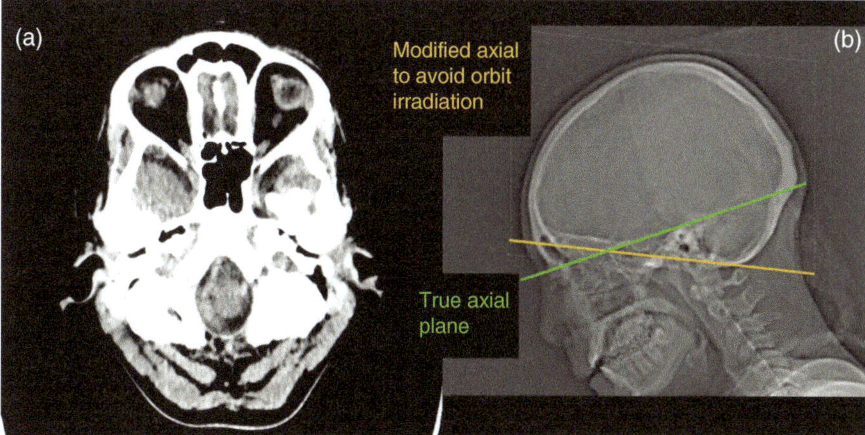

FIGURE 27.3 Modified axial CT (a) and the CT scout view (b) showing the angle of the scan in relation to the skull base.

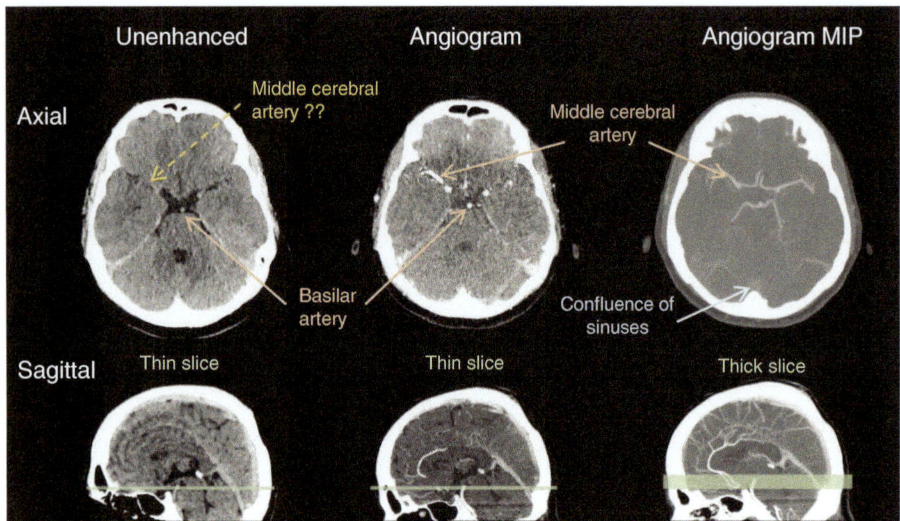

FIGURE 27.5 Normal axial and sagittal CT images in the same patient using three different techniques. The axial slice thickness is shown as the green band on the corresponding sagittal views. Compare the differences between an unenhanced CT head and CT angiogram. *Unenhanced*: the larger blood vessels on unenhanced scans are visible as linear grey structures, provided they are surrounded by CSF which is black. This is demonstrated with the basilar artery. The density of the flowing blood is similar to that of brain tissue, hence it becomes much more tricky to distinguish between the vessel and brain when they are touching (e.g. right MCA dashed yellow arrow). *Angiogram*: intravenous contrast increases the density in the vessels, so they are brighter (i.e. whiter) in relation to the background brain and CSF. Note how much clearer the right middle cerebral artery is on the angiographic image. Invariably there will be some venous contrast present, even on arterial phase imaging. In the example given, the confluence of sinuses can be seen faintly. The straight sinus is also visible on the sagittal images. *Maximum intensity projection* (MIP): this is a visualisation tool which increases the slice thickness and shows the brightest voxel value across the thicker slice. It provides a useful overview of the vasculature and so will be used in this chapter for illustrative purposes to show the course of the arteries.

27.3.4 Correlating the Vascular Anatomy with the CT Image

27.3.4.1 Vessels in Relation to the Skull and Meninges
The internal carotid artery travels in the carotid canal through the skull base, before passing through the cavernous sinus to emerge into the cranial vault (at the middle cranial fossa) to form the circle of Willis (COW) (Figures 27.6 and 27.7).

The vertebral arteries travel through the foramen magnum to enter the skull. They then combine to form the basilar artery (Figures 27.4, 27.6 and 27.8). The dural venous sinuses are often visible on CT angiogram due to early venous enhancement.

Even on an unenhanced scan, it is still worth tracing the course of the vessels (see Figures 27.5 and 27.11). They are more visible when surrounded by a tissue of different density (e.g. fat, fluid or bone). When this is not the case (e.g. they abut against brain parenchyma) then the arteries are very difficult to see without contrast.

Pathology which changes the contour of the vessel may be visible without contrast, for example large aneurysms and calcified atherosclerotic plaques. Although the internal diameter of the vessel cannot be assessed without contrast, if there is a large thrombus within the vessel then it may be visible as an area of increased density (see Head Chapter 29 –Figure 27.9).

27.3.4.2 Cerebrospinal Fluid (CSF) Spaces
The CSF drains from the lateral ventricles inferiorly through the third ventricle, and then to the fourth ventricle before communicating with the extra-axial CSF spaces (Figures 27.9 and 27.10).

The extra-axial spaces are divided into sulci and cisterns. These form a continuous space around the outside of the brain and are usually named after the adjacent brain anatomy. A key reason for checking the cisterns in the acute situation is because they can be effaced by brain herniation and raised intracranial pressure. Hence *their absence may be pathological* (see Head Chapter 29). Beware also that compromise of the vessels and nerves that run within the cisterns can provide helpful localising clinical signs (Figure 27.11).

27.3.5 The Ageing Brain and Ventricles

As we age, the brain tissue reduces in volume (often described as involution). The result is that the CSF spaces, such as the ventricles and fissures, increase in size (Figure 27.12). This is a normal process of ageing and should not be confused with pathology such as hydrocephalus.

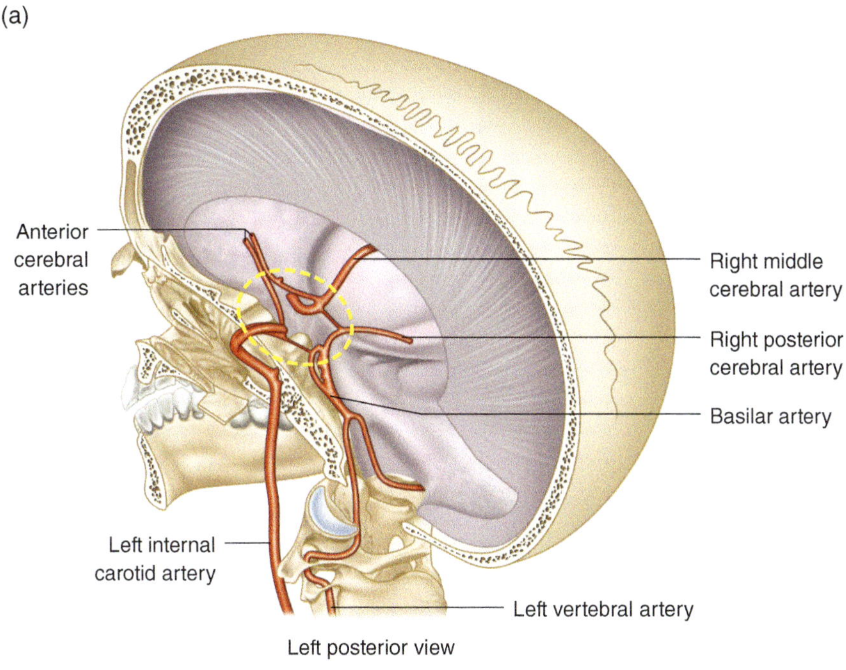

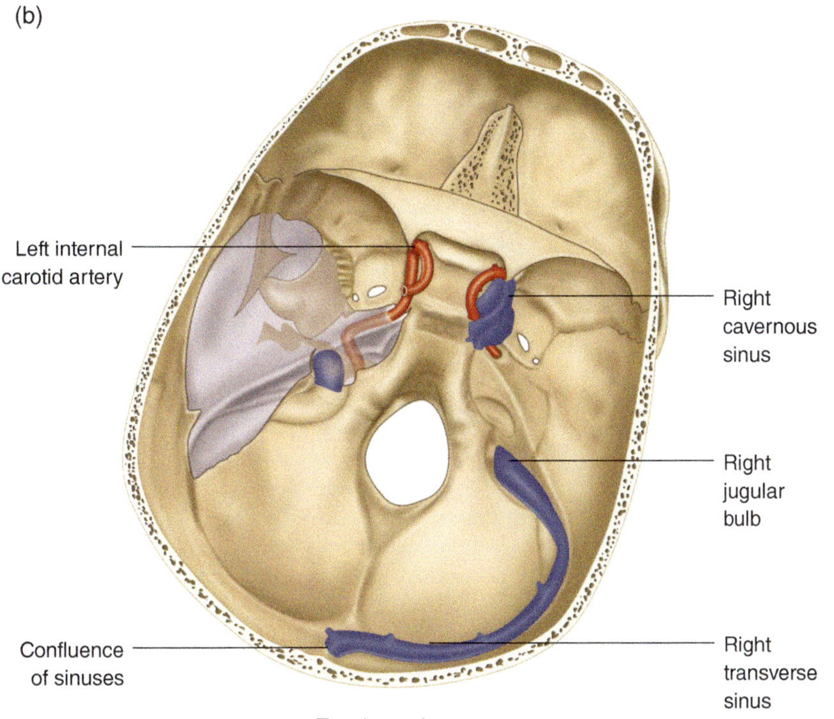

FIGURE 27.6 Intracranial vasculature. (a) Left posterior view. View of the base of skull showing the course of the vertebral arteries, forming the basilar artery. This, in turn, links with the internal carotid to form the COW (yellow circle). (b) Top-down view. Course of the left internal carotid artery through the base of the skull and the location of the right cavernous venous sinus. Both of these lie on the wall of the sphenoid. The right dural venous sinuses are also shown draining into the right jugular bulb via the sigmoid sinus.

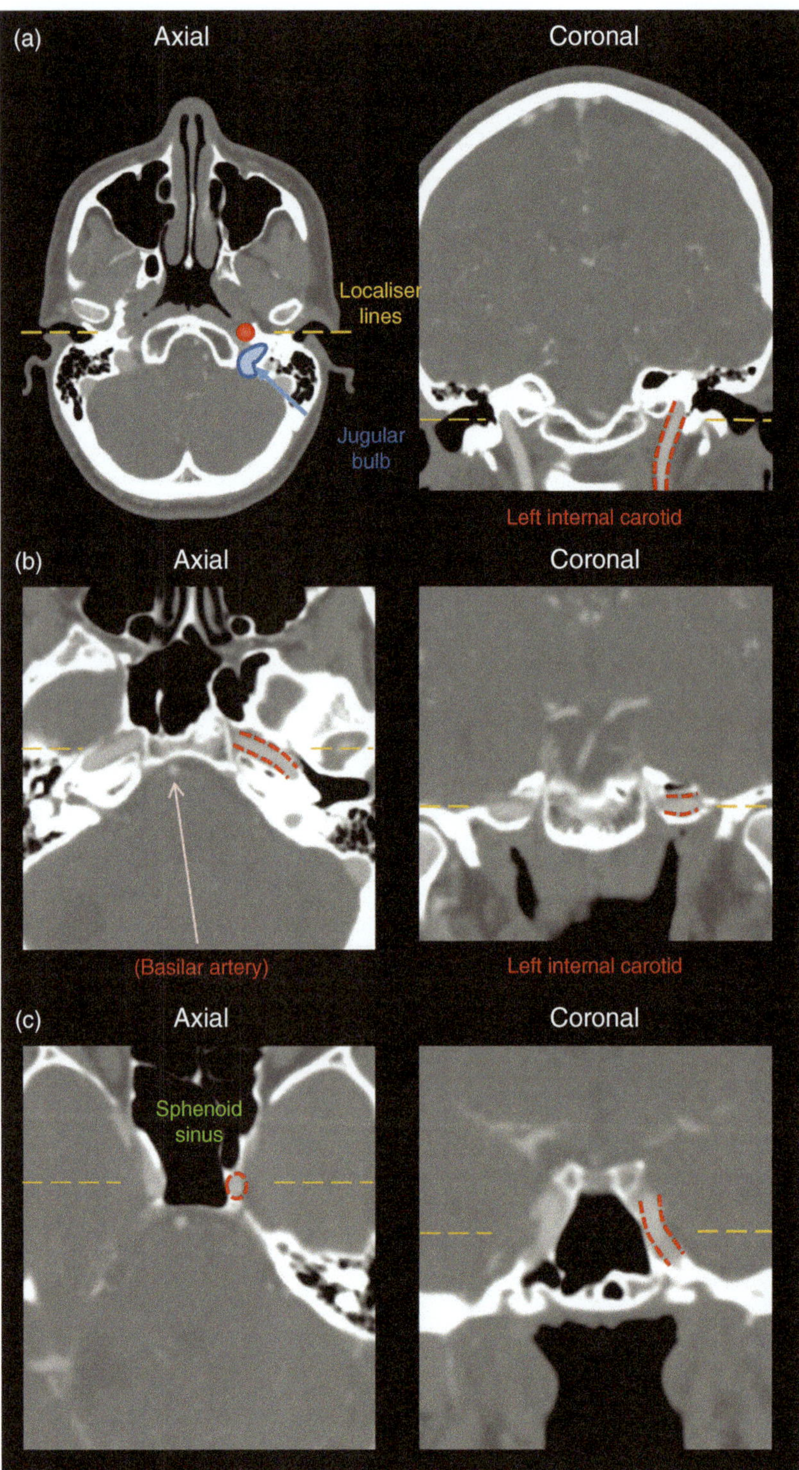

FIGURE 27.7 The internal carotids and carotid canal. CT angiogram on a modified bone window. Axial and coronal slices are displayed. The level of the axial slice is indicated on the coronal views with the localiser lines. The left internal carotid is annotated. (a) The internal carotids enter the skull base through the carotid canal, just anterior to the jugular bulb lying in the jugular foramen. (b) The carotid canals take a horizontal course as they travel medially and anteriorly towards the sphenoid sinus which lies within the sphenoid bone. (c) The carotid canal turns superiorly and the internal carotids run within the cavernous sinus, immediately lateral to the sphenoid sinus. The cavernous sinus is a venous structure and can often be distinguished from the carotid artery if the correct windows are used.

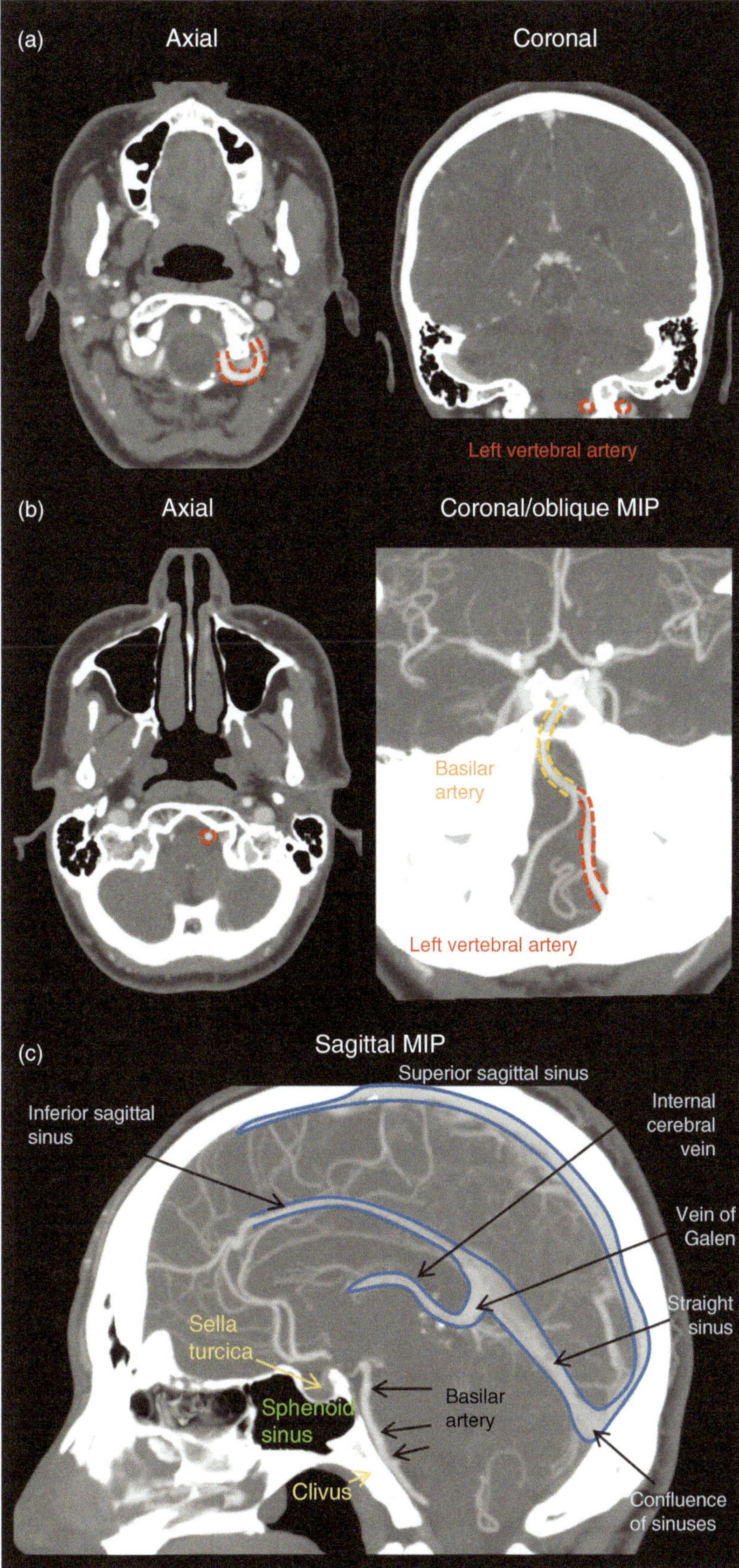

FIGURE 27.8 The vertebral and basilar arteries plus midline venous structures. CT angiogram on a modified bone window in various anatomical planes. Maximum intensity projections (MIP) are used to best demonstrate the course of the vessels (see Chapter 1). (a) The vertebral arteries leave the transverse foramina of C1 and loop posteriorly to enter the foramen magnum. The left vertebral artery is annotated. (b) Typically the right and left vertebral arteries are asymmetrical, one being bigger than the other. They also often take a tortuous, and varying, course before combining to become the basilar artery. This may be to facilitate rotation at C1/C2 without stretching the vessel. (c) The basilar artery runs approximately in the midline, immediately posterior to the clivus. Note, the sagittal plane also gives a good overview of the midline venous structures.

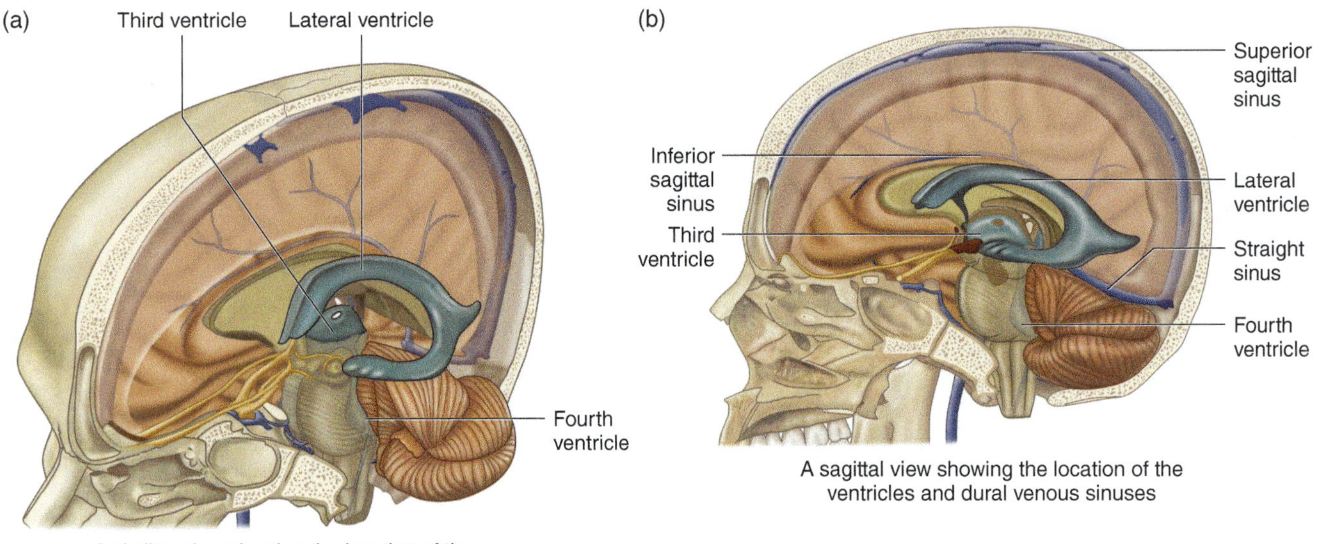

FIGURE 27.9 (a) A skyline view showing the location of the ventricles and venous sinuses. (b) A sagittal view showing the location of the ventricles and venous sinuses.

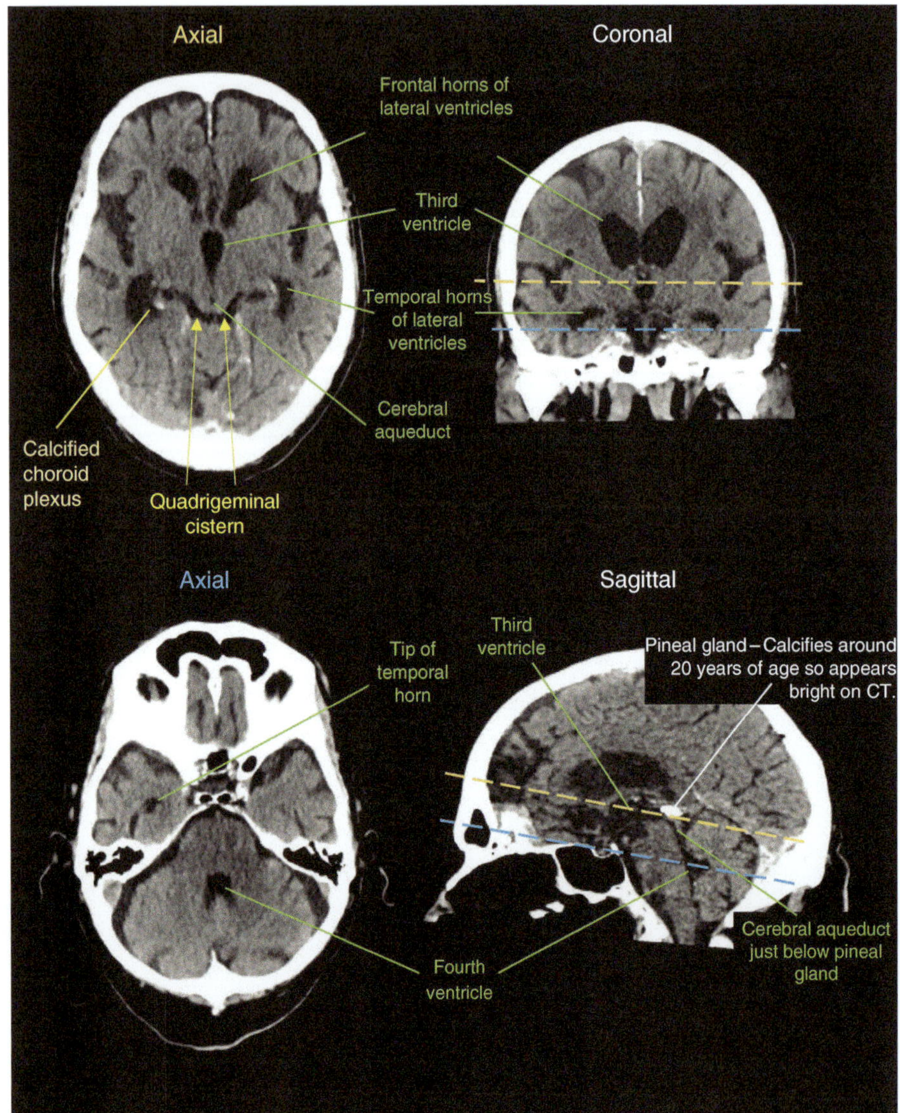

FIGURE 27.10 CT head on brain windows – unenhanced. The level of the axial slices is cross-referenced on the coronal and sagittal views. This is an elderly patient with capacious CSF spaces. Note the ventricles filled with CSF (black in relation to brain tissue). The two lateral ventricles are best seen on axial and coronal slices. In contrast, the midline third and fourth ventricles are more easily visualised on the sagittal plane. It is normal to see calcified choroid plexus inside the ventricles. This should not be mistaken for haemorrhage (see Figure 27.14).

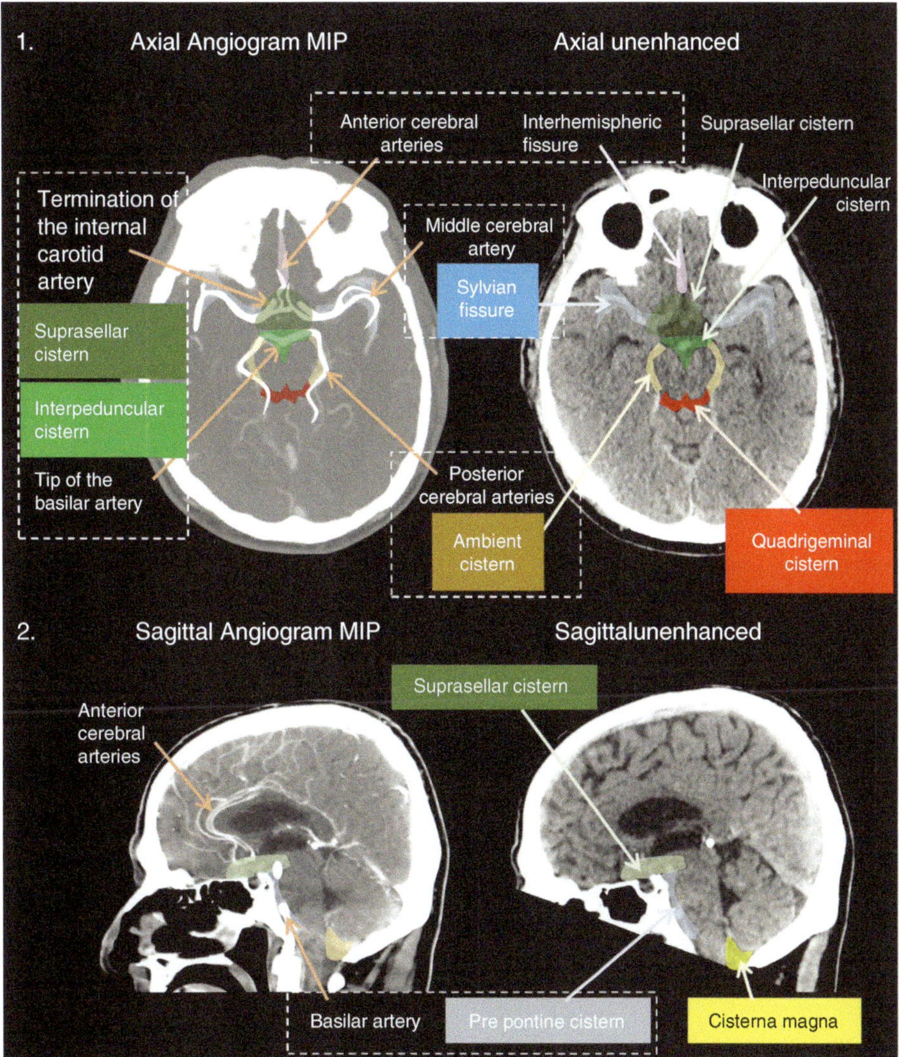

FIGURE 27.11 CT showing the location of the basal cisterns and corresponding cerebral arteries. The white boxes group the artery with its corresponding CSF space. The quadrigeminal cistern contains no artery but is an important review area when checking for brain herniation (see Head Chapter 29 – Figure 29.11). The cisterna magna lies behind the medulla and contains the openings from the fourth ventricle (foramen of *Magendie* in the *midline* and foramen of *Luschka laterally*).

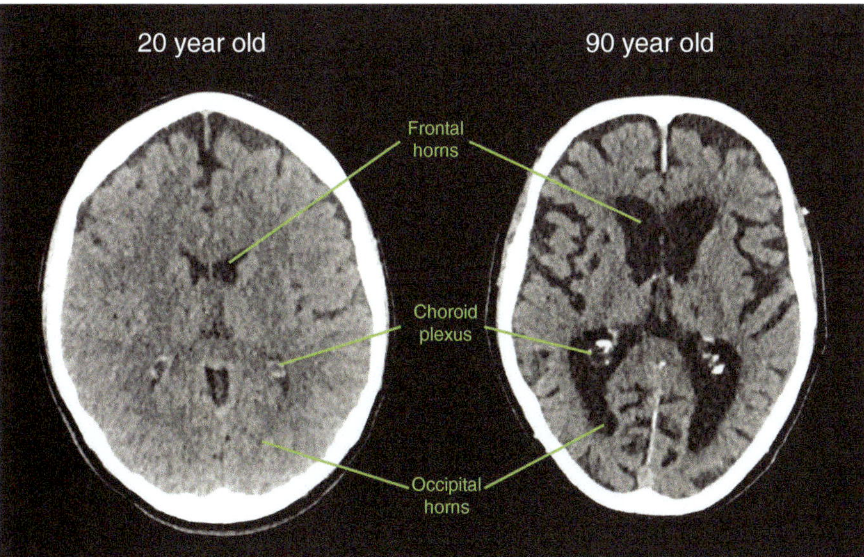

FIGURE 27.12 Axial CT head on brain windows – unenhanced. The paired lateral ventricles are the largest and each have three horns, which are named after their corresponding anatomical lobes. Note how the occipital horns in the young brain are flat and almost impossible to see. The temporal horn cannot be seen in this image (compare with Figure 27.10). The choroid plexus can be seen within the lateral ventricles and is often calcified, making it appear white on CT.

27.4 Review of the Clinical Case

- Why is CT indicated?
- Why is a CT angiogram indicated?
- What is your final diagnosis and definitive management?

27.4.1 Differential Diagnosis

27.4.1.1 Subarachnoid Haemorrhage (SAH)

- A sudden onset of severe headache raises the suspicion of subarachnoid haemorrhage (Box 27.1).
- There may be associated neurology but 50% of patients will have a normal neurological examination.
- Non-contrast CT head is extremely accurate for acute subarachnoid haemorrhage. Provided it is performed within six hours of symptom onset, it can be considered a 'rule out' study. After this time the blood drops in density and is more difficult to spot on CT.
- Lumbar puncture should be considered after this six-hour window, if the patient has a low haematocrit or if the CT head is suboptimal, e.g. due to movement artefact.
- Once the subarachnoid haemorrhage has been confirmed, CTA is used to look for an underlying aneurysmal cause. This is present in around 85% of atraumatic cases.
- Some advocate the use of CTA as an alternative to lumbar puncture to exclude subarachnoid haemorrhage with a negative non-contrast CT head. However, with the prevalence of aneurysms estimated to be 2–5%, an aneurysm found on a CTA may be incidental and unrelated to the cause of headache.

27.4.1.2 Migraine

- The SAH headache can be similar to migraine. A possible distinguishing clue is that in SAH, there is a simultaneous onset of headache, vertigo and vomiting. With migraine the headache may precede the vertigo and vomiting.
- Beware that meningeal irritation (i.e. photophobia and neck stiffness) can occur in severe migraine. It is therefore not pathognomonic of a SAH.

Box 27.1 | Headache Characteristics of a SAH

Remember the **S** of **S**AH: **S**udden; **S**evere; **S**wiftly reaches its peak (seconds to minutes); **S**ustained (i.e. lasts over an hour).

27.4.1.3 Meningitis This can also present with headache, neck stiffness, nausea and vomiting.

27.4.2 Unenhanced CT

Patient A has blood in the subarachnoid space (Figure 27.13).

Even though the bleeding source is not within the ventricular system, the flow of CSF causes the blood to backtrack into the ventricles. The normal choroid plexus can be confused with haemorrhage but a good rule of thumb is demonstrated in Figure 27.14.

If there are small intraventricular bleeds, a blood/CSF fluid level may be seen at the back of the occipital horns in the recumbent patient (Figure 27.15).

27.4.3 CT Angiogram

Patient A has an aneurysm of the left posterior communicating artery (PCOM), which is responsible for the subarachnoid haemorrhage (Figure 27.16).

Patient A had focal neurology due to compression of the oculomotor nerve (i.e. left ptosis, left dilated and sluggish pupil and a left eye which was looking down and out). This occurs due to the close anatomical relationship between the oculomotor nerve and the posterior cerebral artery (Figure 27.17).

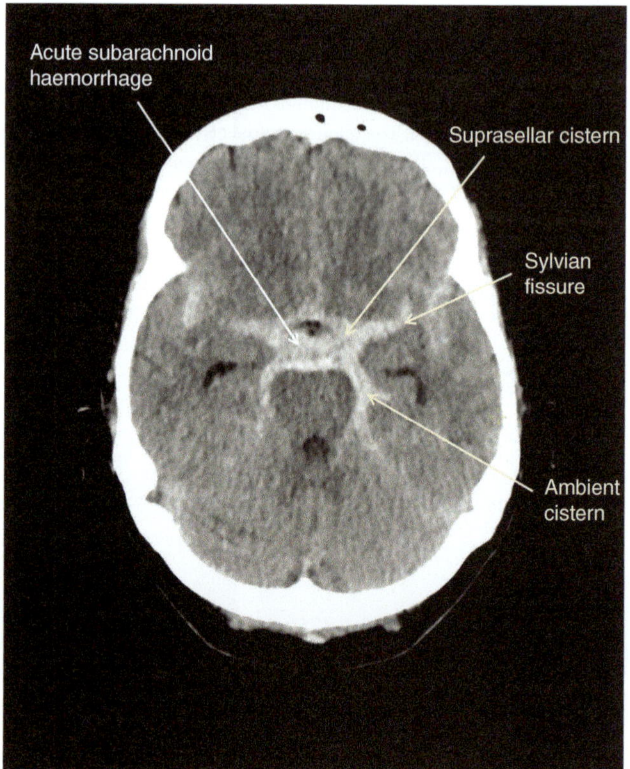

FIGURE 27.13 Patient A. Annotated axial CT head on brain windows. There is an acute subarachnoid haemorrhage, with clotted blood in the suprasellar cistern, sylvian fissures and ambient cisterns.

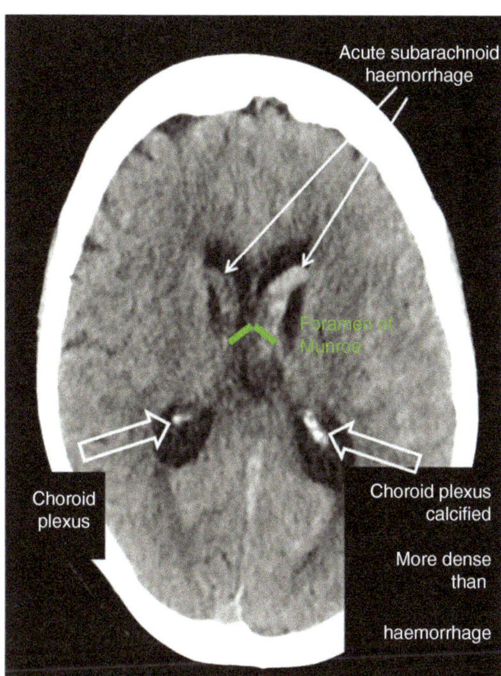

FIGURE 27.14 Patient A. Axial CT head on brain windows at the level of the foramen of Munroe. There is acute subarachnoid haemorrhage in the frontal horns of the lateral ventricles (white arrows). The choroid plexus is often calcified so will appear *more dense* than acute blood clot. It can be seen more posteriorly within the lateral ventricles (hollow arrows) but should never extend more anteriorly than the foramen of Munroe (green lines). *Therefore, if material is seen in the frontal horns then it is almost certainly acute subarachnoid haemorrhage as opposed to normal choroid plexus.*

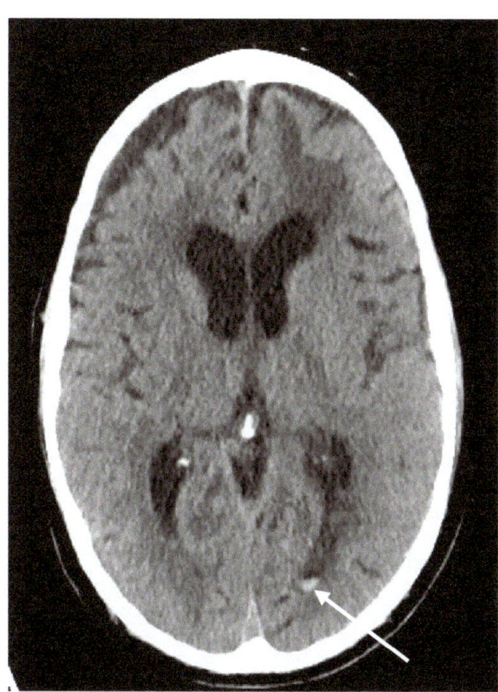

FIGURE 27.15 CT head, brain window – axial view. This is a different patient with intraventricular haemorrhage. There is clotted blood layering in the left occipital horn (white arrow). As blood is denser than CSF, it will tend to collect posteriorly.

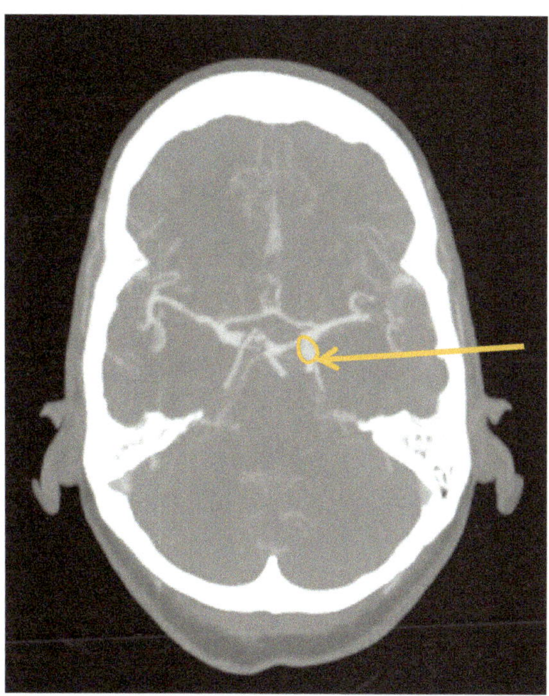

FIGURE 27.16 Patient A. Annotated CT angiogram showing a left PCOM (posterior communicating artery) aneurysm (arrow).

27.4.4 Other Investigations to Consider

- *Magnetic resonance angiography (MRA)*: this is occasionally used if there is an allergy to contrast, but it lacks the resolution of CT and is prone to artefacts.
- *Digital subtraction angiography (DSA)*: this is the gold standard investigation; it allows intervention such as coiling to be performed but is only available in neuro-interventional centres.

27.4.5 Final Diagnosis

Subarachnoid haemorrhage secondary to a left PCOM aneurysm.

27.5 Take-home Message – Imaging in Atraumatic Headache

- Unenhanced CT is the first-line test to exclude subarachnoid haemorrhage and can be used to exclude this diagnosis, provided it is performed within six hours of symptom onset.
- Outside this time window, consider lumbar puncture.
- CT angiogram is used after confirmation of subarachnoid haemorrhage, to look for an underlying aneurysm.

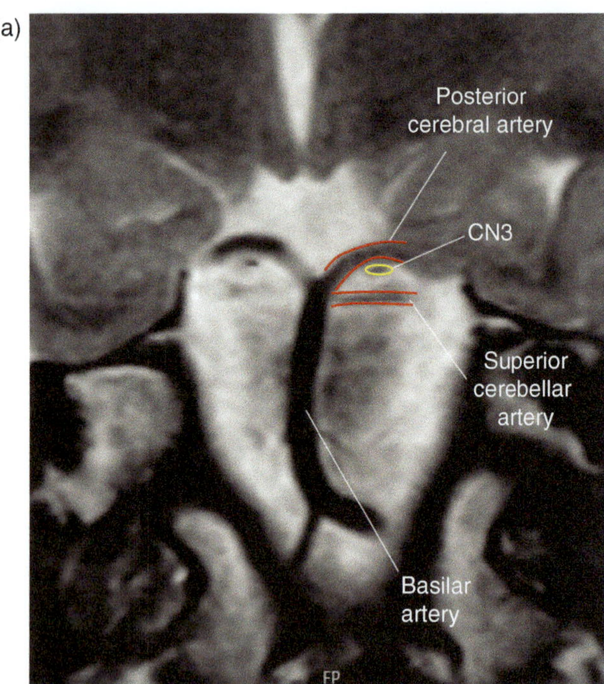

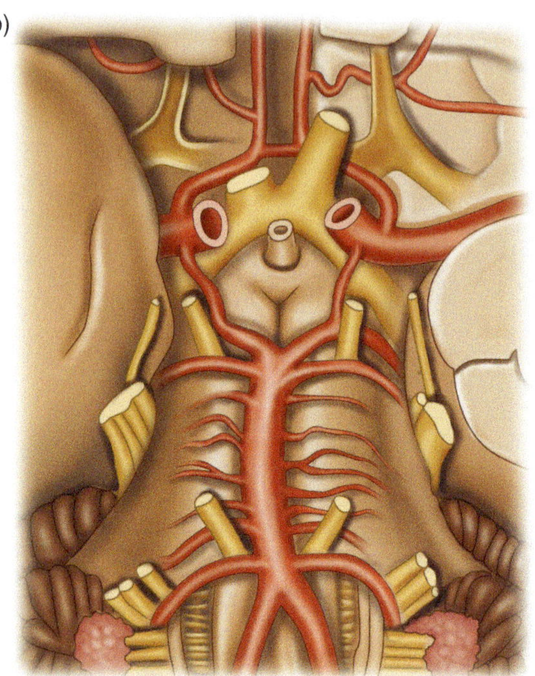

FIGURE 27.17 (a) T2 MRI, modified coronal plane through the basilar tip (see Head Chapter 28 for more information on MRI sequences). (b) Anatomical drawing showing the same relationship. The oculomotor nerve travels between the posterior cerebral artery and the superior cerebellar artery. Aneurysms in this region can press on the nerve, giving rise to the clinical symptoms observed.

Further Resources

Edlow, J.A. and Fisher, J. (2012). Diagnosis of subarachnoid hemorrhage: time to change the guidelines? *Stroke* 43 (8): 2031–2032.

Marcolini, E. and Hine, J. (2019). Approach to the diagnosis and management of subarachnoid hemorrhage. *West J Emerg. Med* 20 (2): 203–211.

Schwedt, T.J., Matharu, M.S., and Dodick, D.W. (2006). Thunderclap headache. *Lancet Neurol* 5 (7): 621–631.

CHAPTER 28

Sudden Weakness

Joshua Lauder[1], Aleksandr Valkov[2], and Peter Driscoll[3]

[1]*East Lancashire Hospitals NHS Trust, University of Central Lancashire and University of Manchester, UK*
[2]*Salford Royal Hospital and University of Central Lancashire, Salford, UK*
[3]*School of Medicine and Dentistry, University of Central Lancashire, Preston, UK*

28.1 Primary Case

28.1.1 Presentation

A 65-year-old male is brough to the Emergency Department by ambulance. One hour previously he developed sudden right-sided weakness. He has remained conscious throughout and has no history of trauma.

28.1.2 PMH (from Wife)

- Hypertension (five years) taking amlodipine 5 mg and ramipril 5 mg.
- Hyperlipidaemia taking atorvastatin 20 mg.
- Smokes 20 cigarettes/day.

28.1.3 Examination

- Chest – no abnormality detected.
- Normal heart sounds on auscultation.
- Glasgow Coma Scale: Eye opening 4; Verbal response 3; Motor response 6 (on left).
- Neurological examination:
  - Global aphasia.
  - Right facial droop.
  - Right hemiplegia (upper limb 0/5 and lower limb 2/5) and decreased tone.
  - Left gaze preference.
  - Unable to test sensation due to aphasia.

28.1.4 CT

In view of this presentation, urgent CT and CT angiogram (CTA) of the head were performed (Figures 28.1 and 28.2).

Clinical Case Questions

- What is your differential diagnosis? Why?
- What is the location of the lesion? Why?
- Why were these types of CT scans requested?
- What is your system for interpreting these images?
- What is your final diagnosis?

28.2 Radiology Self-assessment

28.2.1 Technical

28.2.1.1 MRI

- What are the visual differences between T1 and T2 images?
- What is fluid-attenuated inversion recovery (FLAIR) imaging?
- What is diffusion-weighted imaging (DWI)?

Diagnostic Imaging and Anatomy in Acute Care, First Edition. Edited by Joshua Lauder and Peter Driscoll.
© 2025 John Wiley & Sons Ltd. Published 2025 by John Wiley & Sons Ltd.
Companion website: www.wiley.com/go/DiagnosticImaginginAcuteCare

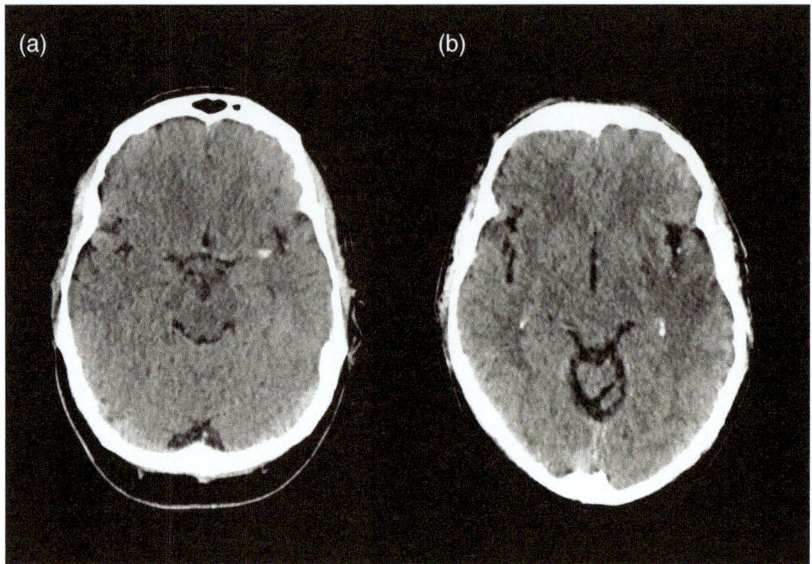

FIGURE 28.1 Patient A. Axial CT head on brain windows at the level of the suprasellar cistern (a) and the third ventricle (b).

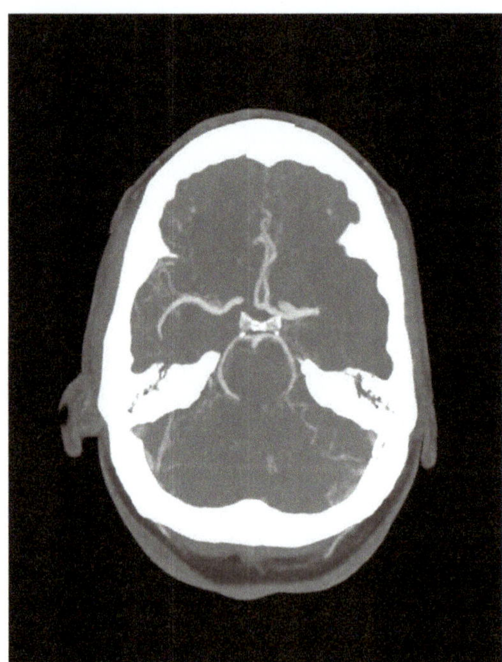

FIGURE 28.2 Patient A. Axial CT angiogram (CTA) of the brain maximum intensity projection (MIP) at the level of the circle of Willis.

28.2.2 Correlation of Gross Anatomy with CT and MRI

28.2.2.1 Vessels

- What do vessels looks like on MRI?
- What is the anterior circulation and where does it run from and to?
- What is the posterior circulation and where does it run from and to?

28.2.2.2 Cerebrum – Grey and White Matter

- How can you distinguish between grey and white matter on CT?
- Can you identify the deep grey matter structures on CT?
- How do you identify the central sulcus on CT?
- Can you find each of the cerebral lobes on CT?
- Can grey and white matter be distinguished on MRI?
- What are the vascular territories on MRI imaging?

28.2.3 Anatomical Variants

- What is a foetal origin of the posterior cerebral artery?

28.3 Key Radiology Review

28.3.1 Magnetic Resonance Imaging (MRI)

MRI is used extensively to view the central nervous system as it can readily identify the difference between grey and white matter, as well as CSF and vessels (see Introduction Chapter 1 for an overview of MRI imaging).

Several sequences are commonly used in neuro MRI including T1, T2, FLAIR (Figure 28.3) and DWI (Figure 28.4).

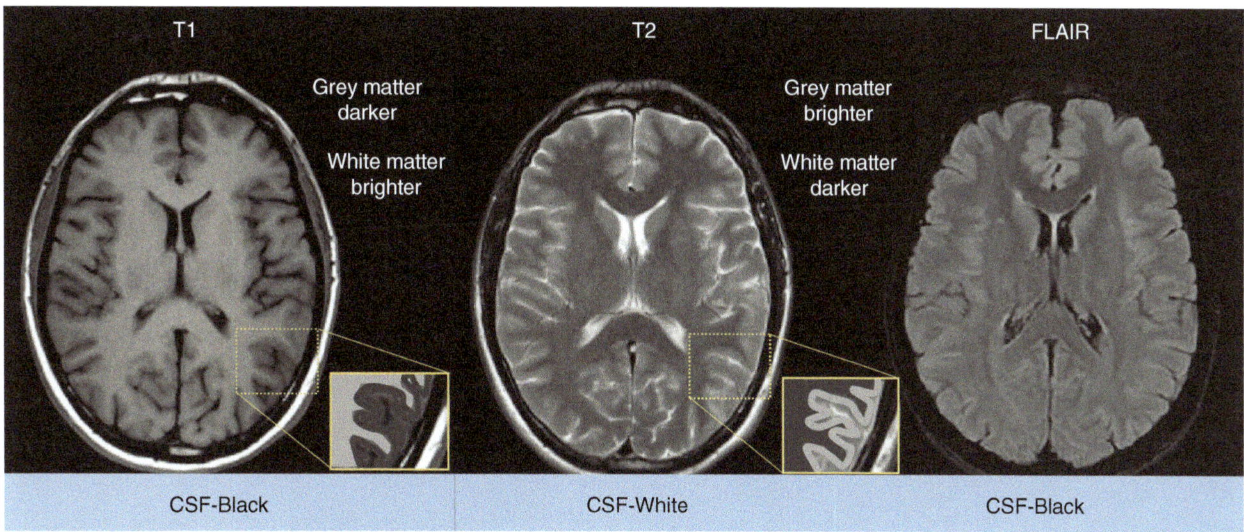

FIGURE 28.3 Axial MRI head, T1, T2 and FLAIR (fluid-attenuated inversion recovery) sequences. *T1*: this is often referred to as the anatomical sequence because the shade of the grey and white matter corresponds to the name (i.e. grey matter is darker than white matter). Fluid is always dark on T1, hence the CSF appears black. This sequence can be used to look for haemorrhage, which is bright on T1 in the acute and subacute phase (1–7 days). See Introduction Chapter 1 for appearance of blood on MRI. *T2*: this is one of the most useful sequences. Fluid is bright so the CSF will be white. Pathological processes like oedema will also be bright. The intensity of the grey and white matter is reversed on this sequence (i.e. grey matter is brighter than white matter). *FLAIR*: this sequence is identical to T2 except that the fluid has been suppressed, making the CSF black. This can be useful as cortical or periventricular abnormalities become more obvious due to increased contrast between the abnormality and the adjacent CSF.

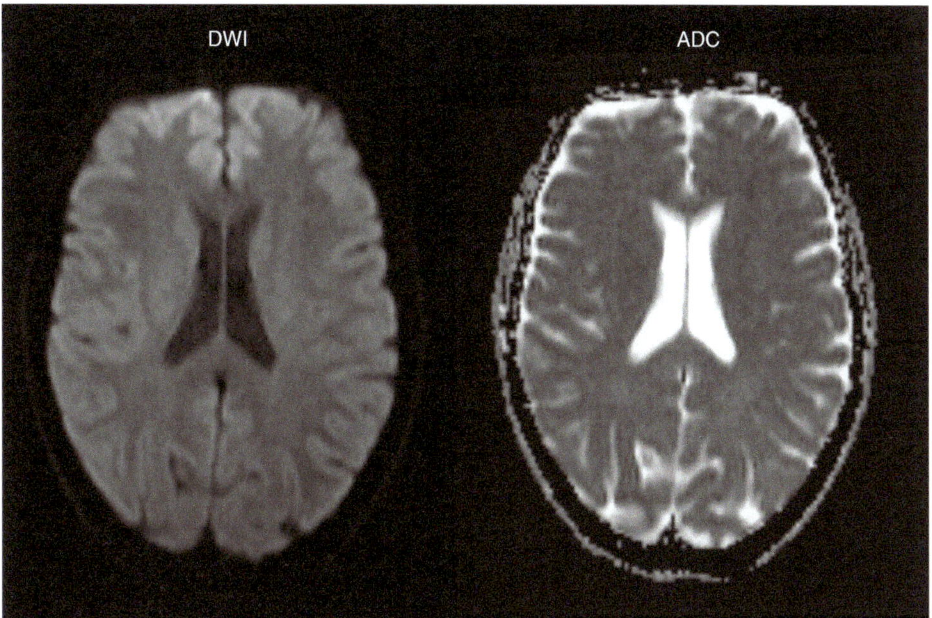

FIGURE 28.4 Axial MRI head, diffusion-weighted imaging (DWI), apparent diffusion coefficient (ADC) sequences. DWI shows the relative movement of water molecules on a microscopic level. Certain pathologies result in restricted diffusion so this is a useful sequence to characterise abnormalities previously identified on other sequences. However, it has poor spatial resolution compared to other sequences and is prone to artefacts at the skull base so should not be used in isolation. The DWI sequence must always be viewed in conjunction with the ADC. This is because bright areas on the DWI can be caused by an artefact called 'T2 shine-through'. The ADC is required to exclude this as an explanation and confirm true diffusion restriction. (This concept is better elicited with an example – see Figure 28.13).

28.3.2 Correlation of Gross Anatomy to CT and MRI (Figure 28.5)

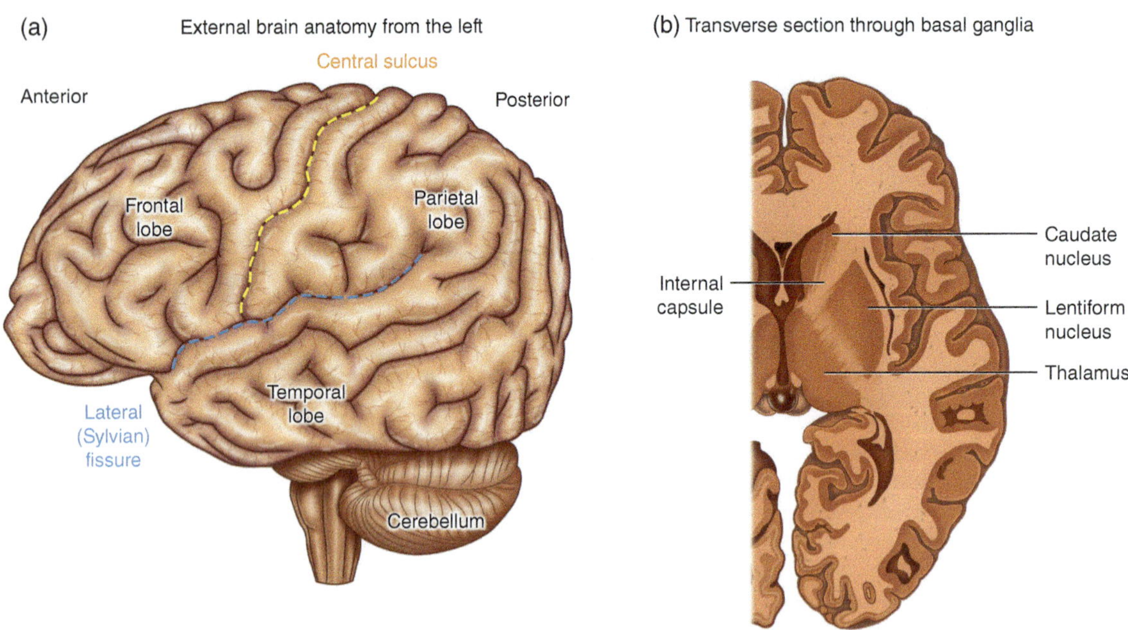

FIGURE 28.5 (a) External surface of the brain seen from the top and left side. The main sulci are marked. The occipital lobe is mostly hidden round the posterior aspect of the brain. (b) Transverse section through the cerebral hemisphere at the level of the basal ganglia. The figures show the key landmarks to look for when viewing the CT and MRI scan.

28.3.2.1 Cerebrum – Grey and White Matter (Figure 28.6)

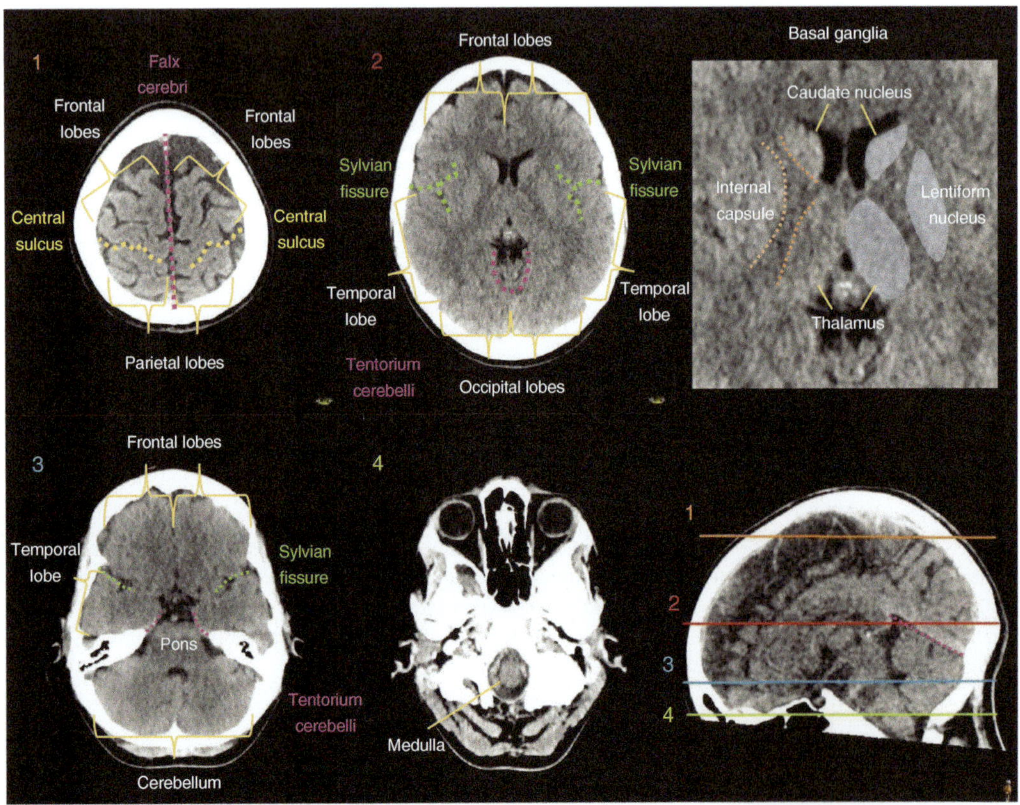

FIGURE 28.6 Axial CT on brain windows: brain anatomy (images 1–4). Sagittal view shown to demonstrate the planes. The central sulcus is a key landmark for separating the frontal and parietal lobes. The grey and white matter can be vaguely distinguished on CT. This is much easier on MRI (see Figure 28.3).

28.3.2.2 Vessels To review the anatomy of the cerebral arteries, see Head Chapter 27 – Figure 27.11.

A limited assessment of the vessels is possible on a standard MRI brain scan. This is because of an artefact called 'flow void' (Figure 28.7).

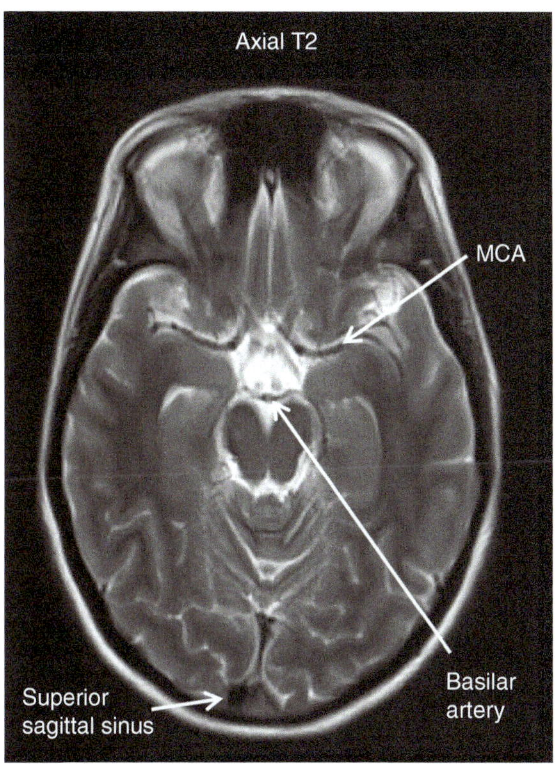

FIGURE 28.7 Axial MRI brain, T2 sequence. Normally vessels are black on T2, as demonstrated by the MCA and basilar arteries. This results from an artefact caused by the movement of the blood called 'flow void'. It can be used as an indicator of vessel patency but does not have the same diagnostic accuracy as dedicated angiographic imaging. Note that there should also be a flow void in the superior sagittal sinus. Loss of this could indicate a dural venous thrombus.

28.3.2.3 Vascular Territories (Figure 28.8)

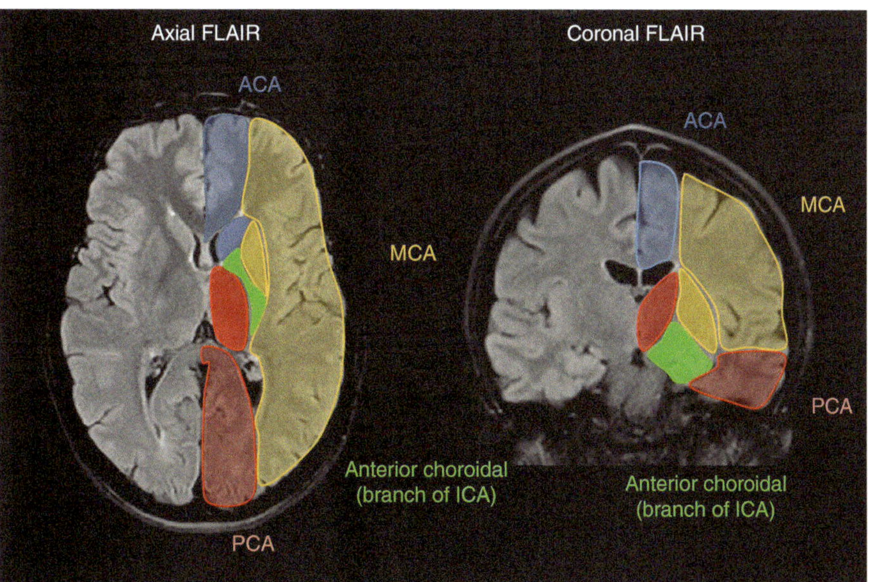

FIGURE 28.8 MRI head, FLAIR sequence, axial and coronal slices. Annotation showing the major anterior circulation vascular territories. The same distribution can be applied to a CT scan. The anterior choroidal artery is a branch of the ICA, near its termination. ACA, Anterior cerebral artery; MCA, middle cerebral artery; PCA, posterior cerebral artery; ICA, internal carotid artery.

28.3.3 Anatomical Variants

28.3.3.1 Foetal Origin of the Posterior Communicating Artery (Figure 28.9)

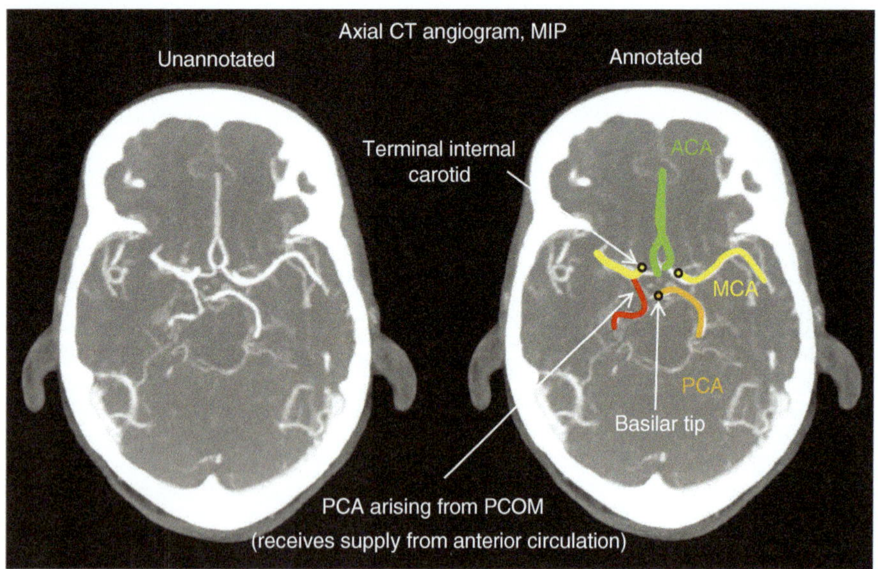

FIGURE 28.9 Axial CT angiogram of the brain, maximum intensity projection (MIP), unannotated and annotated. In this case there is a persistent foetal origin to the right posterior cerebral artery (PCA). This means the PCA receives its supply from the posterior communicating artery, rather than the basilar artery. The clinical significance of this is that a large terminal internal carotid thrombus could cause ischaemia in the posterior cerebral artery territory. ACA, anterior cerebral artery; MCA, middle cerebral artery.

28.4 Review of the Clinical Case

- Why is CT head indicated?
- Why is CTA indicated?
- What is your final diagnosis and clinical management?

28.4.1 Differential Diagnosis

As with all neurological cases, the clinical aims are to:

- Localise the site of the lesion.
  - Hemiplegia and aphasia suggest a lesion involving the frontal, parietal and temporal lobes of the contralateral hemisphere (Table 28.1).

- Identify the cause.
  - This depends on the speed of onset of symptoms (Table 28.2). A one-hour onset in the absence of trauma is highly suggestive of a vascular cause (stroke).

28.4.1.1 Stroke (Box 28.1) Eighty percent of strokes are ischaemic in nature; this type will be confined to a single vascular territory (see Figure 28.8). Twenty percent of strokes are haemorrhagic and may involve more random regions of the brain.

TABLE 28.1

Cerebral Sites Associated with the Patient's Presenting Signs.

Sign	Site
Global aphasia	Left temporal and parietal area
Right facial droop	Left precentral gyrus
Right hemiplegia (upper limb 0/5 and lower limb 2/5) and decreased tone	Left precentral gyrus and premotor area
Left gaze preference	Left frontal eye field

TABLE 28.2

Speed of Onset and likely Neurological condition.

	Acute	Subacute	Chronic
Time of onset	Minutes – days	Days – weeks	Months – years
Likely causes	Vascular	Infection	Neoplasm
	Trauma	Haematoma (SDH)	Degenerative disease[a]
	Hypoxia[a]		
	Hypoglycaemia[a]	Vasculitis	Vasculitis
		MS	MS

MS, multiple sclerosis; SDH, subdural haemorrhage.
[a] *These* causes will tend to cause more global symptoms, rather than focal neurology.

28.4.2 Unenhanced CT

An unenhanced CT scan was performed initially. The main aim of this is to exclude intracranial haemorrhage but it can also help to diagnose ischaemic stroke (Figure 28.10).

It is possible to approximately age an infarct on CT. In the hyperacute stage, there may be no visible changes to the brain tissue on CT. In some cases there may be subtle loss of the grey/white matter differentiation and/or sulcal effacement. Over the next week the infarct will become a large hypodense area, representing oedema. In the chronic stage, the brain tissue will die, leaving an area of encephalomalacia which fills with CSF (Figure 28.11).

28.4.3 CT Angiogram (CTA)

In cases where mechanical thrombectomy is considered, it is vital to perform a CTA at the same session as the unenhanced CT. This is more time efficient, which is critical if mechanical thrombectomy is to be successful.

To decide which patients are eligible for mechanical thrombectomy, the time of onset of symptoms, the modified Rankin score (mRS) and the National Institutes of Health Stroke Scale (NIHSS) scoring systems are used. Local protocols differ and guidelines change regularly so consult with your designated stroke lead (see Further Resources for further information).

CTA provides a detailed view of the arteries in the brain and neck to help confirm a treatable proximal thrombus and to plan the procedure (Figure 28.12).

28.4.4 MRI in Stroke

MRI is extremely sensitive for stroke so can be used in equivocal cases. The DWI sequence is the most useful (Figure 28.13). Identifying these small cortical and lacunar infarcts can help manage secondary prevention.

28.4.5 Final Diagnosis

Acute left MCA thrombus.

28.5 Management

In this case the patient was sent for an urgent mechanical thrombectomy and normal flow was returned to the MCA (Figure 28.14).

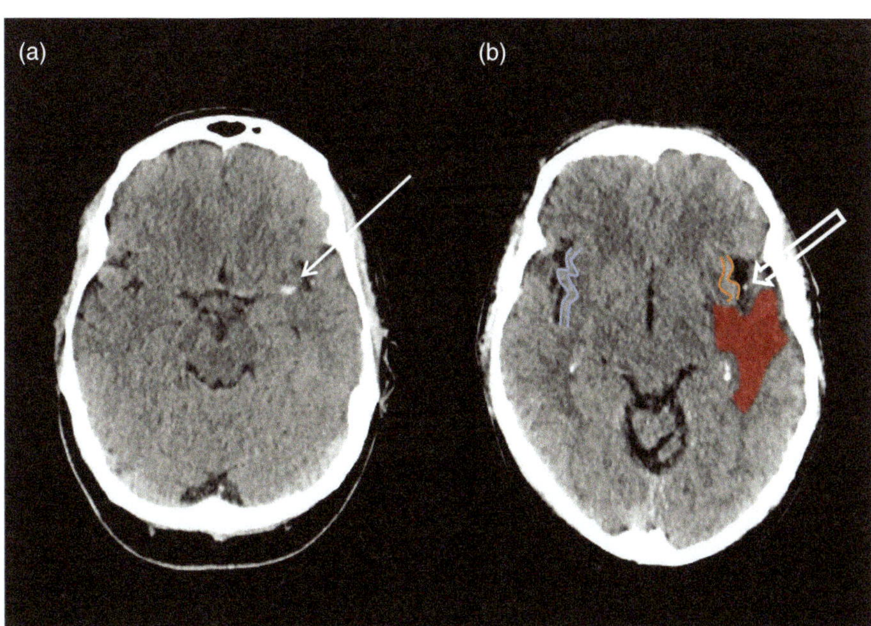

FIGURE 28.10 Patient A. Axial CT head on brain windows at the level of the suprasellar cistern (a) and the third ventricle (b). There is an intraluminal thrombus in the left middle cerebral artery which appears white. At the level of the CoW this will be oriented horizontally and appear as a line (white arrow). Higher up in the Sylvian fissure, the vessel travels vertically so will appear as a dot (hollow arrow). There is a subtle hypodense change in the left temporal lobe and posterior aspect of the insular cortex (red area). This represents cytotoxic oedema and is early evidence of cerebral ischaemia. Compare the intact right insular ribbon (blue) with the left which is lost posteriorly (orange).

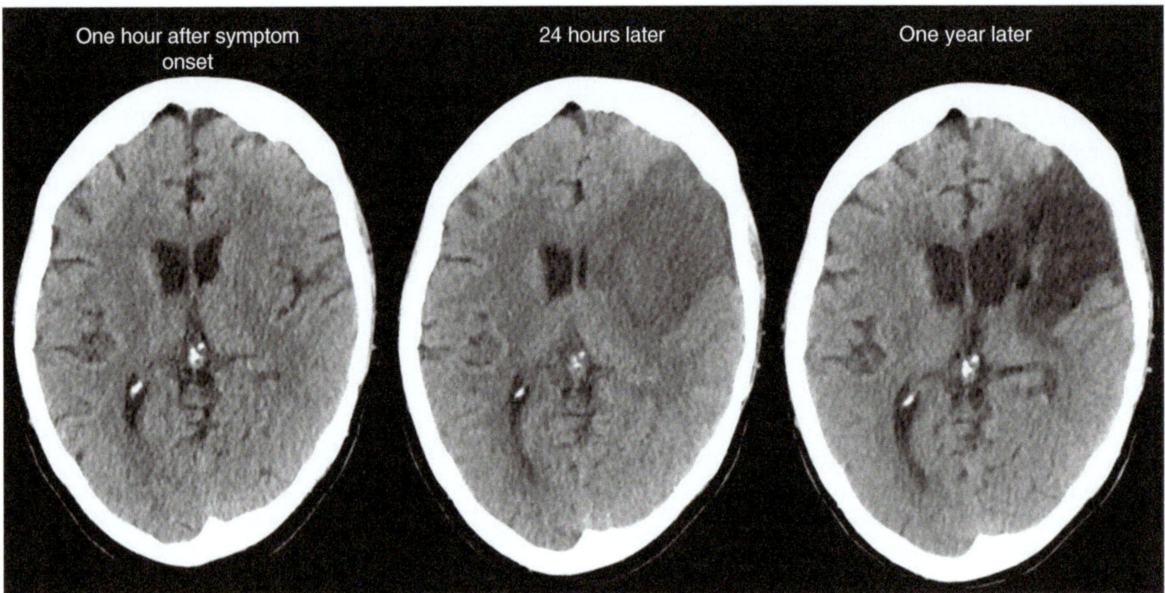

FIGURE 28.11 Ageing an infarct. Axial CT head on brain windows. At initial presentation the CT confirms there is *no haemorrhage*. There is subtle loss of grey/white matter definition in the left frontal lobe representing a hyperacute infarct. Twenty-four hours later, the ischaemic area has become hypodense, representing cytotoxic oedema. There is slight compression of the left frontal horn because of the swelling. One year later, the brain tissue has died, resulting in encephalomalacia. The CSF fills the space so it appears hypodense. There is now compensatory enlargement of the left frontal horn to fill the empty space.

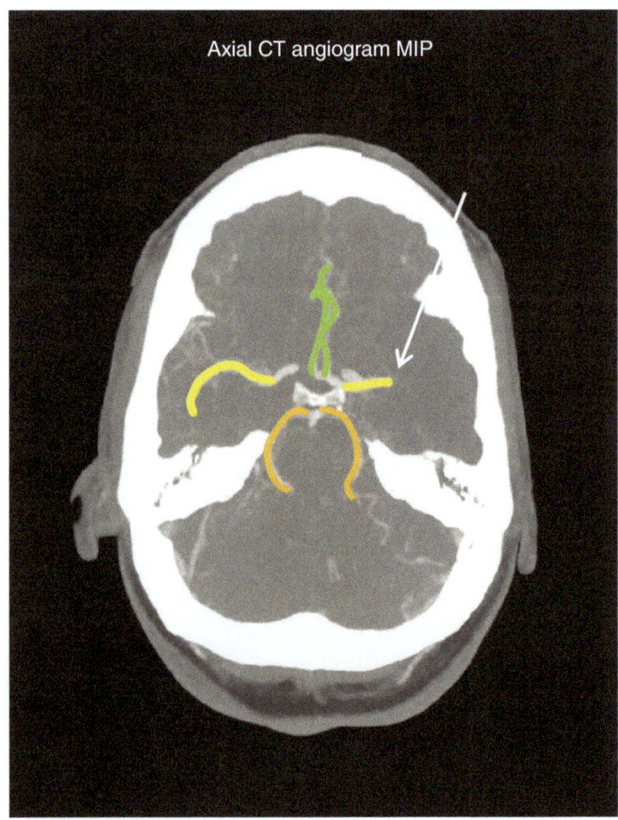

FIGURE 28.12 Patient A. Axial CT angiogram of the brain MIP at the level of the CoW. There is a large thrombus in the left middle cerebral artery which shows an abrupt cut-off (white arrow) compared to the contralateral side (highlighted in yellow). The anterior cerebral arteries are shown in green and lie in the interhemispheric fissure. The posterior cerebral arteries are shown in orange sund travel through the ambient cistern.

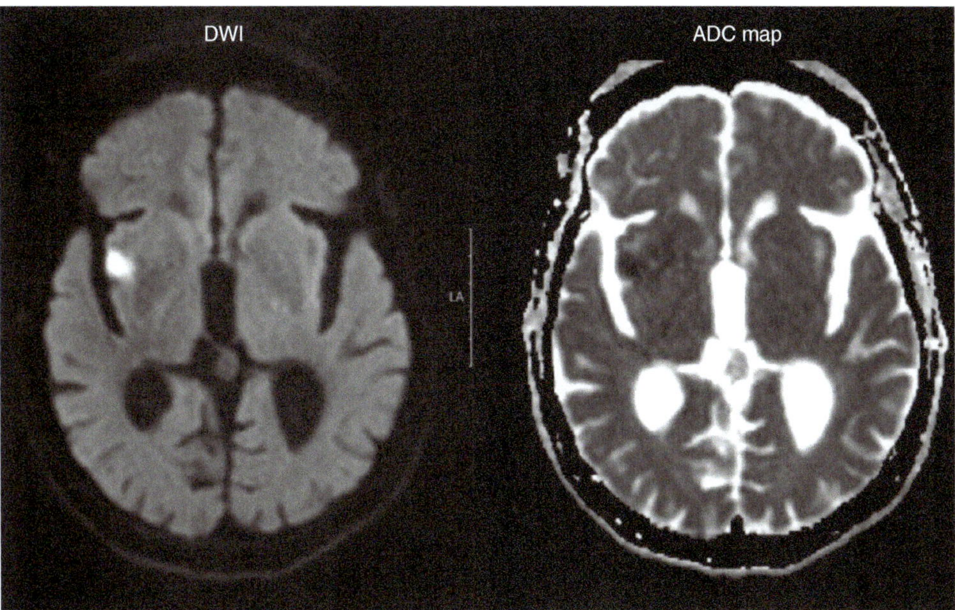

FIGURE 28.13 Axial DWI and ADC sequences, MRI brain. As the brain changes are difficult to spot on CT, MRI is often used to identify small areas of infarction. This example shows a different patient with left facial droop and dysarthria. DWI shows a small focus of restricted diffusion in the right insular cortex (white area). The ADC shows corresponding low signal (dark area), which proves this is real diffusion restriction and not 'T2 shine-through'. Consequently this confirms the presence of an acute infarct. No abnormality was visible on CT.

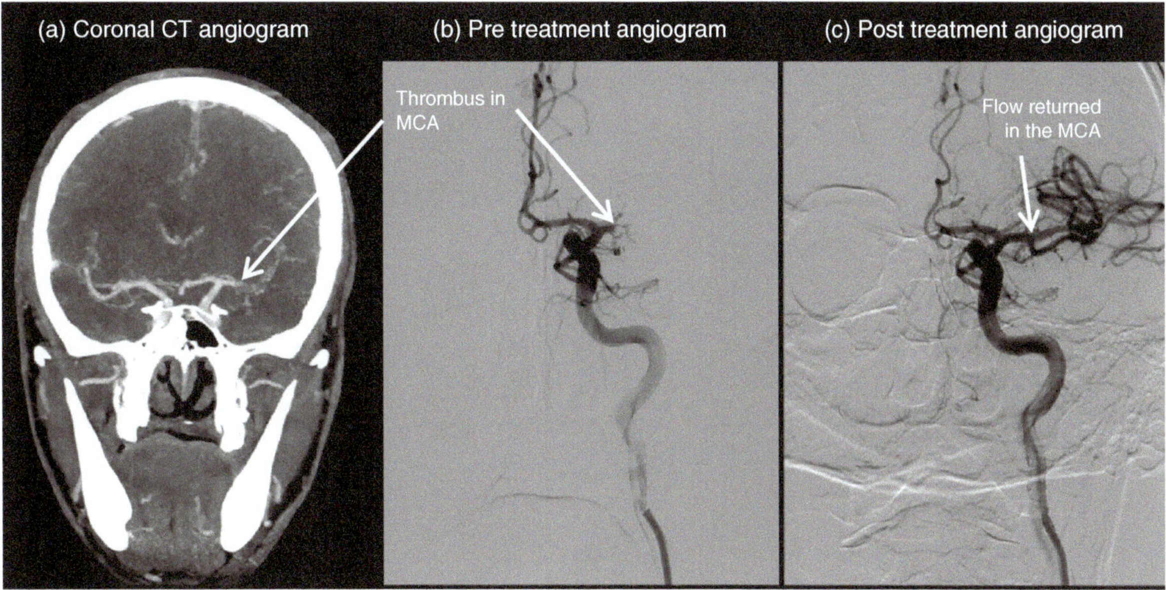

FIGURE 28.14 Patient A. CT head, coronal MIP fluoroscopic-guided mechanical thrombectomy. The coronal CT angiogram (a) is given to show the location of the thrombus in the MCA. This is the same view as the following fluoroscopy images. The left internal carotid artery is cannulated and dye injected (b). Digital subtraction is applied so the bones of the skull cannot be seen, just the vessels of interest. On this image, the MCA does not fill with contrast due to a large proximal thrombus. The thrombus is aspirated and another contrast run is performed (c). Now the MCA and its branches fill with contrast.

Further Resources

Stroke Engine is a useful website for current guidelines in stroke: https://strokengine.ca

Modified Rankin Scale: https://strokengine.ca/en/assessments/modified-rankin-scale-mrs

NIHSS: https://strokengine.ca/en/assessments/nihss

Vanacor, C., Isolan, G., Yu, Y. et al. (2021). Microsurgical anatomy of language. *Clin Anat* 34: 154.

Li, S. and Francisco, G. (2015). New insights into the pathophysiology of post-stroke spasticity. *Front Human Neurosci* 9: 192.

CHAPTER 29

Head Injury

Joshua Lauder[1], Aleksandr Valkov[2], and Peter Driscoll[3]

[1]*East Lancashire Hospitals NHS Trust, University of Central Lancashire and University of Manchester, UK*
[2]*Salford Royal Hospital and University of Central Lancashire, Salford, UK*
[3]*School of Medicine and Dentistry, University of Central Lancashire, Preston, UK*

29.1 Primary Case

29.1.1 Presentation

Patient A is a 27-year-old male who is brought to the Emergency Department having been involved in a fight. During the altercation he sustained a head injury.

29.1.1.1 History of Presenting Complaint According to witnesses, the patient was found on the street about one hour ago. He had been involved in a fight with several people. The weapons used appeared to be feet, fists and baseball bats. No other information is available

29.1.2 Examination

- Bruising and soft tissue swelling in the right temporal and periorbital areas (Figure 29.1).
- Chest – no abnormality detected.
- Normal heart sounds on auscultation.
- Glasgow Coma Scale: Eye opening 2; Verbal response 4; Motor response 3 on both sides.
- Eyes:
  - Right scleral haemorrhage with no posterior margin.
  - Pupils: right 6 mm diameter and less responsive than left (3 mm diameter).

Modified early warning signs (MEWS):

- Respiratory rate 16 rpm.
- SpO_2 92% on room air.
- Tympanic temperature 36.5 °C.

- HR 90 bpm regular.
- BP 150/90 mmHg.
- Confused.

29.1.3 CT

An urgent, unenhanced CT of the head was performed (Figure 29.2).

Clinical Case Questions

- What head trauma do you suspect? Why?
- Where do you think these injuries are located? Why?
- Why is an unenhanced CT of the head the investigation of choice in this case?
- What is your system for image interpretation? What abnormalities are visible?

29.2 Radiology Self-assessment

29.2.1 Technical

29.2.1.1 Blood on CT

- What does clotted blood look like on CT?

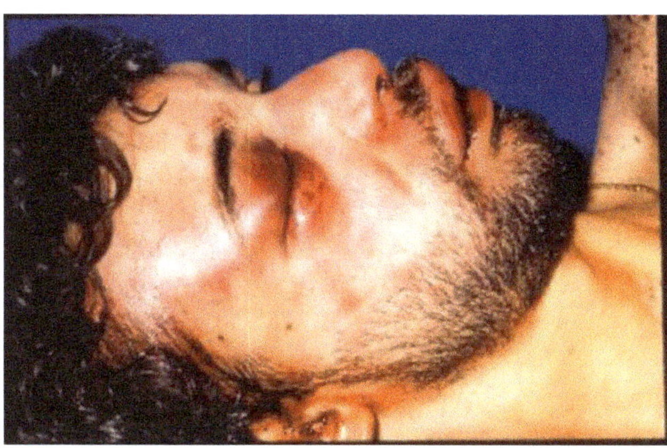

FIGURE 29.1 Patient A. Head injuries sustained during an assault.
Source: Driscoll et al. (2023)/John Wiley & Sons.

29.2.2 Correlation of Gross Anatomy to CT

29.2.2.1 Scalp

- What does the scalp look like on CT?
- In which layer do scalp haematomas tend to collect?

29.2.2.2 Skull

- How can you identify the bones making up the skull vault on CT?

- What do sutures look like on CT?
- How can meningeal vessels be identified on CT?
- Which parts of the skull should be aerated?

29.2.2.3 Vessels

- Where does the middle meningeal artery enter the skull and what does this look like on CT?

29.2.2.4 Meninges

- Where are the falx cerebri and tentorium cerebelli? How can these be identified on the axial and coronal plane?
- How do the dural folds compartmentalise the intracranial cavity?

29.3 Key Radiology Review

29.3.1 Scalp Anatomy

The predominant layer of the scalp visible on imaging is the cutaneous tissue (Figure 29.3). This has a fat density which extends down to the outer surface of the skull. Haematomas following trauma most often collect in the subgaleal (also called subaponeurotic) compartment and will appear as high density between the fatty cutaneous tissue and the skull (see Figure 29.8).

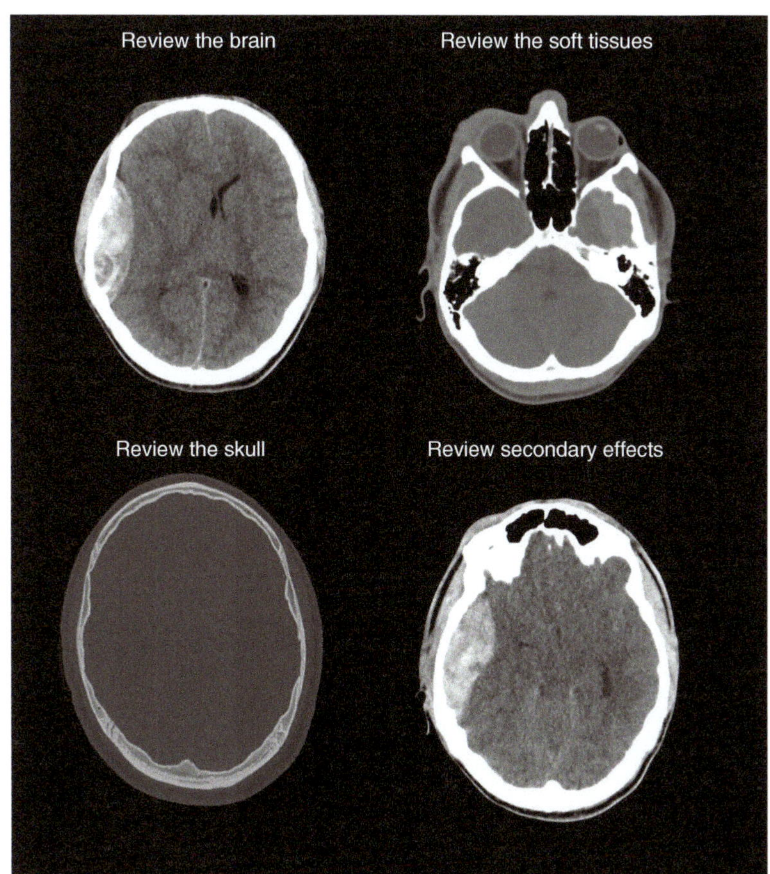

FIGURE 29.2 Patient A. Selected axial CT slices. Review the brain – axial CT head on brain windows. Review the soft tissues – axial CT head on soft tissue windows. Review the skull – axial CT head on bone windows. Review secondary effects – axial CT head on brain windows.

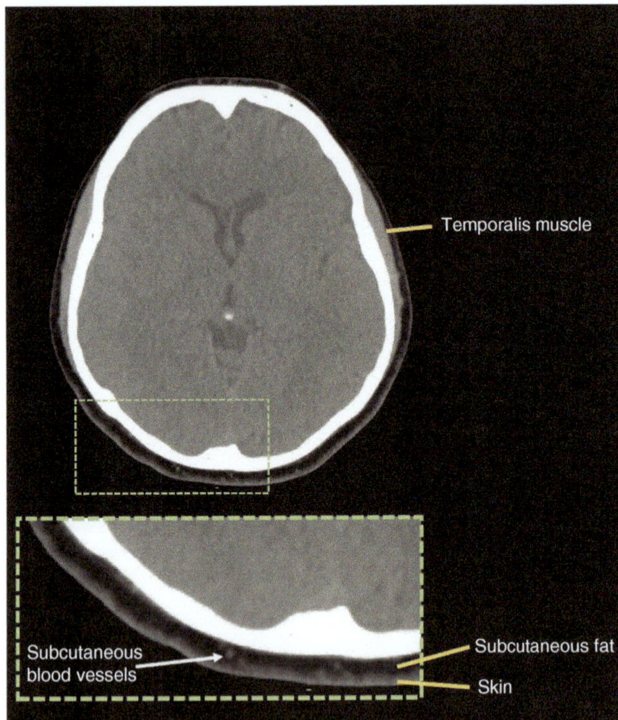

FIGURE 29.3 Normal scalp anatomy on CT. This is an axial CT on a soft tissue window. With this window, the brain has poor contrast and appears a bland grey, while the cutaneous fat layer of the scalp is more apparent. It is normal to have blood vessels coursing through the cutaneous layer of the scalp (white arrow). When there is a scalp haemorrhage, blood tends to collect deeper, immediately superficial to the periosteum of the skull. This is termed a subgaleal (or subaponeurotic) haematoma (see Figure 29.8). Note the location of the temporalis muscles. These need to be distinguished from a haematoma. In addition to its position, another helpful clue is the right and left symmetry.

29.3.2 Skull CT Anatomy

The bones making up the neurocranium can be identified on a CT by their location, particular features (e.g. sinuses) and adjacent sutures (Figures 29.4 and 29.5). When viewing the latter, it is important to distinguish the joint from a fracture. The key is knowing their location and appearance. The sutures' distinguishing features are the symmetry between right and left sides and the convoluted overlapping of the bones (see sagittal suture on Figure 29.6). One practical use of 3D reconstructions is to appreciate the suture anatomy in contrast to a fracture (see Figures 29.6 and 29.10).

29.3.3 Pterion

This is the name given to the 'H-shaped' collection of sutures seen in the temporal area (Figure 29.7a).

> ### Question
> What are the four bones which join at the pterion? Frontal, temporal, sphenoid and parietal.

In about 70% of people, the centre of the pterion is approximately 2.5 cm above the centre of the zygomatic arch (Figure 29.7b).

The bone thickness at this point is around half a centimetre but its true thickness is less where it is grooved by

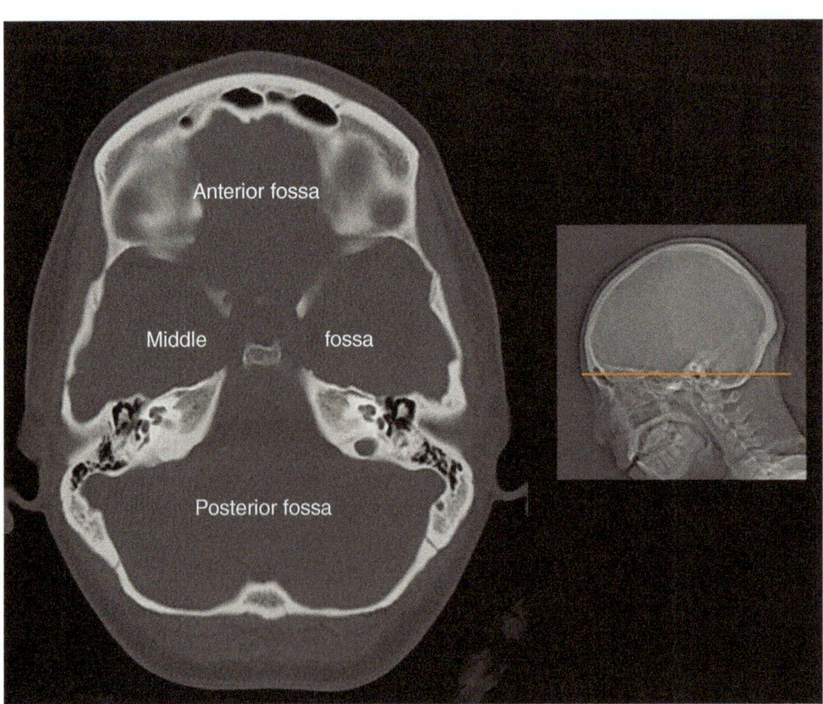

FIGURE 29.4 Axial CT head on bone windows, at the level of the skull base. The three cranial fossae are visible.

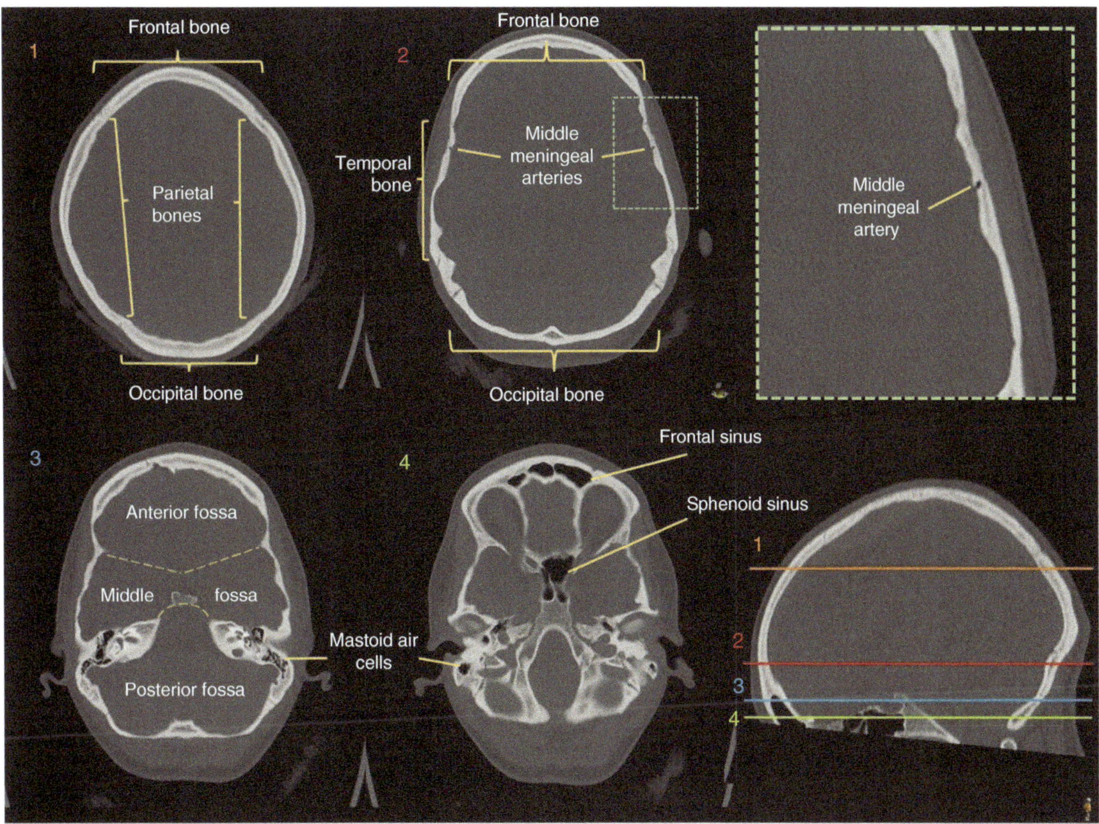

FIGURE 29.5 Axial CT on bone windows to illustrate the skull anatomy at four levels (images 1–4). The bottom right image shows the relative position of these planes on a sagittal view. The indentation of the inner table of the skull vault by the middle meningeal artery can be seen on the CT image (image 2). The aerated portions of the skull are labelled in images 3 and 4.

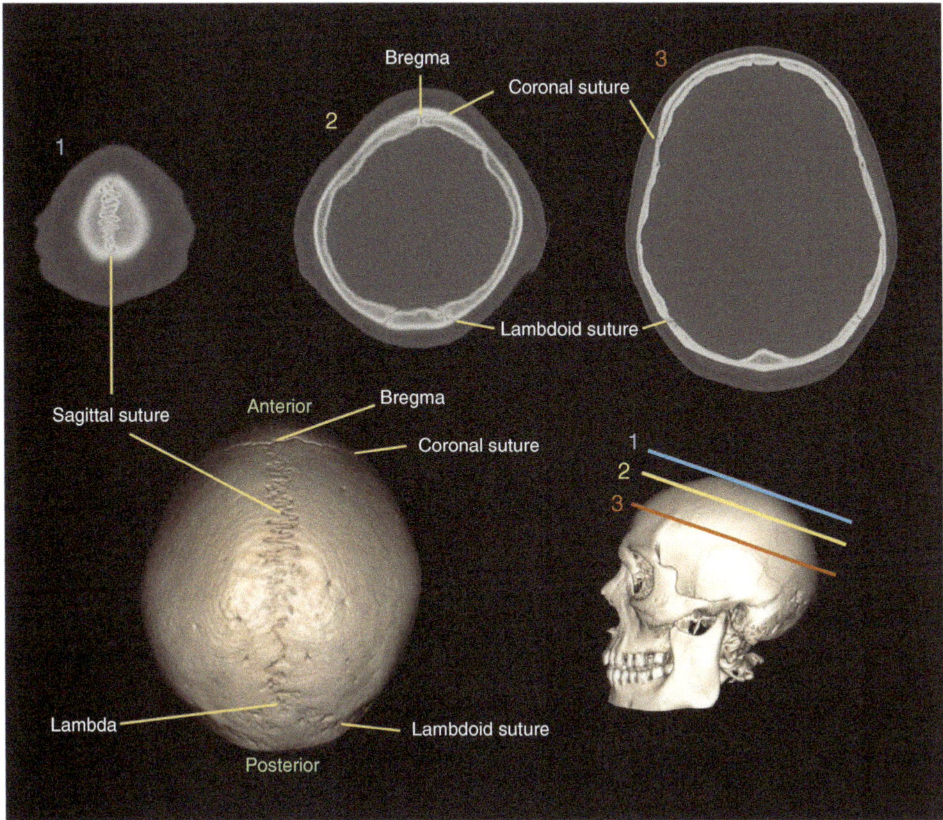

FIGURE 29.6 CT head showing suture anatomy. Images 1–3 are axial slices on bone windows at the corresponding numbered levels from the vertex downwards. A top-down 3D view of the skull is also shown for cross-reference. The sagittal suture shows the classic convoluted, overlapping appearance of the fused bones.

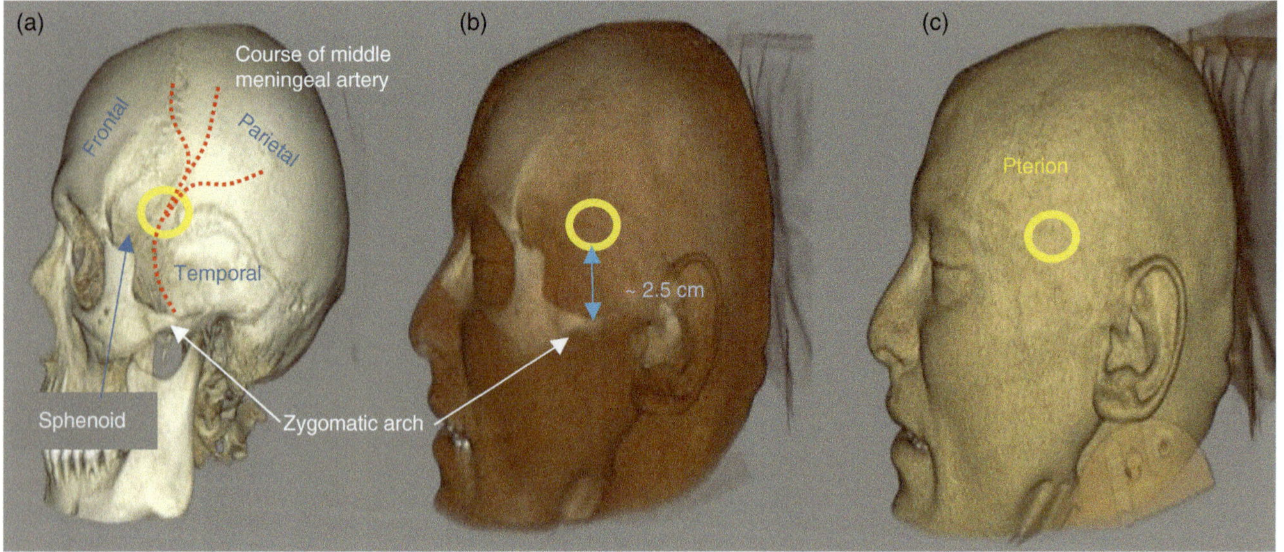

FIGURE 29.7 A 3D rendering going from progressively superficial from (a) skull to (b) soft tissues, to (c) skin showing the location of the pterion. The locations of the four bones making up the pterion are shown (frontal, parietal, sphenoid and temporal).

the middle meningeal artery. Due to this close relationship, a pterion fracture runs the risk of tearing these vessels. The highest chance lies within a 1 cm diameter circle on the centre of the pterion (Figure 29.7c).

29.3.4 Vessels

Even on an unenhanced CT, the cerebral arteries will be visible, provided they are surrounded by CSF (see Head Chapter 27 – Figure 27.5). The meningeal arteries can be seen on CT as they lie immediately deep to the skull, leaving an impression on the inner skull cortex (see Figure 29.5).

29.3.5 Meninges

Review the chapter on subarachnoid haemorrhage (Head Chapter 27) to appreciate the CT anatomy of the falx cerebri and tentorium cerebelli. This will become important when considering the way the brain herniates through the narrow passages created by the folds (see Head Chapter 27 – Figures 27.4 and 27.10).

29.4 Review of the Clinical Case

- What head trauma do you suspect? Why?
- Where do you think these injuries are located? Why?
- Why is an unenhanced CT of the head the investigation of choice in this case?
- What is your system for image interpretation? What abnormalities are visible?

29.4.1 Differential Diagnosis

Patient A has sustained a significant head trauma with a resulting lowered GCS. This is an indication for a CT head (see NICE head injury guidelines).

Head injury can give rise to intracranial haemorrhage. The four main types are characterised by their depth related to the meningeal layers. These tend to have different clinical features.

- *Extradural*: lie just under the skull and are usually related to skull fractures. They are often caused by arterial bleeding from the meningeal arteries. For this reason, they can grow rapidly, causing a fall in consciousness shortly after the head injury. Classically, it is therefore taught that there is a lucid period between the initial stunning immediately after the injury and the subsequent deterioration. However, this classic triad is uncommon.
- *Subdural*: lie under the dura and are usually the result of venous bleeding from bridging veins. This type is more common in the elderly and alcoholics where the brain involution causes the veins to be stretched.
- *Subarachnoid*: this occurs at similar sites to intracerebral haemorrhage stated below. It can result in hydrocephalus in the subacute stage after injury.
- *Intracerebral*: this will usually occur directly under the site of injury (i.e. the coup), on the opposite side of the brain (i.e. the contracoup) or at the inferior part of the brain where it impacts the floors of the cranial fossae.

Whichever type of haemorrhage occurs, the important factor is how much space the bleeding takes up and whether it results in **brain herniation** or **hydro-cephalus**. These features can exacerbate the intracranial pressure and lead to deterioration.

29.4.2 Unenhanced CT

29.4.2.1 Symmetry When reviewing the CT, use asymmetry as a big clue to pathology. The brain and skull are usually symmetrical about the midline. The only caveat to this is that CT scans are often taken in an oblique plane due to patient positioning. Most modern PACS systems allow correction of this when viewing scans on the ward or in the Emergency Department.

29.4.3 Review the Brain – Brain Window

Patient A has an acute extradural haematoma (Figure 29.8). This is confined by the sutures of the skull which causes it to form a biconvex or lens shape. Acutely clotted blood is dense (i.e. white) in comparison with the brain and CSF but will not be as dense as bone or calcium.

29.4.4 Review the Soft Tissues – Soft Tissue Window

Scalp haematomas are not in themselves life-threatening unless they are causing significant blood

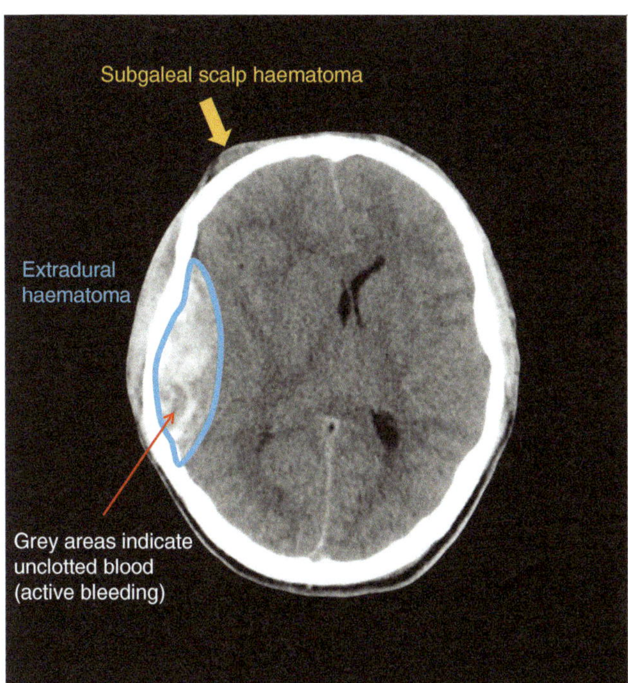

FIGURE 29.8 Patient A. Axial CT on brain windows. Right-sided extradural haematoma (blue area). The areas of lower density in the haematoma suggest unclotted blood (red arrow). This is a marker of active bleeding and so an indication that the haematoma may continue to increase in size. There is also a subgaleal scalp haematoma in the right frontal region (big orange arrow).

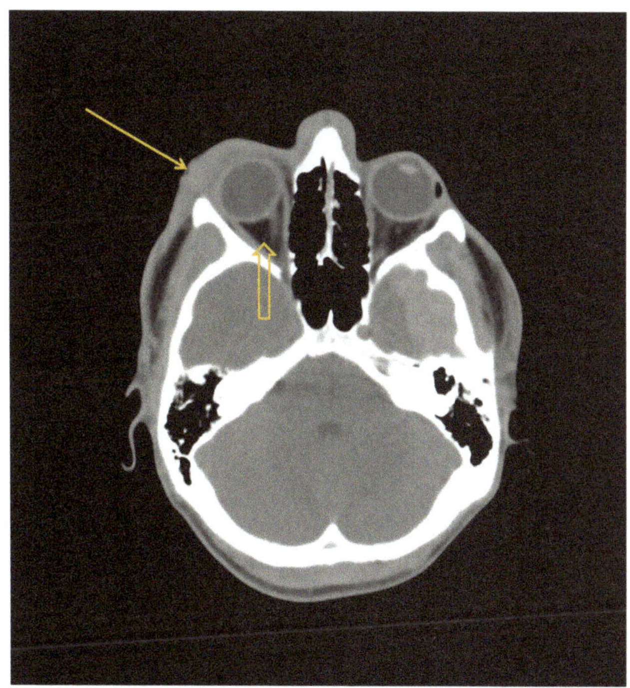

FIGURE 29.9 Patient A. Axial CT on soft tissue windows. There is a right-sided periorbital scalp haematoma (arrow). Reviewing the orbital fat reveals no associated orbital haematoma (hollow arrow).

loss. Nevertheless, they are useful to identify on imaging as they can herald an underlying skull fracture or brain contusion. When located around the eye (Figure 29.9), it is also important to check for orbital haematomas (not shown here).

29.4.5 Review the Skull – Bone Window

As the thickness of the cranial bones varies, the presence of a linear fracture does not automatically mean there will be significant underlying primary brain injury. However, its location can be important. For example, a linear fracture around the pterion increases the risk of intracranial haemorrhage, even if minimally displaced (Figure 29.10; see also Figure 29.7).

29.4.6 Review Secondary Effects – Brain Window

29.4.6.1 Secondary Brain Injury This results *after* the primary brain injury due to factors acting in isolation or in combination (Box 29.1). These mainly cause injury through a lack of oxygen delivery and tissue perfusion, either locally (in the case of a large haematoma) or globally (in generalised loss of circulating blood to the brain, called hypoxic ischaemic encephalopathy). Consequently, they are often correctable, or avoidable, by appropriate resuscitation. It is estimated that up to 30% of deaths after head injury are due to secondary injury, many of which are preventable or treatable within the Emergency Department.

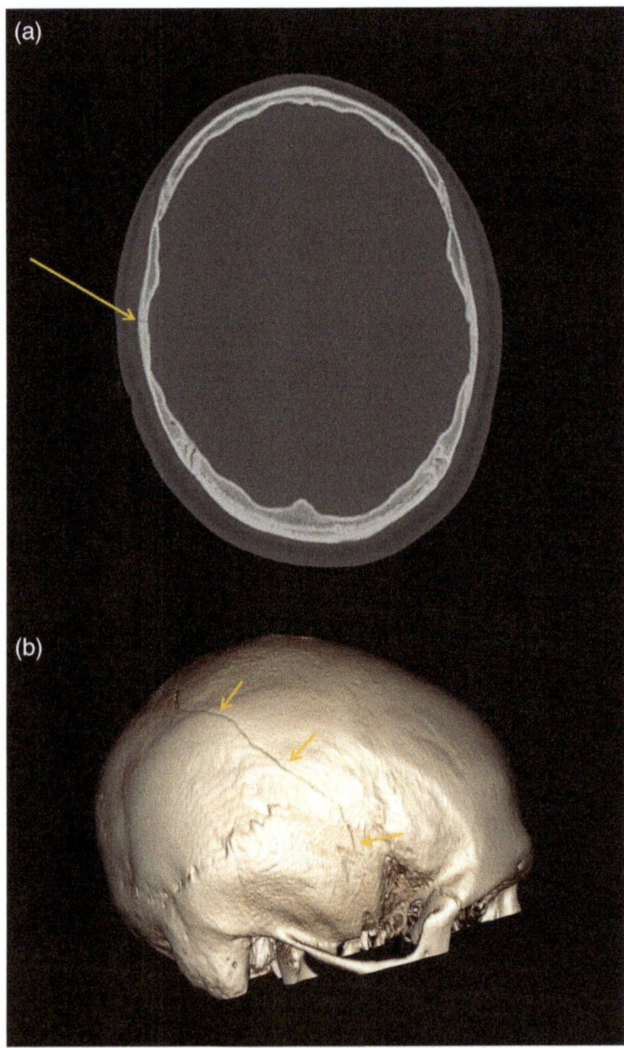

FIGURE 29.10   Patient A. (a) Axial CT on bone windows. (b) 3D reformat of skull. Subtle linear right parietal and temporal skull fracture (arrow). This extends through the pterion. The 3D reformat can be useful to differentiate between fractures and sutures (see Figure 29.6).

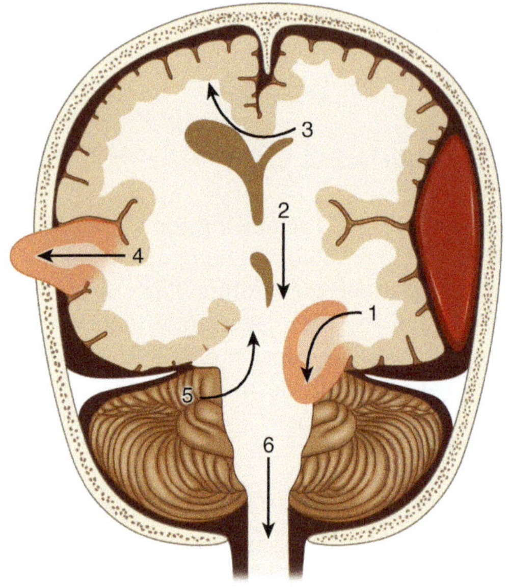

FIGURE 29.11   Types of brain herniation. 1 Uncal; 2 downwards transtentorial; 3 subfalcine; 4 transcranial; 5 upward transtentorial; 6 tonsillar herniation. ***Source:*** RupertMillard/wikipedia Commons/ CC BY 3.0.

Box 29.1 | Main Causes of Secondary Brain Injury

- Hypoxia, i.e. an airway or breathing problem causing a fall in PaO_2.
- Hypovolaemia, i.e. a circulatory problem causing a fall in cerebral perfusion pressure (CPP).
- Raised intracranial pressure, i.e. an intracranial problem causing a fall in CPP.
- Hypoglycaemia.
- Infection.

29.4.6.2 Brain Herniation and Hydrocephalus As the adult brain is contained in a closed box, any increase in intracranial pressure from haematomas or swellings will force the contents through openings. This is known as 'brain herniation' (Figure 29.11). There are several types, and if the pressure rises are unchecked, they can result in hydrocephalus and/or brain ischaemia.

29.4.6.3 Subfalcine Herniation (Midline Shift) This occurs early with unilateral supratentorial pressure increase (Figures 29.12a and 29.13). It seldom produces any clinical effect but it can be detected on the CT scan.

29.4.6.4 Downward Transtentorial Herniation If supratentorial pressure increases further, the midbrain and diencephalon are vertically displaced downwards through the tentorial hiatus (Figure 29.12b). Both pupils may dilate due to the stretching of CN III. Brainstem ischaemia, with progressive dysfunction, also occurs from mechanical distortion, stretching and tearing of the basilar perforating vessels.

29.4.7 Final Diagnosis

Acute right extradural haematoma secondary to a linear skull fracture which involves the pterion. There is subfalcine herniation to the left and downwards transtentorial herniation. This requires urgent referral to neurosurgery.

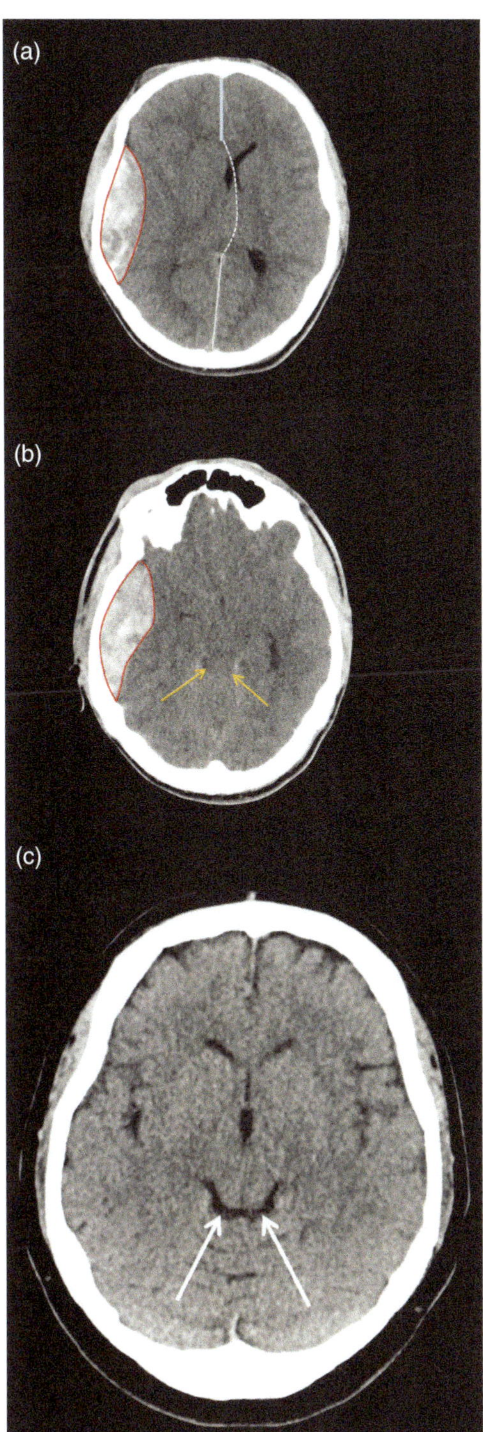

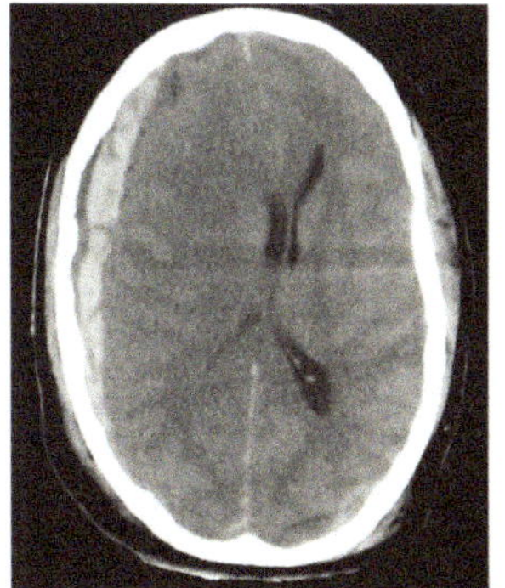

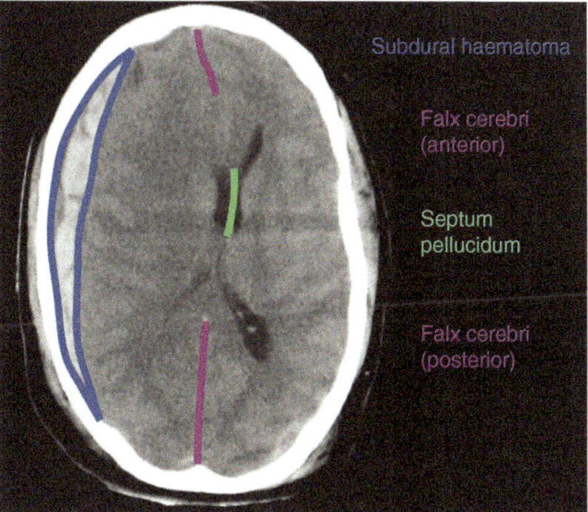

FIGURE 29.13 Axial CT on brain windows, showing an acute right-sided subdural haematoma. Note its crescent shape and the fact that it crosses the coronal suture. The septum pellucidum is a useful midline structure to appreciate as its deviation can be a sign of brain herniation.

29.5 Other Types of Brain Haemorrhage

29.5.1 Subdural Haematoma

In contrast to an extradural haematoma, a subdural haematoma is crescent shaped (Figure 29.13). The reason for this is that it is not confined by the sutures, but instead only limited by the dural folds (i.e. falx cerebri and tentorium cerebelli). In some cases, it extends along these folds but should not cross them.

29.6 Take-home Message – Imaging in Atraumatic Headache

Unenhanced CT is the first-line test to exclude subarachnoid haemorrhage and can be used to exclude this diagnosis, provided it is performed within six hours of symptom onset.

FIGURE 29.12 Patient A. Axial CT on brain windows at the level of the (a) septum pellucidum and (b) quadrigeminal cistern. Image (a) shows subfalcine herniation to the left, which is unlikely to cause symptoms. A more concerning finding is the loss of the quadrigeminal cistern on image (b) (normal appearance shown in (c)). This suggests transtentorial herniation and can precipitate obstructive hydrocephalus. (c) Example of the normal quadrigeminal cistern. This is also called the neurosurgical smile as its presence keeps the neurosurgeon happy.

Further Resources

Driscoll, P.A., Goode, P.N. and Skinner, D.B. (2023) ABC of major trauma: Rescue, resuscitation with imaging, and rehabilitation. Hoboken, NJ, USA: Wiley Blackwell.

NICE head injury guidelines: www.nice.org.uk/guidance/ng232

INDEX

Note: *Italic* page numbers refer to *figure* and **Bold** page numbers reference to **tables**.

A

abdominal aortic aneurysm (AAA), 144
  imaging of, 144
  ultrasound and CT images of
    infrarenal, *146*
abdominal pain:
  clinical case review, 131–136
  key radiology review, 131
  primary case, 130
  radiology self-assessment, 131
abdominal X-ray (AXR), 130, *131*, *132*, *134*
Achilles tendon, 38, *40*
  abnormal ultrasound, *38*
  normal long axis ultrasound, *39*
  rupture, 40, *41*
acromioclavicular joint dislocation, 34
active decision, 5
acute back pain. *See also* back pain
  clinical case review, 154–156
  key radiology review, 152
  primary case, 151
  radiology self-assessment, 151–152
  sagittal MRI and CT of lumbar spine, *156*
  spinal alignment, *153*
acute bacterial endocarditis, 99
acute coronary syndrome (ACS), 107
acute dyspnoea:
  clinical case review, 81
  diagnosis, 81
  key radiology review, 77–78
  primary case, 77
  radiology self-assessment, 77
acute epididymo-orchitis, 62, *62*
acute gout, 17
acute shortness of breath, 111
  clinical case review, 113–115
  correlation to anatomy, 113
  key radiology review, 112–113
  primary case, 111

radiology self-assessment, 112
adequacy, alignment, bones, cartilage,
    soft tissue system (AABCS system for
    extremity X-ray), 22
adhesions, 133
ageing brain, 183–184
airway, 85
airway, apparatus, breathing, circulation
    and dense tissue approach (AABCD
    approach for CT thorax), 85
airway, breathing, circulation, diaphragm and
    everything else system (ABCDE system
    for CXR), 78
alignment, bones, cartilage, soft tissue (ABCS
    approach), 167–168
anatomical planes and orientation in
    radiology, 3, *3*
anatomical sequence (T1 MRI), 8, *195*
anatomical variants, 194, 198
anechoic (ultrasound terminology), 11, *47*
ankle pain:
  clinical case review, 40–42
  key radiology review, 38
  primary case, 37–38
  radiology self-assessment, 38
  Simmonds test, 37, *38*
anterior interventricular artery. *See* left
    anterior descending (LAD)
aortic/aorta:
  axial and coronal CT angiogram, *146*
  dissection, 145
  normal CT angiogram, *145*
  ultrasound of, 144
apparent diffusion coefficient (ADC), 10,
    11, *183*, *189*
appendicitis, 54, 56
artefacts, 5, 10
  edge, 12
  metal, 10

movement, 5–6, *7*, 10
  photon starvation, 6
arthritis, 17
arthropathies, 17
atelectasis, 86
atrial fibrillation (AF), 99
axial and coronal CT KUB of kidneys, *141*
axial CT:
  of abdomen with IV contrast, soft tissue
    window, *129*
  angiogram, *194*, *198*
  on bone windows, *208*
  on brain windows, *207*, *209*
  with contrast on soft tissue windows, *94*, *96*
  KUB at level of bladder, *141*
  on lung windows, *69*, *72*
  on lung window, soft tissue window and
    bone window, *68*
  of mid-abdomen with contrast,
    131, *132*, *135*
  post contrast slices of abdomen, *133*
  slices, *203*
  on soft tissue windows, *68*, *97*, *207*
  of thorax on bone windows, *75*
  thorax on lung windows, *68*
  of thorax on soft tissue windows, *74*
  of upper abdomen with contrast, *120*, *122*
axial CT head:
  angiogram maximum intensity projection
    image, *182*
  on bone windows, *204–205*
  on brain windows, *182*, *194*, *196*, *199–200*
axial CT thorax:
  on bone windows and mediastinal
    windows, *86*
  on lung windows and axial PET/CT, *88*
  on soft tissue windows, *105*
axial MRI brain, T2 sequence, *197*
axial planes, 2, *3*